THE DOUBLE BLIND GUIDE TO PSYCHEDELICS

A ROAD MAP TO TRIPPING, MICRODOSING & BEYOND

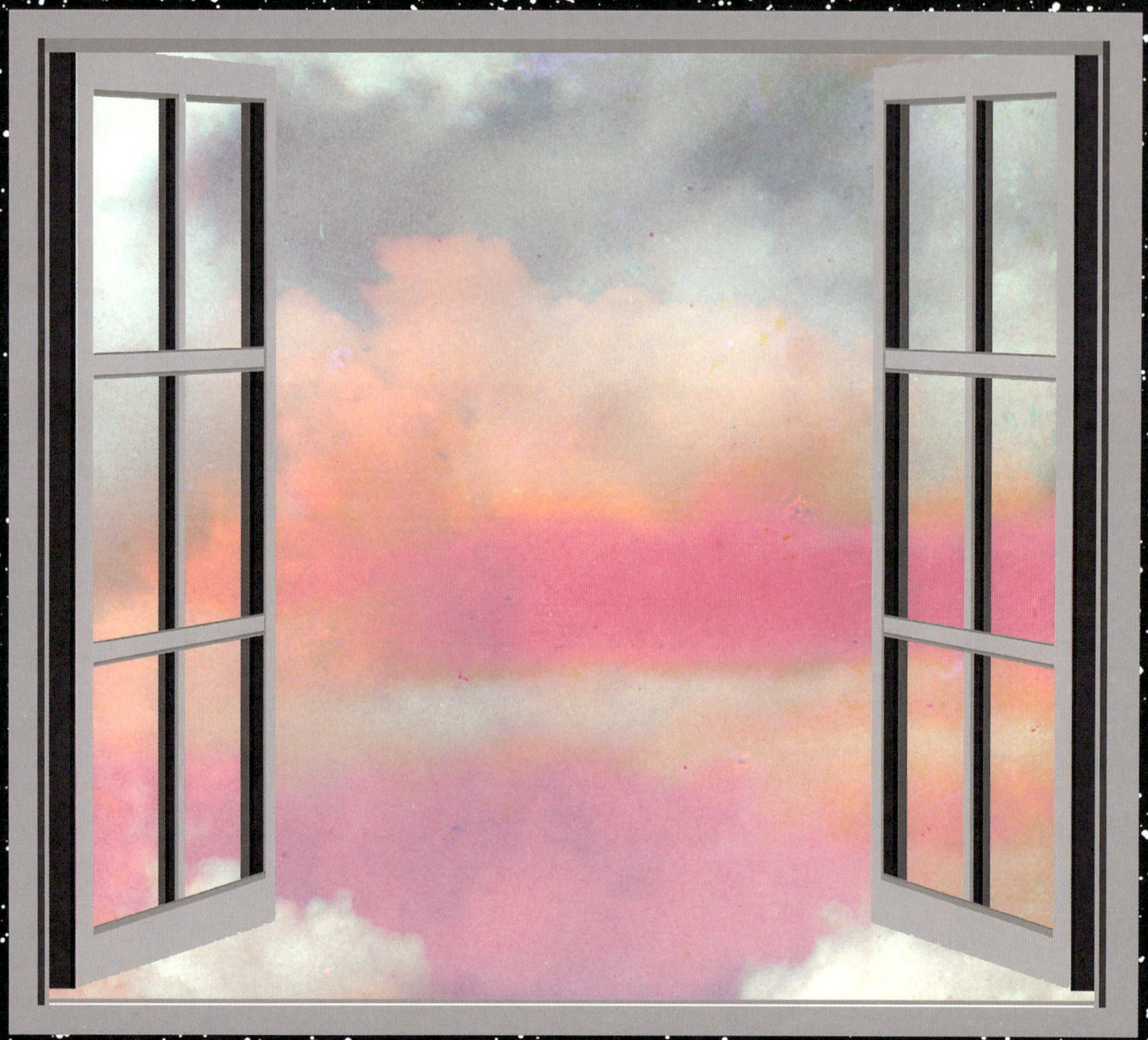

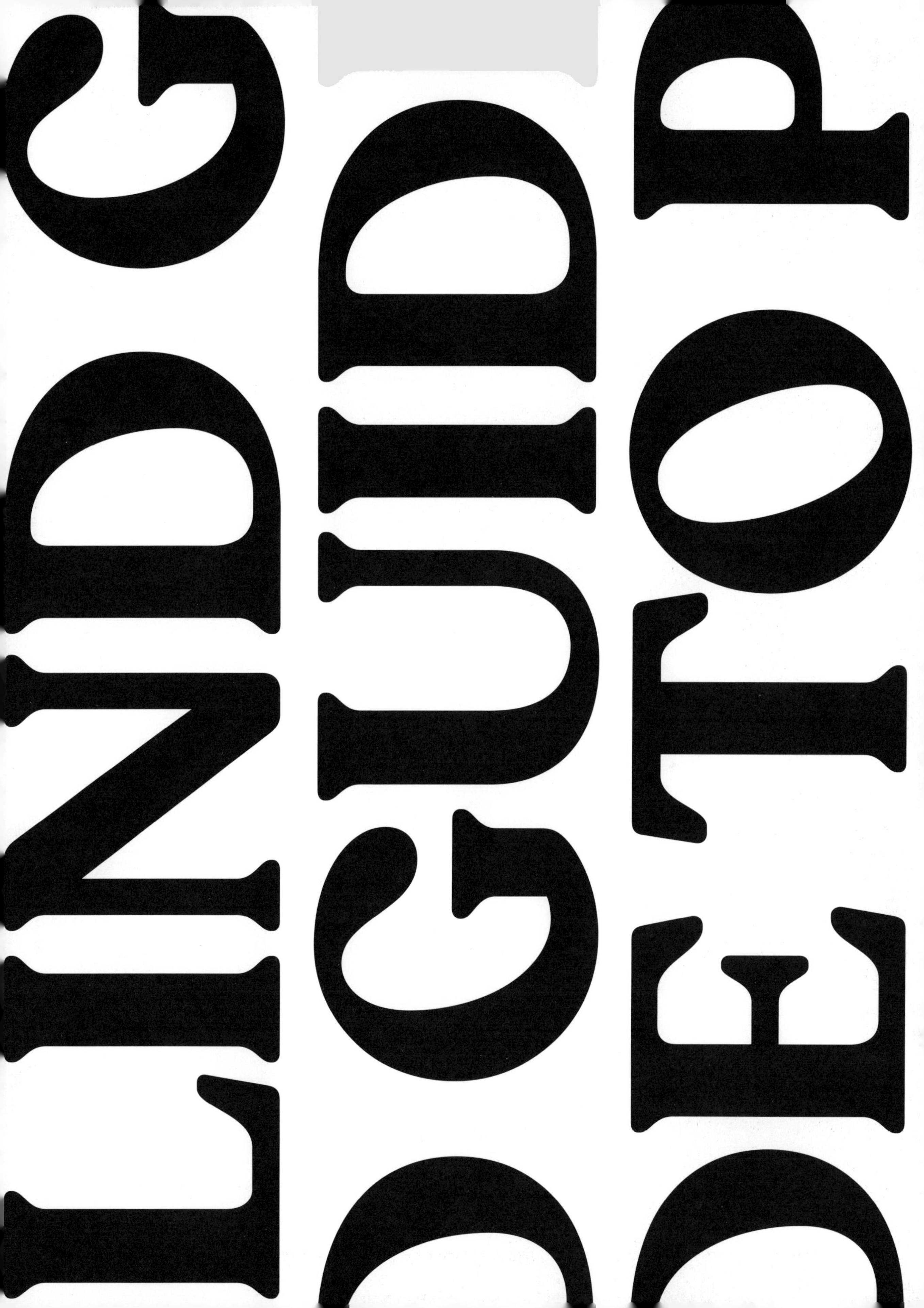

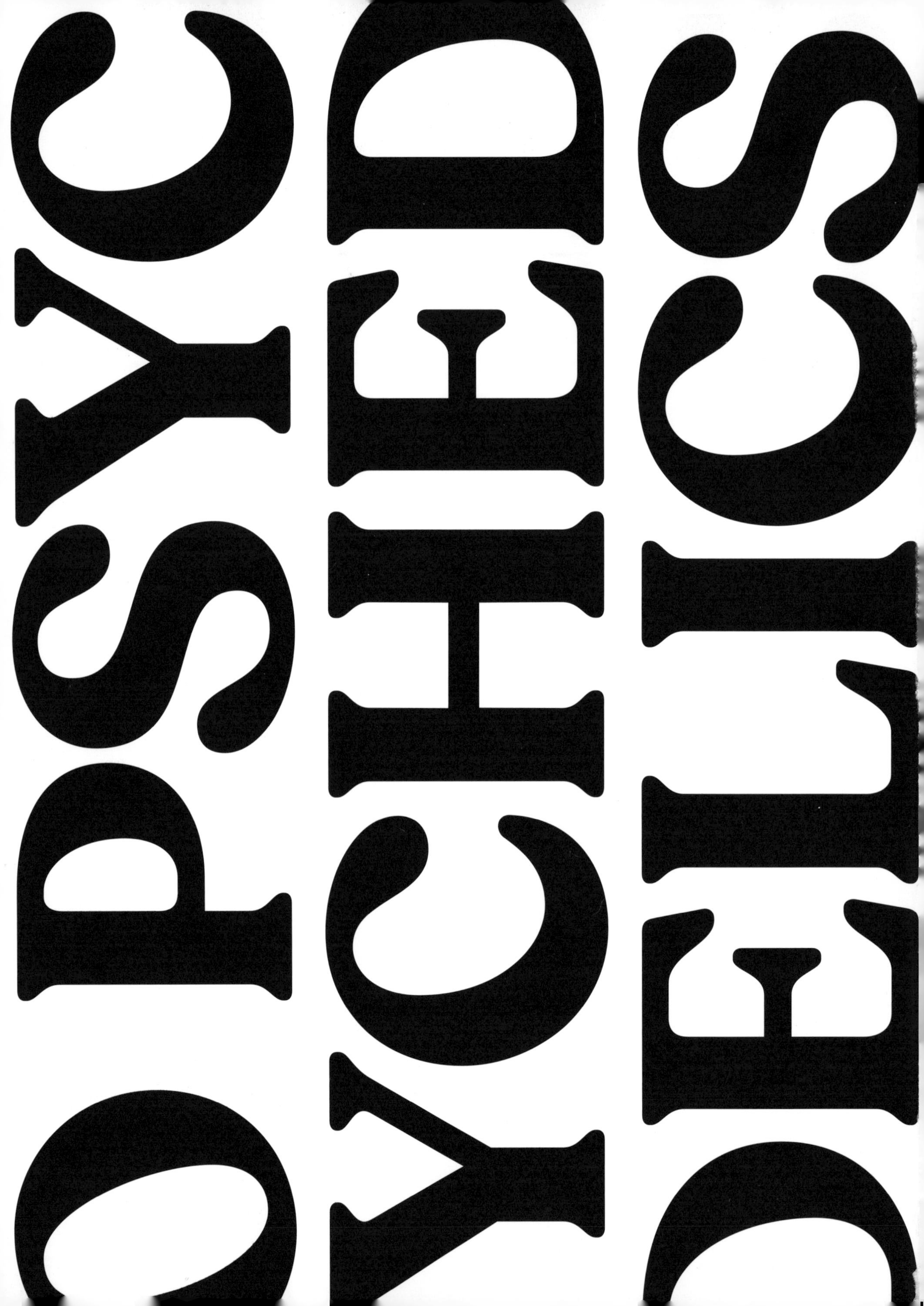

THE DOUBLE BLIND GUIDE TO PSYCHEDELICS

A ROAD MAP TO TRIPPING, MICRODOSING & BEYOND

SHELBY HARTMAN MADISON MARGOLIN

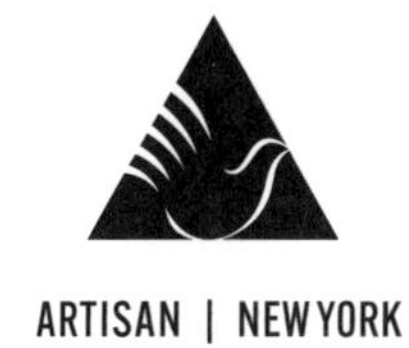

ARTISAN | NEW YORK

For art credits, turn to page 222, which functions as an extension of this page.

Library of Congress Cataloging-in-Publication Data is on file.

ISBN 978-1-64829-179-1

Design by David Good and Jack Dunnington

Published by Artisan,
an imprint of Workman Publishing,
a division of Hachette Book Group, Inc.
1290 Avenue of the Americas
New York, NY 10104
artisanbooks.com

Printed in China (APO) on responsibly sourced paper

First printing, March 2026

10 9 8 7 6 5 4 3 2 1

To all the people, living and passed, who have devoted their lives to helping others heal with these medicines and preserving the knowledge around them

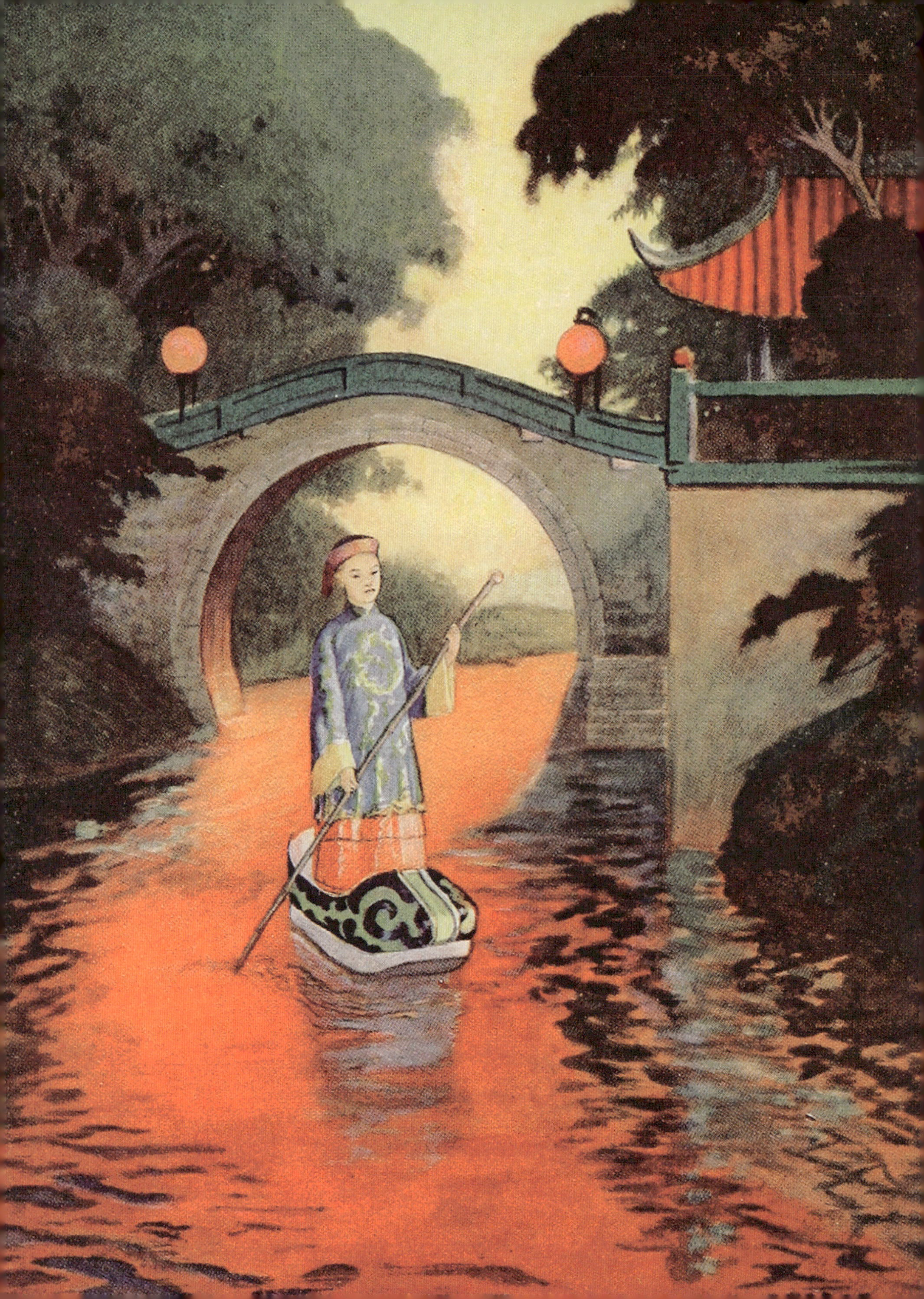

CONTENTS

PREFACE

It's hard to believe how far DoubleBlind has come since we began in 2019. It started as a passion project—a print magazine that we were literally packing into envelopes and driving to the post office ourselves, with the help of our parents. When we had the idea for DoubleBlind, it wasn't because psychedelics were gaining exponential traction in the mainstream (although they were). At the time, we were both reporting on cannabis and psychedelics for *VICE*, *Rolling Stone*, *LA Weekly*, *Playboy*, and other publications, and we were lit up by the idea that psychedelics could be a jumping-off point to tell stories about many of the most prescient issues of our time.

We called up the best journalists and photographers we knew and sold them on the dream. Our pitch was that the places we were all already writing for—major magazines and newspapers—were covering psychedelics, but they were mostly talking about research into the uses of psychedelics for mental health. We wanted to report on that, but also to utilize the growing interest in psychedelics as a lens into other topics: a pharmaceutical industry that requires companies to invest hundreds of millions of dollars into drugs, only to often make them inaccessible; the growing interest worldwide in yoga, meditation, and other spiritual practices; the pitfalls of the criminal justice system; and many others.

We wanted to tell an even bigger story, too, about how psychedelics might propel us to be more conscientious global citizens. We wanted to help people understand how psychedelics can be connected to a larger framework that spans from their potential for conflict resolution to how they might awaken people to the climate crisis. We wanted to center the voices of Indigenous stewards who have preserved the knowledge around many of these plants and fungi for millennia. And we wanted to talk honestly about the risks and limitations of psychedelics, rather than romanticizing them as a silver bullet for the mental health crisis or the world's systemic problems. (They may be one tool for addressing the challenges humanity faces today, but they're certainly not a panacea.)

Though it felt like we birthed DoubleBlind, it quickly took on a life of its own. Hundreds of thousands of people came to our website, without any promotion, in the first week we started publishing. The original vision was just a print magazine, but soon we were invited to speak at Harvard, SXSW, and dozens of psychedelic conferences. And we were getting queries from thousands of people who wanted advice on how to journey on psychedelics. We heard from mothers with postpartum depression who wanted to microdose, veterans who wanted to go to the Amazon and try ayahuasca to help them process their trauma, baby boomers who hadn't tripped for decades but now wanted to come back to psychedelics for mental health, and people from a wide variety of backgrounds who were simply interested in exploring the nature of consciousness or deepening their spiritual paths. People didn't want just journalism from us—they wanted education, community, and support. So we began to put out classes and workshops with leading therapists, researchers, and Indigenous healers whom we knew from our reporting. To date, we've had thousands of people graduate from our classes.

This book serves as a compendium of all the best wisdom we've gathered along the way about how to engage with psychedelics. It includes practical tips on how to take psychedelics, within the context of our reporting about the ethics of turning these substances into legal medicines; the Indigenous use of plant medicines; the politics of the psychedelic industry; and much more. We also get into risks and contraindications, and we feel it's important to name here that, as with almost everything in this world, there are limitations to the safe use of psychedelics. Every person and every journey is different, so it's important to seek individualized and professional support, especially if you have a history of mental health distress. It's important, too, to be aware of the laws in your areas and the potential consequences of partaking in these experiences in the current legal climate.

Our intention for this book, as is the case for the rest of our work, is to support you on your path of healing and growth, but also to help you understand the ecosystem of stakeholders and traditions within which psychedelics are situated. In doing so, we hope to imagine a future in which psychedelics are available to all who need healing, for many generations to come. And we hope that each journey can be understood as an opportunity not only to find greater inner peace but to contemplate how that inner peace might be leveraged to allow each of us to show up with greater care in the world.

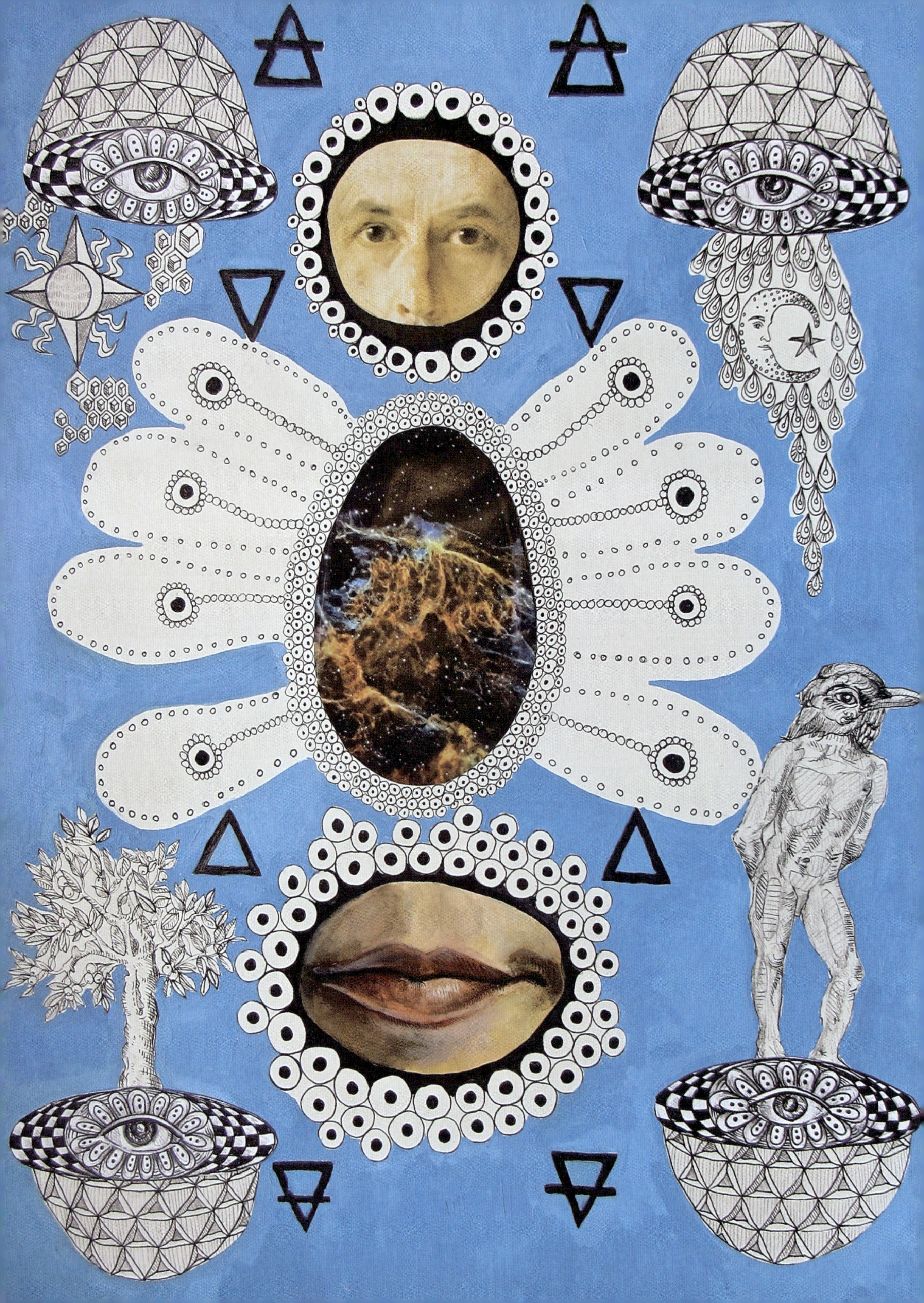

INTRODUCTION

Welcome aboard the spaceship. In the psychedelic community, people often say that the moment you commit to taking a psychedelic is the moment your trip begins. This is because just the prospect of taking a psychedelic can stir up a lot of emotion: fear, excitement, hope. And, as we'll discuss in this book, all of these emotions are a starting point for investigating your inner world. But before we dive into the depths of these mind-altering experiences, let's start by defining our terms.

What Even Is a "Psychedelic"?

There's a lot of debate about what does and doesn't qualify as a psychedelic. When people think of psychedelics, often the first substances that come to mind are LSD and shrooms. But what about ketamine? MDMA (or ecstasy)? Cannabis? It depends on how you define *psychedelic* and who you ask.

The term *psychedelic*, derived from the Greek words *psyche* (soul, self, spirit) and *delos* (manifest, apparent), etymologically translates to "mind-manifesting." *Psychoactive*, by contrast, is a broader term. It refers to any substance that changes brain function and results in alterations in perception, mood, consciousness, cognition, or behavior. This includes psychedelics but also encompasses substances like caffeine, alcohol, and antidepressants. These psychoactive, but not psychedelic, substances change how you feel, but they don't necessarily bring forth content living within your unconscious for processing. All psychedelics are psychoactive, but not all psychoactive substances are psychedelic.

As Albert Hofmann, the scientist who first synthesized LSD, described it in an interview with *The New York Times* just shy of his one hundredth birthday, acid is "medicine for the soul"—and the same could perhaps be said of all psychedelics. More recently, on the *Psychedelic Medicine Podcast*, psychedelic pharmacologist Ben Malcolm, a.k.a. Spirit Pharmacist, suggested that a more apt term for this class of substances would be *psychosomatodelics* because they magnify not only what's happening in the mind but the sensations living within our bodies, which can be a powerful portal into understanding what needs to be healed.

Generally speaking, one common way a psychedelic can be defined is by what it does neurologically. LSD, shrooms, and DMT—often referred to as "classic psychedelics"—are grouped together because they interact with the 5-HT2A receptors in the brain. MDMA, ketamine, and cannabis, however, each spur psychoactivity in their own unique way. That said, if we're defining a psychedelic simply by its ability to take the user on

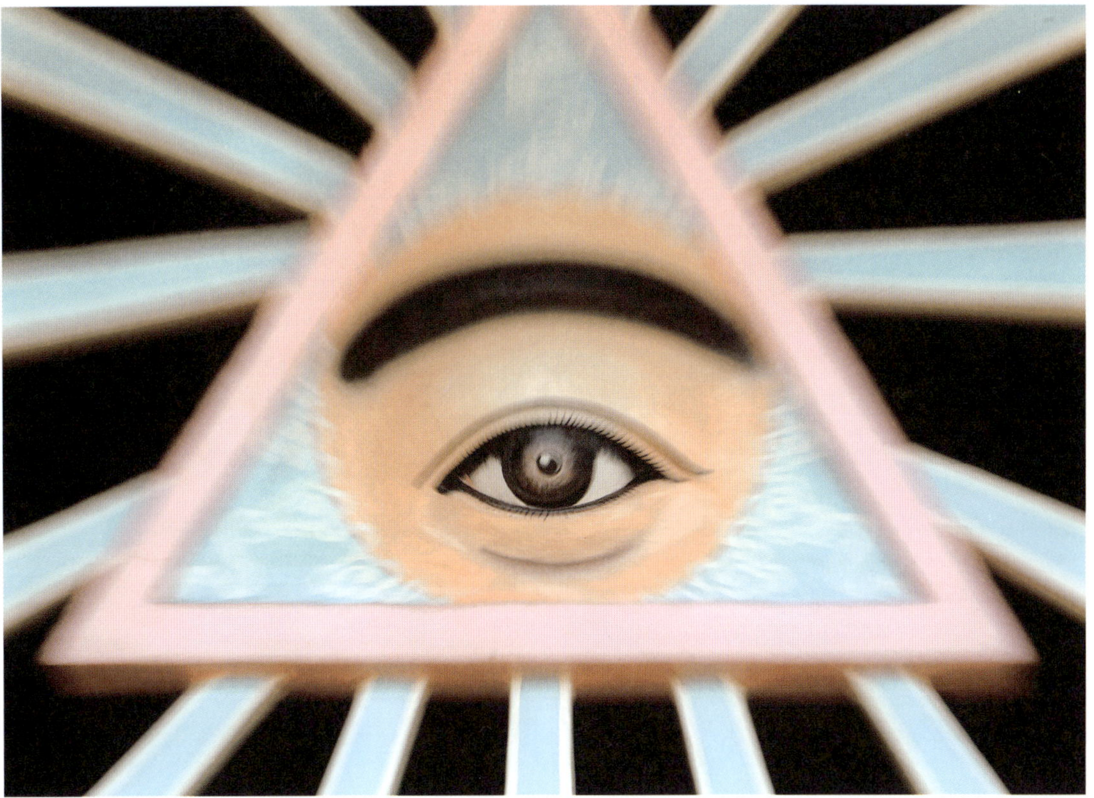

a journey of consciousness that can fuel healing (as we do), then what's included in this category becomes much broader. In this book, we chose the latter definition because we wanted to cover all the substances that are most commonly being investigated for their therapeutic potential within the psychedelic movement right now in order to help you assess which experience might be best for you.

In addition to *psychedelic*, people use a number of other terms for these substances (see page 14). These terms are important to consider because each implies the intention behind a psychedelic's use, whether it be religious, therapeutic, or recreational. For example, some Indigenous communities feel strongly that their ancestral sacraments—such as ayahuasca and peyote—should not be taken out of their traditional contexts and turned into pharmaceutical medicines for mental health. Meanwhile, some therapists, researchers, and doctors working within the Western medical framework feel that psychedelics shouldn't be taken recreationally.

---

somatics
noun

the study and exploration of the body as perceived from within, focusing on the internal experience of movement, sensation, and bodily awareness

Somatics is rooted in the idea that the mind and body are interconnected, and how we move or hold ourselves physically can deeply affect our emotional and psychological state. In recent years somatic therapy, which prompts a person to reflect on the sensations in their body instead of analyzing their thoughts, has grown in popularity, particularly as a tool to help people prepare for and process their psychedelic experiences.

There's also a contingent of "psychonauts" (i.e., people who frequently trip on psychedelics) who feel that there's much healing to be had outside the clinic, on dance floors, at festivals, and beyond. At DoubleBlind, we say the only "wrong way" to use a psychedelic is if you're causing harm to yourself or other people in the process. (This includes taking a psychedelic in a context where you or others are not safe psychologically or physiologically as well as disregarding the requests of Indigenous communities with ties to these medicines—more on this later.) Otherwise, we don't take a position on the "right way" to journey—and that's why, in our reporting and throughout this book, we generally default to the neutral terms *psychedelics* or *substances*.

But we're not overly rigid with the terms we use, because we know that it's impossible to confine these experiences, even if they're approached with a very particular intent. Indeed, someone can do a psychedelic in a clinical context for their mental health and end up having a deeply mystical experience that inspires them to embark on a spiritual path (in fact, that's not uncommon). On the flip side, someone can take acid or shrooms at a festival to have fun and end up unintentionally healing psychological distress. This isn't to say that the intention with which you approach these substances doesn't make a difference—it can make a massive difference—but there's an inherent element of unpredictability that comes along with these experiences, too.

WHAT'S IN A NAME?

A number of terms are used to describe psychedelics.

ENTHEOGEN

You may have heard the words *psychedelic* and *entheogen* used interchangeably, but it's helpful to make a distinction. *Entheogen* means "generating the divine within," and it refers to any substance, be it cannabis, wine, ayahuasca, or psilocybin (the most prominent psychedelic compound in magic mushrooms), that carries spiritual potential. The people who use this word often do so because they believe that there's a mystical or divine component at play when someone goes on a journey with these substances and that the healing can be attributed to more than just a rewiring of neurological patterns.

MEDICINE

Psychedelics are sometimes referred to as medicines to highlight their therapeutic potential and ability to treat a range of ailments, from anxiety and depression to substance dependence and PTSD. People who are adamant about the term *medicines* seek to distinguish psychedelics from substances that are more commonly used in recreational contexts and have a higher potential for abuse or dependence.

DRUG

Given their status as federally illegal and their use in recreational settings, psychedelics are also sometimes called drugs. Some psychedelic advocates actually prefer the term because they feel passionately that psychedelics should be legal in recreational contexts, from festivals to camping.

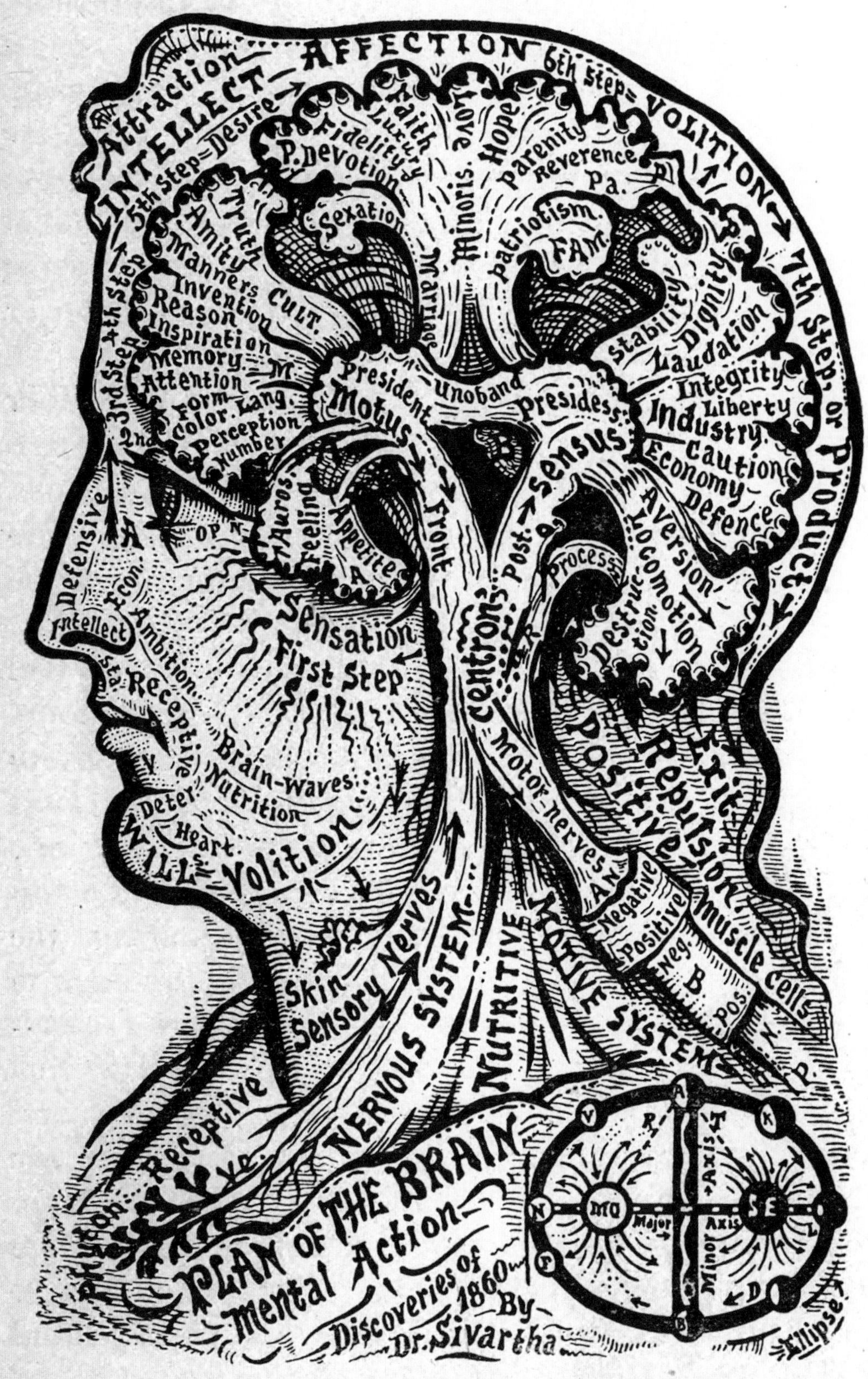
PLAN OF THE BRAIN
Mental Action
Discoveries of 1860 By
Dr. Sivartha
AFFECTION
Attraction
INTELLECT
5th step=Desire
6th step=VOLITION
7th step, or Product
Faith
Luxury
Fidelity
P. Devotion
Love
Hope
Parenity
Reverence
Pa.
Truth
Amity
Manners
Sexation
Minoris
Marriage
Patriotism
FAM.
Stability
Dignity
Invention
Reason
CULT.
Inspiration
Memory
Attention
Form
Color
Lang.
Perception
Number
4th step
3rd step
2nd
President
Unoband
Motus
Presides
Laudation
Integrity
Liberty
Industry
Caution
Economy
Defence
Sensus
Aversion
Locomotion
Destruction
Process
Post.
Front
Appetite
Feeling
Auros
Defensive
Econ
Intellect
Ambition
Sensation
First Step
Receptive
Centrons
Positive
Repulsion
Exit
Brain-Waves
Nutrition
Deter
Heart
WILL
Volition
Motor-nerves
Negative
Positive
Neg.
B
Pos.
Muscle Cells
Skin
Sensory Nerves
NERVOUS SYSTEM
NUTRITIVE
MOTIVE SYSTEM
Receptive
MO
SE
Major Axis
Minor Axis
Ellipse

Psychedelics Weren't "Discovered" in the '60s

We always like to remind folks at DoubleBlind that psychedelics weren't invented in the twentieth century—even if the word *psychedelic* and concepts like "tripping" are relatively new. Records of human use of psychoactive plants, fungi, and animals date back millennia, spanning cultures around the world, for purposes ranging from therapeutic to spiritual to recreational.

Of course, when we're talking about consumables imbibed thousands of years ago, much is based on speculation. That said, there is compelling evidence that from the ancient Amazonian rainforests to the vibrant cities of the Middle East and the glittering temples of India, mind-expanding, soul-stirring psychedelics have shaped beliefs and rituals since long before they were encountered by curious travelers.

In Europe, some scholars have hypothesized that prehistoric cave art dating as far back as 10,000 BCE indicates the use of psilocybin mushrooms in rituals (the drawings look like mushrooms, but they may be something else). In India, soma, a potentially psychoactive drink, is mentioned in the Rig Veda, an ancient Vedic text from 2000 BCE, although there's a lot of debate online about what was really in it. Many blogs also point to the use of "kykeon" in the Eleusinian Mysteries (secret initiation rites in Greece in 1500 BCE to 400 CE) as proof of ancient psychedelic use, but it's worth noting that one of the most persuasive arguments is that kykeon actually contained opium. And if you're geeky about shrooms, you may have heard that Siberian shamans have long used the *Amanita muscaria* mushroom and that it even has ties to the origin of Santa Claus, but we're sorry to inform you that this info, while fun, is pretty dubious.

More definitively, the use of hashish has a deep history among devotees of the deity Shiva, known for his dominion over yoga and mind-altering substances. In the Middle East, there's evidence of the use of psychedelic substances like the DMT-containing acacia plant in the ancient temple of Jerusalem, thought by some to be connected to prophecy. Bwiti, an animist belief system based on ancestor worship and animism of the forest-dwelling Punu and Mitsogo peoples of Gabon, has incorporated iboga (*Tabernanthe iboga*), a psychoactive root bark, into its rituals for at least centuries.

In the Americas, Indigenous cultures have long revered plant medicines like ayahuasca and peyote as sacred. The Mazatec people in Oaxaca, Mexico, have been conducting sacred mushroom ceremonies, referring to the fungi as "holy children," for centuries (if not millennia). The *Codex Magliabechiano*, a mid-sixteenth century manuscript, shows Mictlantecuhtli, god of the Mexican (Aztec) underworld, approaching a man taking mushrooms, which may have contained psilocybin (pictured below). The Wixárika people in Mexico have been using peyote in spiritual ceremonies for guidance and healing for at least 15,000 years, and in the nineteenth century, peyote found its way north along trade routes to many tribes in what is now the United States.

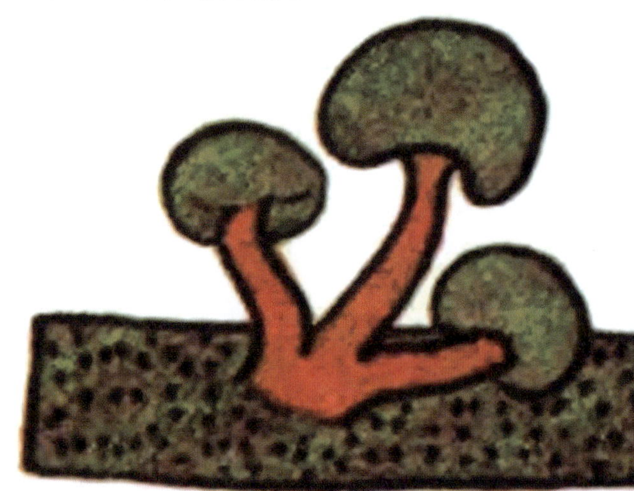

Across the globe, evidence points to a deep connection between humanity and psychedelic substances, suggesting a shared human desire to transcend ordinary experience and access other realms of consciousness. This is a story that goes beyond mere experimentation; it reflects a fundamental human impulse to connect with the divine, to explore consciousness, and to experience the sacred dimensions of existence.

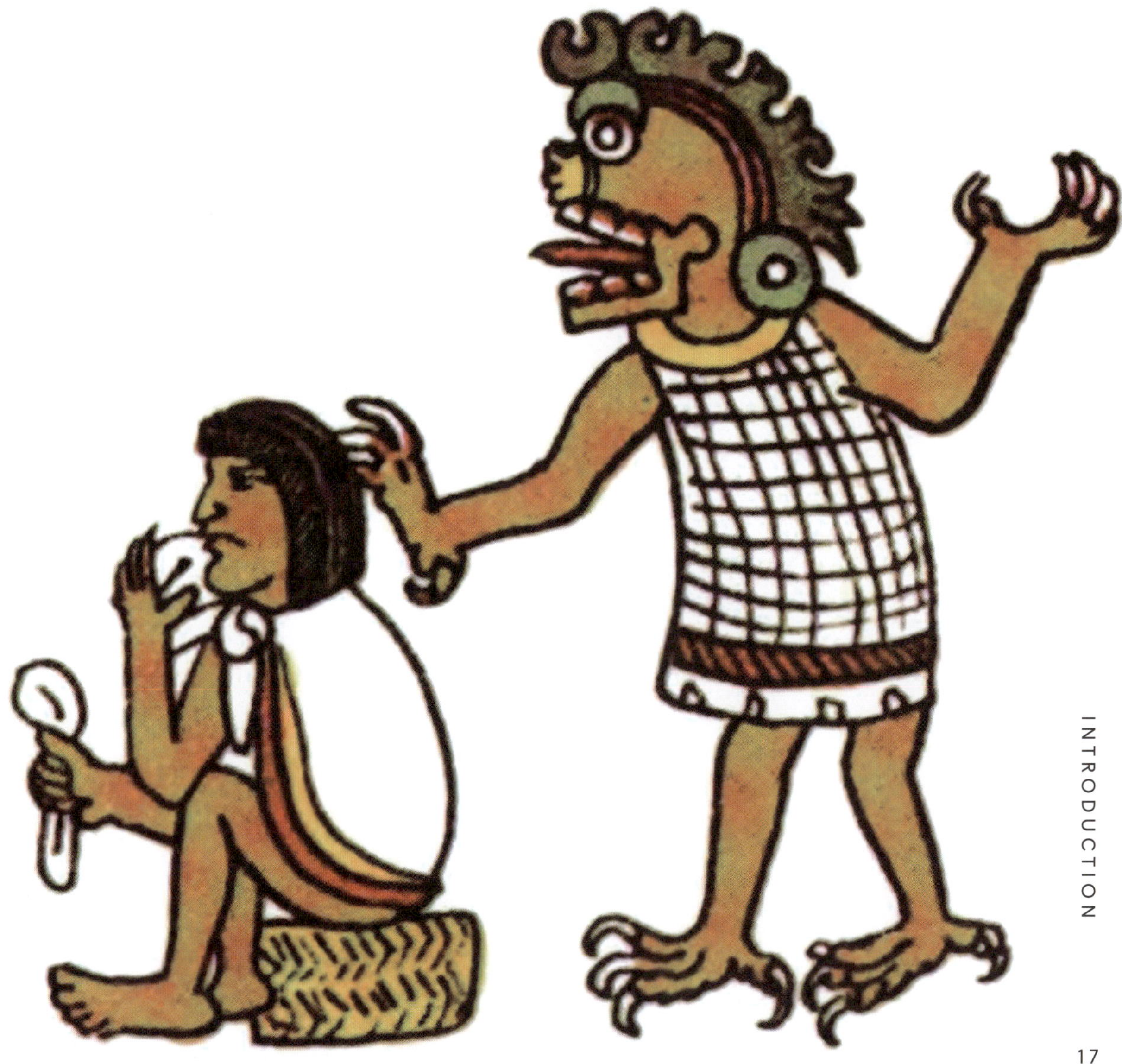

Psychedelics in the Modern Era: A Timeline

1912

The Merck pharmaceutical company synthesizes MDMA (3,4-methylenedioxymethamphetamine) for the first time as part of a pharmaceutical research project.

1938

Albert Hofmann synthesizes LSD while working at Sandoz Laboratories.

1943

Hofmann accidentally absorbs LSD, discovering its powerful psychedelic effects.

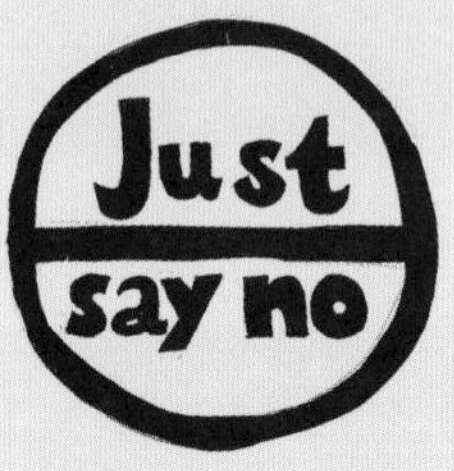

1975

Sasha Shulgin resynthesizes MDMA and explores its potential therapeutic applications.

1985

MDMA is officially classified as a Schedule I substance and outlawed, despite its therapeutic potential.

1986

Rick Doblin founds the Multidisciplinary Association for Psychedelic Studies (MAPS), aiming to overturn MDMA prohibition and explore its therapeutic use.

2000

Johns Hopkins University receives US government approval to study psilocybin's effects on end-of-life distress in cancer patients, marking the beginning of the modern psychedelic renaissance.

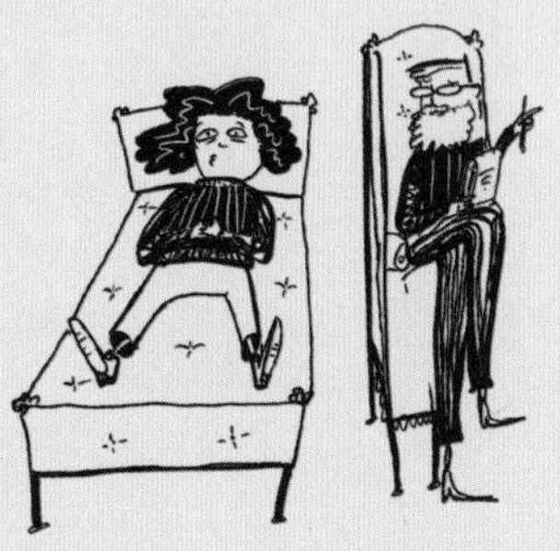

2020

Oregon becomes the first state to legalize psilocybin therapy, with Colorado following in 2022.

2023

Compass Pathways advances clinical trials for psilocybin as a treatment for depression.

2024

The FDA rejects MDMA-assisted therapy for PTSD, though MAPS continues its advocacy.

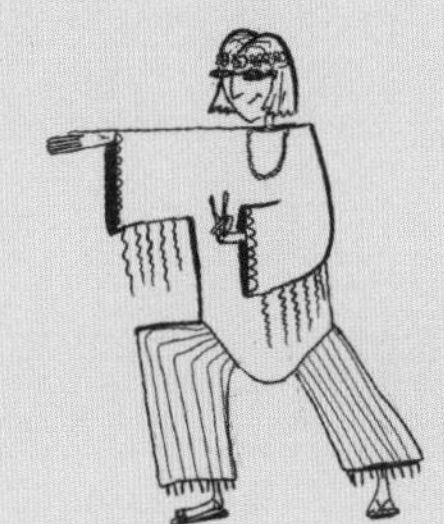

1955

María Sabina, a Mazatec shaman, introduces psilocybin mushrooms to amateur ethnomycologist R. Gordon Wasson.

1957

Wasson writes about his experience with psychedelic mushrooms in *Life* magazine, introducing psilocybin mushrooms to a Western audience.

1960s

Psychedelics are embraced by the counterculture in the United States, Canada, Europe, and beyond for spiritual exploration, creativity, and rebellion.

1970

President Richard Nixon signs the Controlled Substances Act, classifying psychedelics like LSD and psilocybin as Schedule I drugs. This legislation effectively halts psychedelic research in the United States.

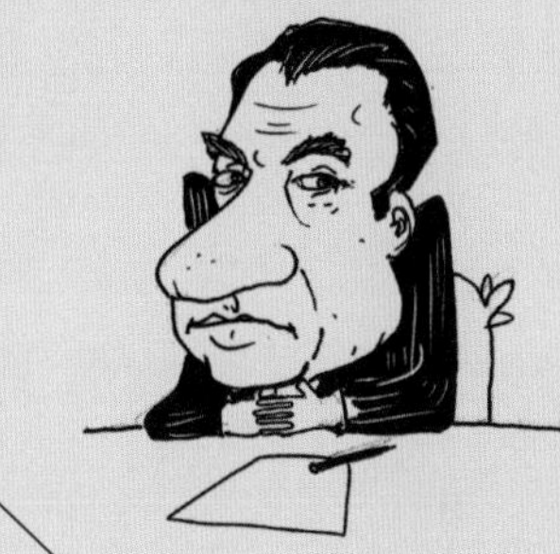

2016

Compass Pathways, a psychedelic pharmaceutical company, transitions from a nonprofit to a for-profit entity, signaling that psychedelics may not be immune from traditional pharma models that prioritize profit over access.

2018

Michael Pollan's *How to Change Your Mind* revitalizes public interest in the therapeutic use of psychedelics.

2019

Denver, Colorado, becomes the first US city to decriminalize psilocybin mushrooms, and is followed by Oakland, California, starting a national decriminalization movement.

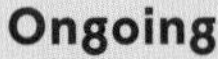

Ongoing

Decriminalization movements, therapeutic research, and legalization efforts expand globally, signaling a new era for psychedelics.

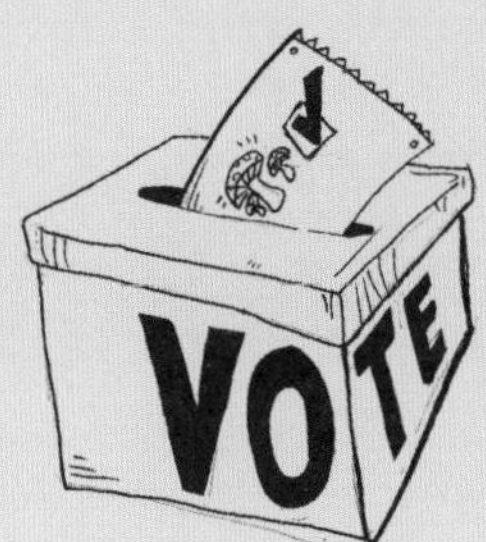

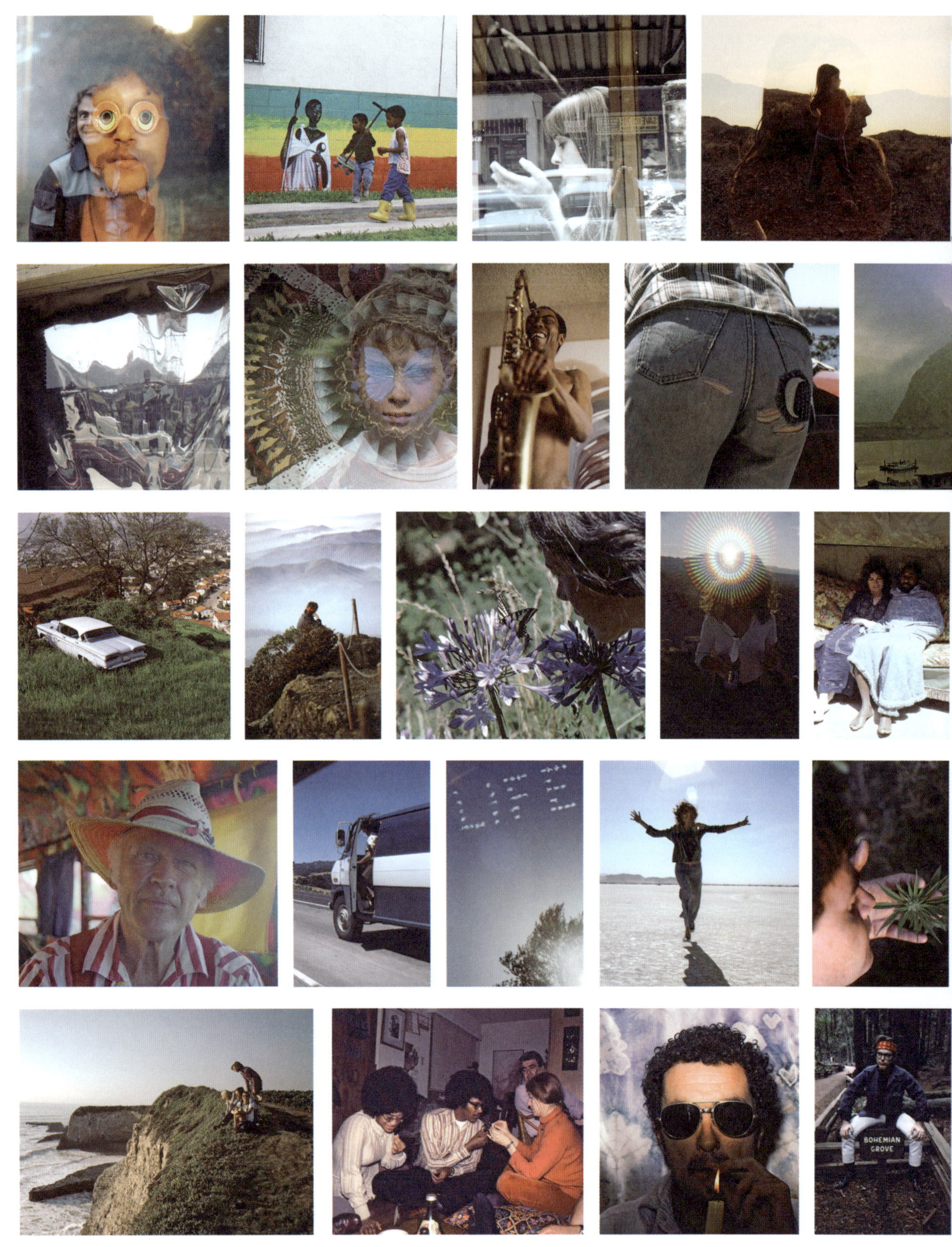

Over the course of forty years, photographer Roger Steffens captured his ever-revolving circle of Rastas, beatniks, musicians, artists, gonzo journalists, friends, and family, publishing his work under the name "The Family Acid."

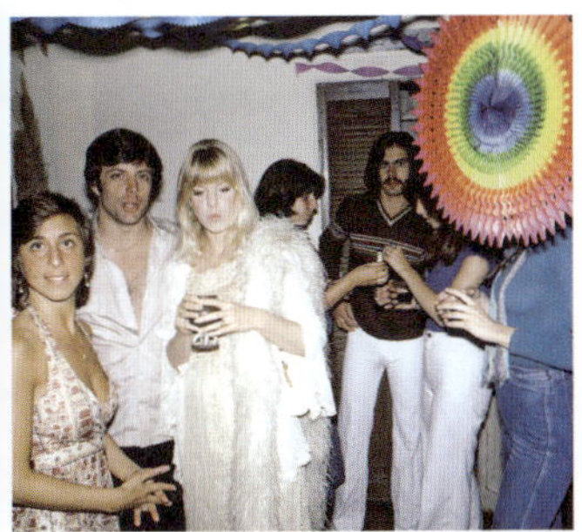
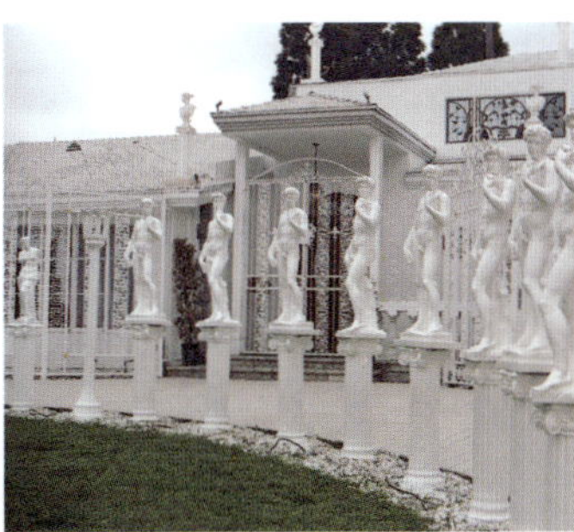
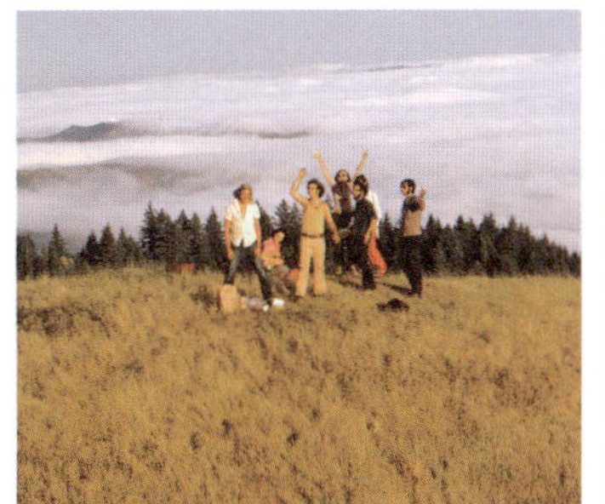
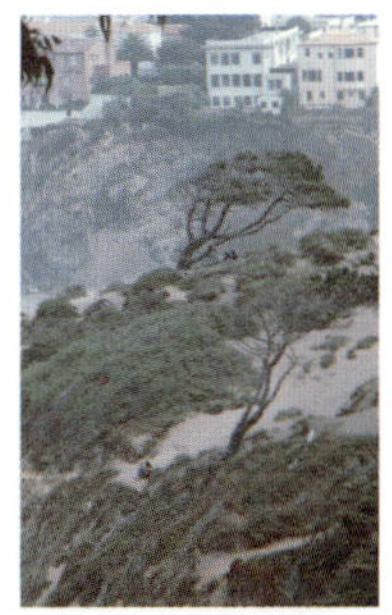
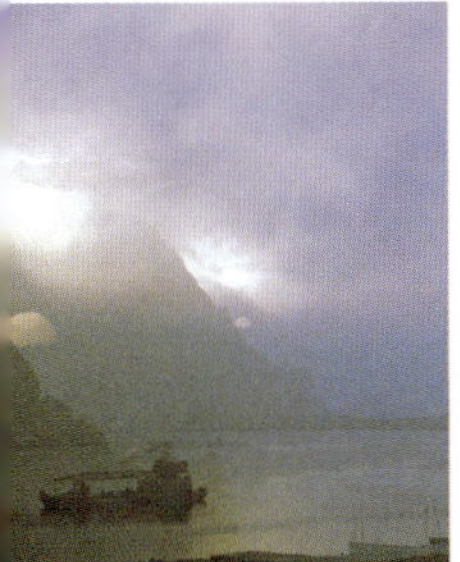
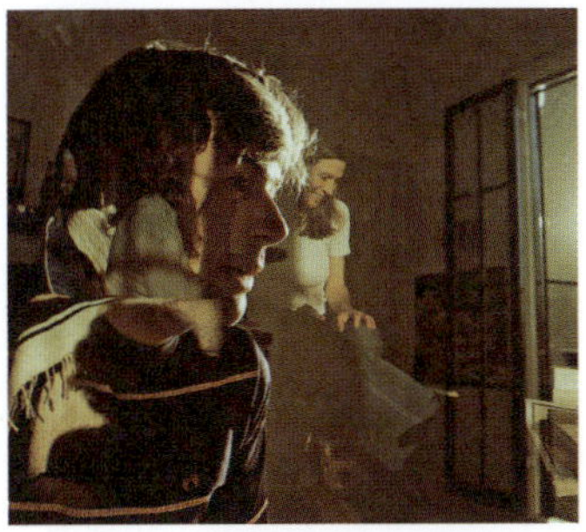
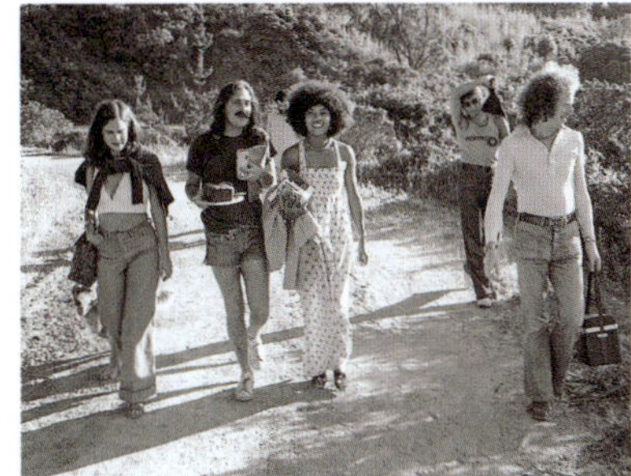
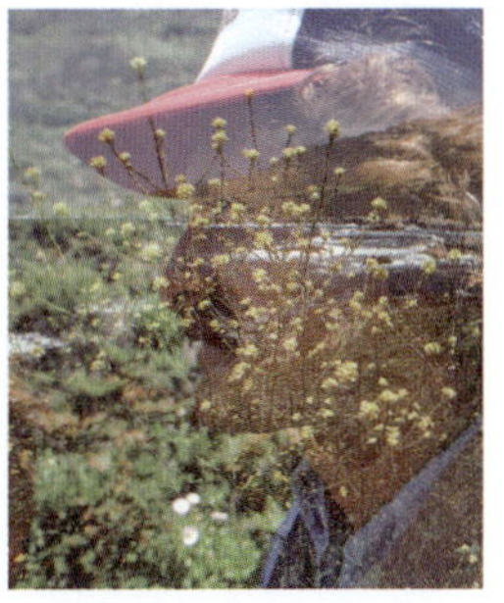
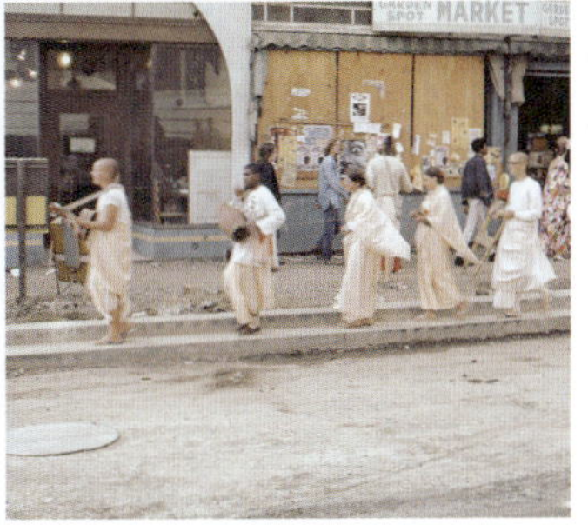
SPOT
MARKET
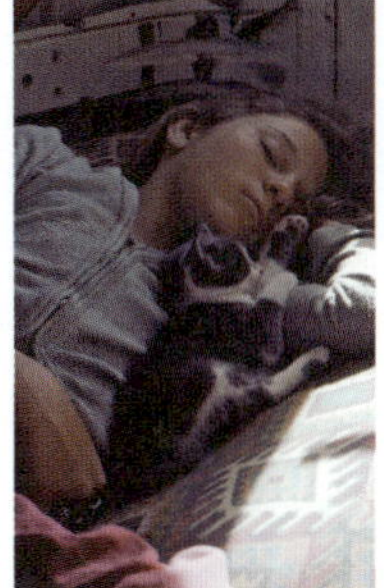
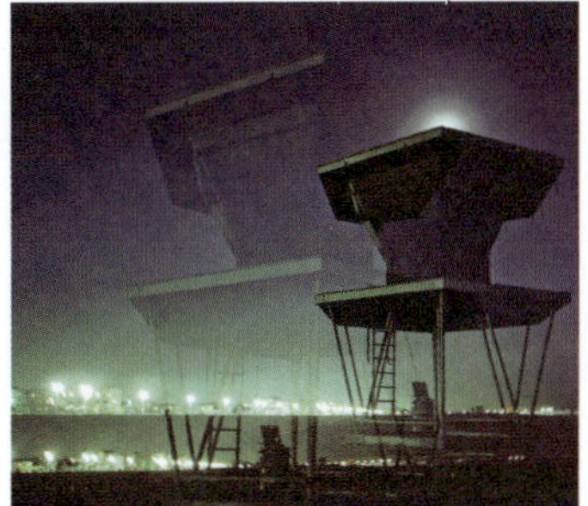
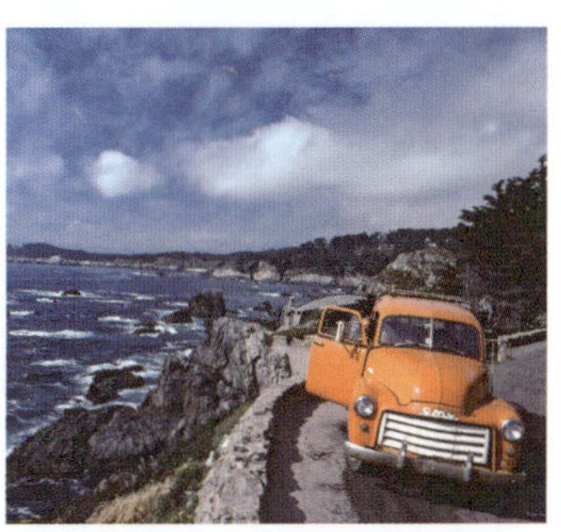
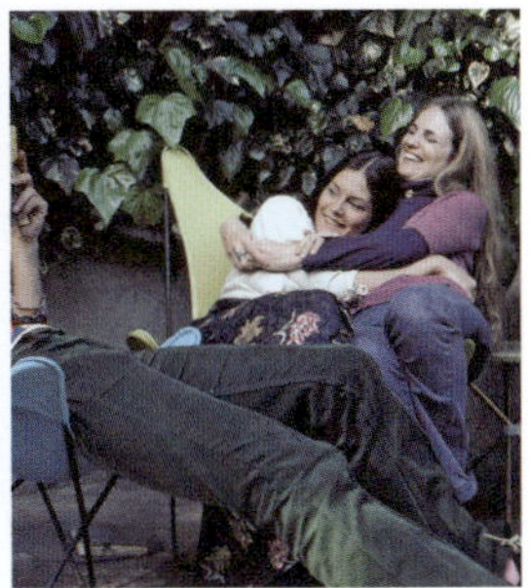
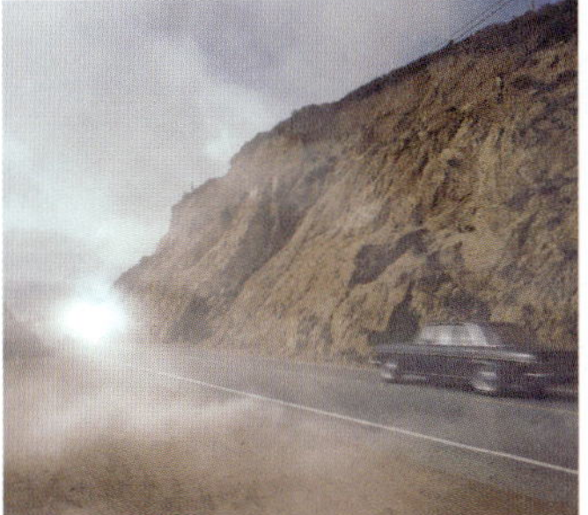
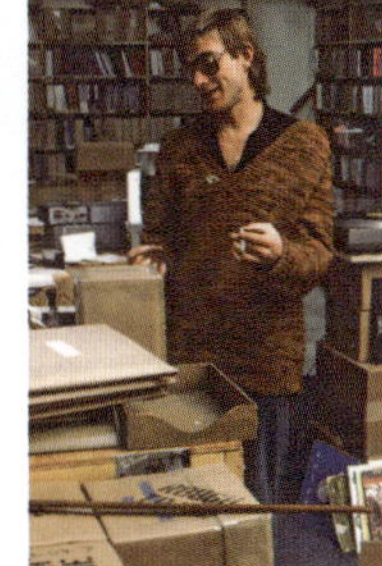
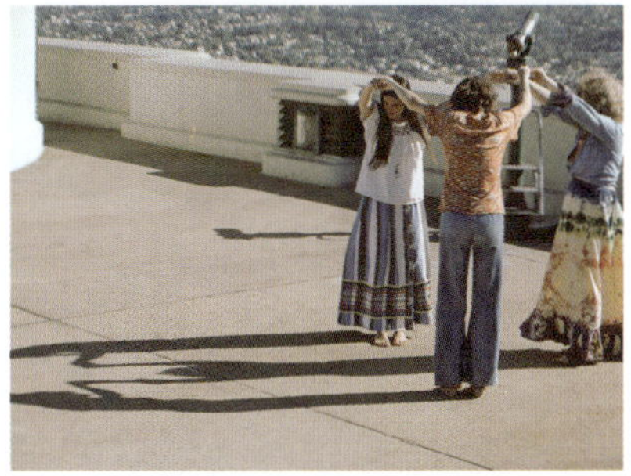
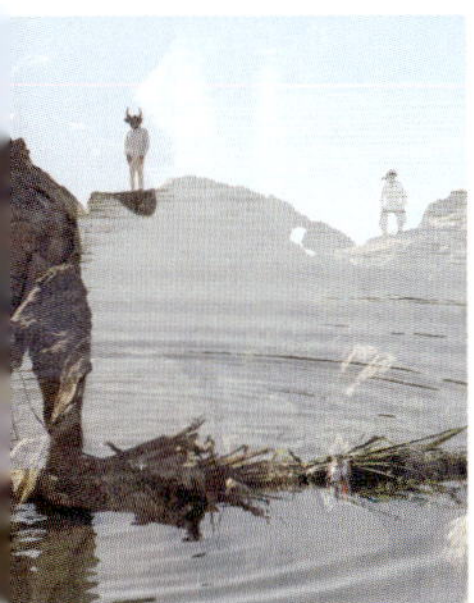
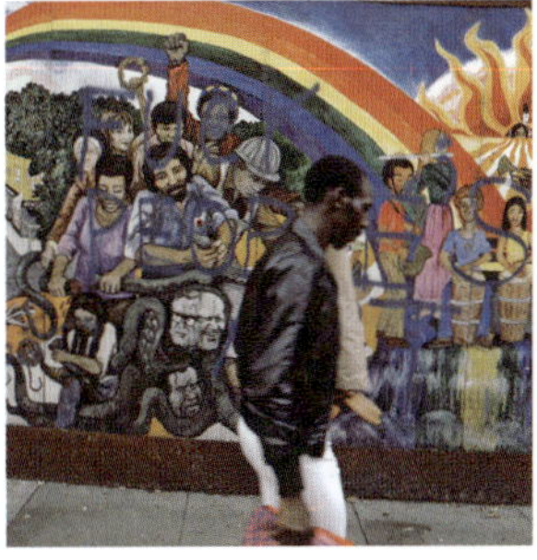
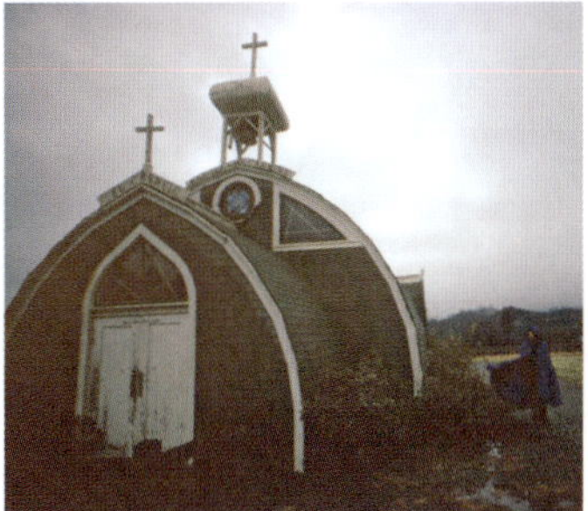
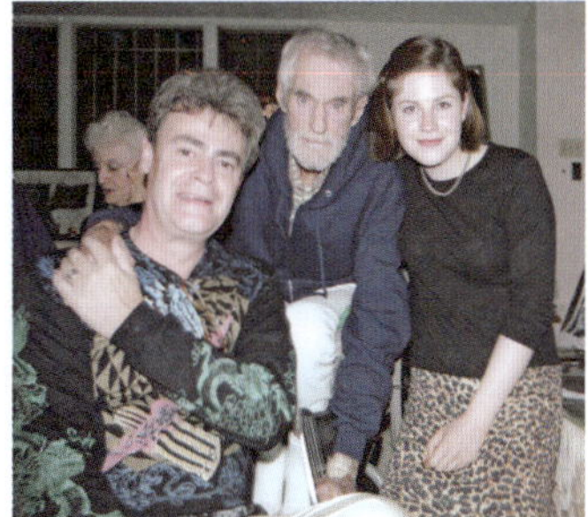

The Psychedelic Revolution, in Waves

The modern psychedelic movement began to take shape in the mid-twentieth century with the work of researchers like Albert Hofmann, who first synthesized LSD, and Harvard researchers like Richard Alpert (later known as Ram Dass) and Timothy Leary, who popularized the use of psychedelics in the counterculture movement of the 1960s. Indeed, once the Harvard administration saw that Leary and Alpert's research had gone too far (dosing undergrads and tripping alongside their subjects), the duo were expelled, and Leary in particular went on to lead a generation of flower children in a psychedelic-fueled movement defined by his tagline "turn on, tune in, drop out."

This first wave of psychedelic research and experimentation in the United States led to a cultural overhaul, with artists, therapists, scientists, mystics, and others making waves in the areas of music, art, literature, philosophy, and even religion. Artists like the Beatles and Jimi Hendrix; authors like Aldous Huxley and Ken Kesey; and even Rabbi Zalman Schachter-Shalomi, father of the Jewish Renewal movement, all were turned on by these mind-bending substances, going on to influence anyone who engaged with their work and leadership.

But it wasn't all rainbows and paisleys. In addition to inspiring art and ideologies that centered peace and love, psychedelics have a dark history of being used by ideological extremists, from Nazis who experimented with mescaline on people in concentration camps to white supremacists who proliferated conspiracy theories that influenced the founding of QAnon.

When President Richard Nixon clamped down on these substances with his War on Drugs, beginning in 1971, the psychedelic research boom came to a halt and experimentation went underground. In the media, psychedelics like LSD were painted as demonic substances that would send people into states of mania and psychosis, a far cry from earlier headlines telling a whimsical story of healing and magic. But this shift, fueled by fears of addiction, social unrest, and cultural upheaval, led to the suppression of research, the stigmatization of psychedelic users, and the incarceration of millions of people, disproportionately affecting communities of color.

MDMA, sometimes referred to as ecstasy (although they're not quite the same—more on that later), continued to proliferate a bit longer, slipping under the radar of government officials as a psychedelic that also had profound healing potential. Much of the research with MDMA in the 1970s flourished under the auspices of Bay Area chemist Alexander "Sasha" Shulgin and the many therapists who used this so-called "love drug" in couples therapy. But as MDMA made its way out of therapy offices and onto the dance floors of the rave scene in the 1980s, it too became outlawed. One year after the DEA banned MDMA, an eager young scientist from Harvard, Rick Doblin, started a then-small grassroots nonprofit called MAPS, the Multidisciplinary Association for Psychedelic Studies, working to legalize MDMA for post-traumatic stress disorder.

This was, arguably, the beginning of the second wave of psychedelic research—with MAPS leading the way on clinical trials to prove the therapeutic value of MDMA and other psychedelics. In the early 1990s, scientist Rick Strassman became the first person to acquire government approval for human research with psychedelics, and by the early 2000s, Johns Hopkins University had received approval to study psilocybin—the primary psychoactive ingredient in mushrooms. The momentum has been growing exponentially since, leading some to dub this moment as the "Psychedelic Renaissance."

Berkeley, California, in August 1972

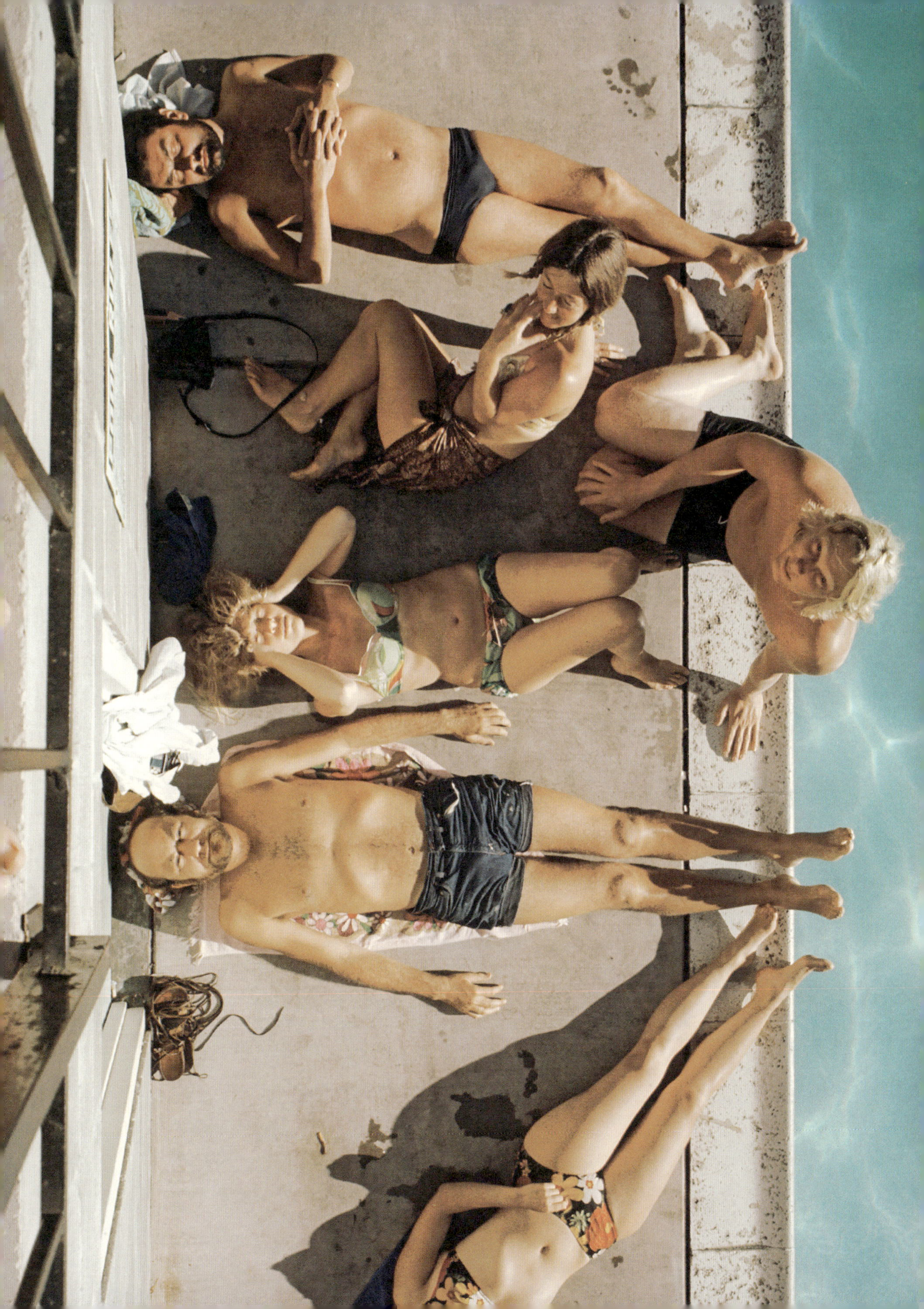

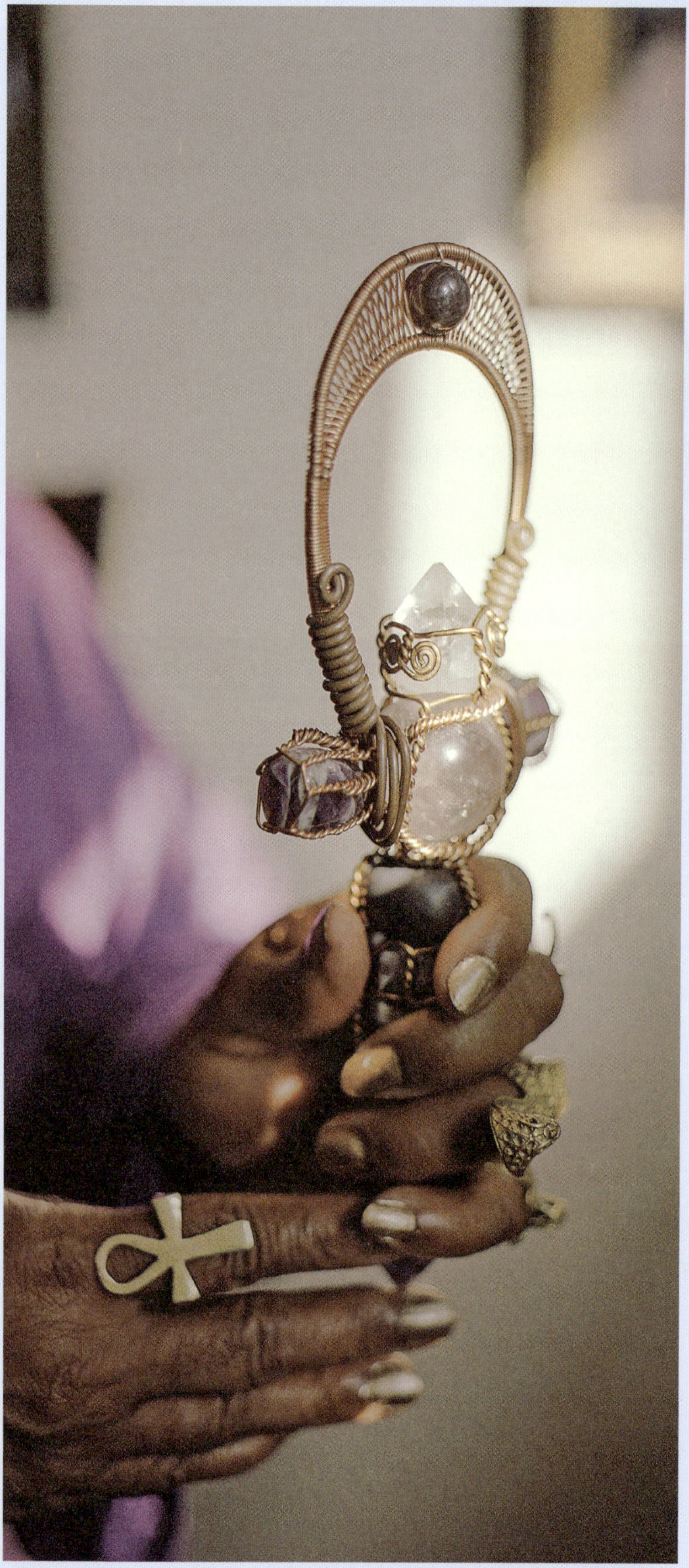

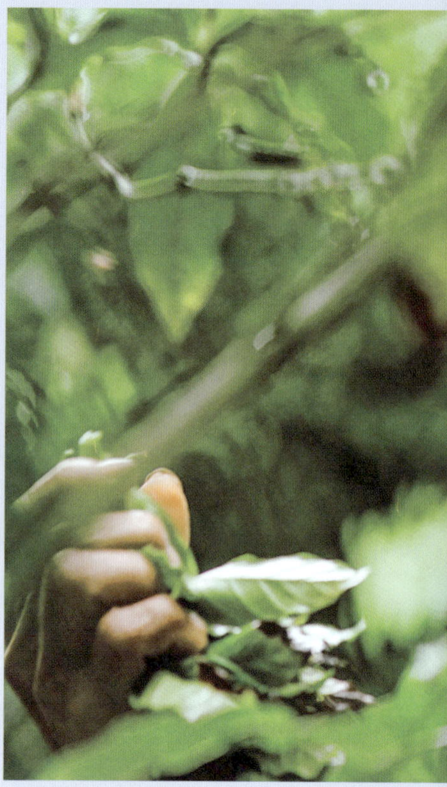

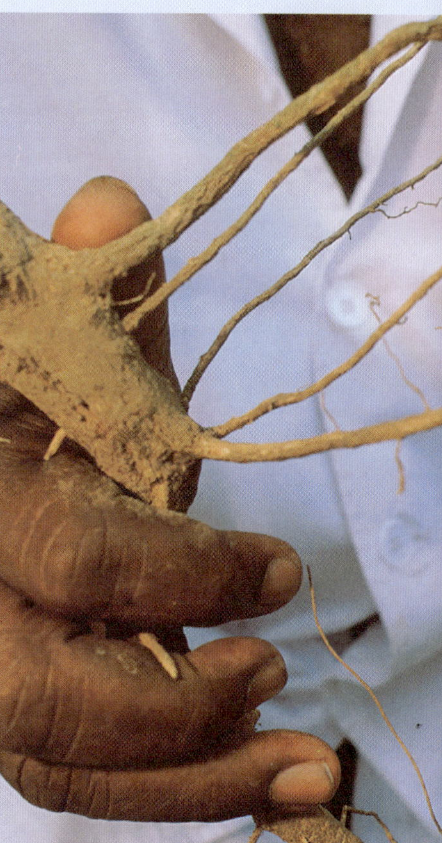

Ayana Iyi, a leader in Detroit's psychedelic community, holding an Egyptian ankh that she uses in ceremony, gifted to her by her late husband, Baba Kilindi Iyi

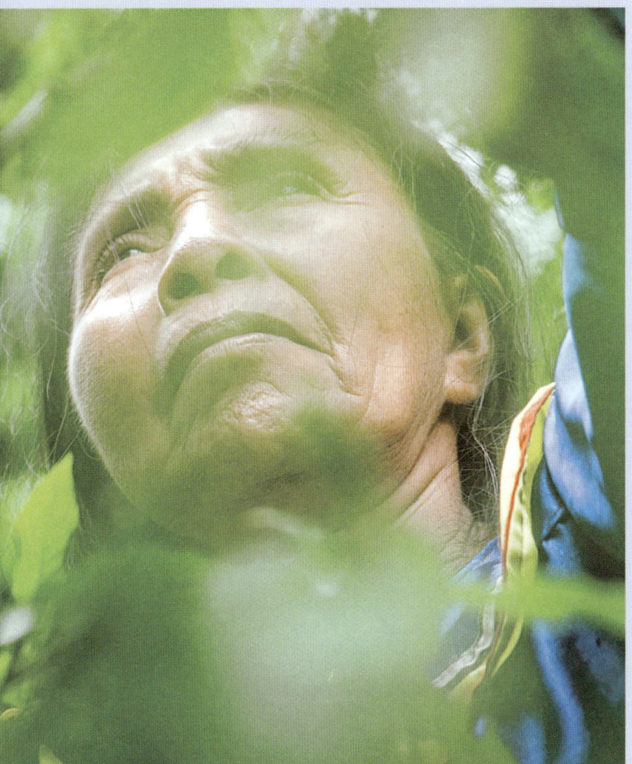

Maestra Rojelia collecting chacruna leaves on the grounds of the Temple of the Way of Light

BEYOND THE JOURNEY

PSYCHEDELICS ARE NOT A "WHITE PEOPLE THING"

In the past decade, there's been a growing number of psychedelic ceremonies and community events led by and for people of color. Many among this new generation of psychedelic leaders say they grew up thinking psychedelics were a "white people thing." This is largely attributable to the US War on Drugs and the increased risk for people of color to be open about their use of illegal substances.

But these healers and community organizers are reclaiming psychedelics not as drugs that were "discovered by" or "invented by" white researchers in the 1950s, but as tools that have been utilized by Indigenous communities around the world for millennia. They highlight the ancient, storied use of these plant medicines, from psilocybin mushrooms to iboga, a powerful psychedelic that comes from the iboga tree in Gabon. Some of the groups they support include Oakland Hyphae (an organization based in Oakland, California, that does mushroom testing and educational events for the BIPOC community), Black People Trip, Black People Need Psychedelics, and the Psychedelic Liberation Training.

Alongside these community efforts, researchers such as clinical psychologist Monnica Williams are working to design more inclusive clinical trials. In a review of past studies, Dr. Williams found that more than 80 percent of participants in psychedelic trials going back to 1993 have been white—and this is, in part, attributed, she hypothesizes, to the lack of psychedelic therapists of color who are able to support BIPOC participants in feeling seen and supported. "People are looking at the researchers," Dr. Williams says, "and going, 'The researchers are not like me, so they may not understand my problems.'" Since Williams's study, organizations such as MAPS have been actively working to assess their clinical trial design and recruit more therapists of color into their trainings.

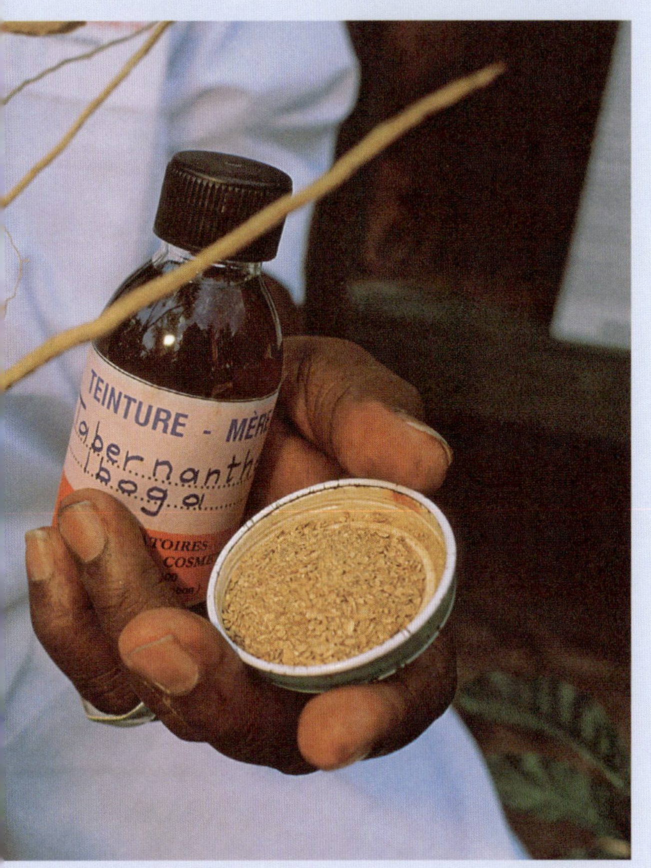

Professor Jean-Noel Gassita holding iboga root, tincture, and powder, the latter two which he made in Libreville, Gabon

The Future Is Now

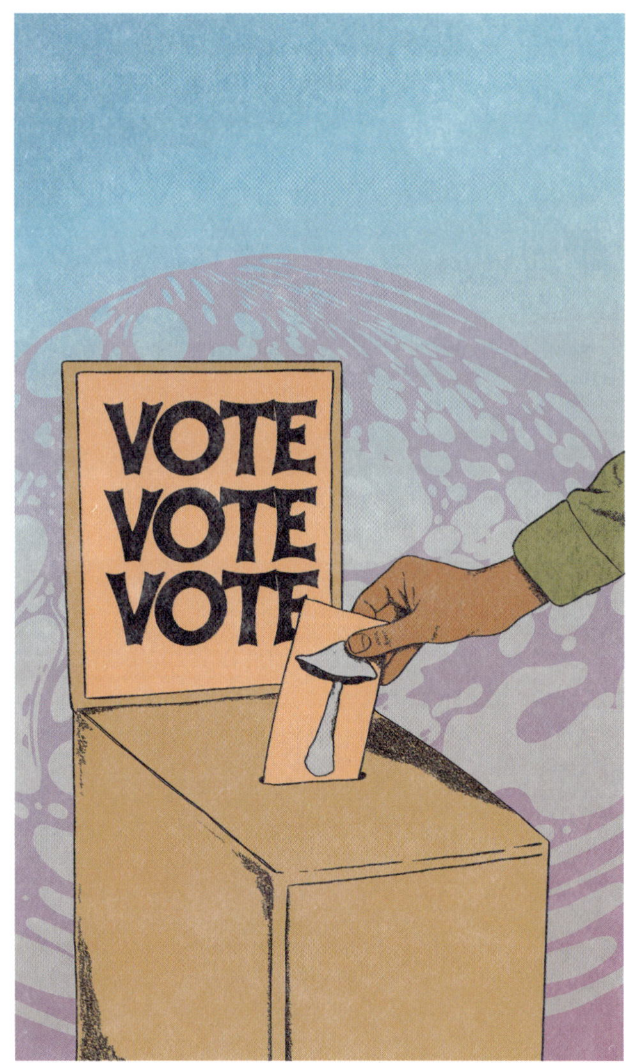

Today, the psychedelic movement is thriving, even amid setbacks, including the unexpected rejection of MDMA for post-traumatic stress disorder by the US Food & Drug Administration (FDA) in 2024. Hundreds of millions of dollars are being invested in for-profit psychedelic drug development, and a wave of psychedelic reform is sweeping across the country, with cities and states decriminalizing or legalizing psychedelic substances for therapeutic and personal use.

The psychedelic movement is about more than policy change and drug development, of course; it's a movement fueled by a desire for deeper meaning, a yearning for connection, and a longing for a more just and equitable world. These days, it might seem that everyone and their mother is microdosing mushrooms or running to the next ayahuasca ceremony. (Yes, microdosing moms is now a thing.) Indeed, psychedelics are becoming more accepted in mainstream society, as medicines in clinical research, as tools for expansion, spirituality, and wellness, and as alternatives to alcohol in recreational settings. With the rise of a new generation of psychedelic explorers, researchers, religious professionals, and advocates who are pushing the boundaries of traditional thought and challenging the status quo, the psychedelic movement is moving faster than public education—and that's where this book comes in.

The DoubleBlind Guide to Psychedelics is designed to be a comprehensive, fun, and accessible guide to the world of psychedelic substances, written for everyone, whether you're a seasoned psychonaut or a newbie just beginning to consider the possibilities. In these pages, you'll find information on how to decide if and when you want to journey, what psychedelic you might want to use for your journey, and how to make sense of the experience once it's over. Chapters focused on a particular substance will cover the fundamentals, such as dosage and what to expect. Woven throughout these practical tips, you'll find information for going "beyond the journey"—cultural and political factoids to help you situate your journey within this moment in psychedelic history. Yes, this book is an opportunity to explore the transformative potential of psychedelics, but we hope that it also serves as a call to integrate the psychedelic ethos and consciousness into life-at-large to effect a more compassionate, healed, and magical world.

CHAPTER 1

WHICH PSYCHEDELIC IS RIGHT FOR YOU?

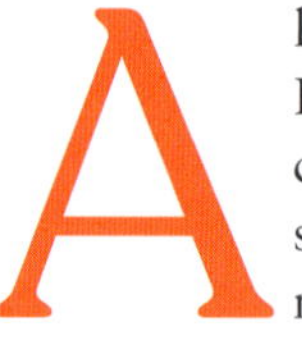ll right, it's the moment you've all been waiting for. Let's get into the psychedelics you're likely to be choosing from when you journey. Countless substances qualify as "psychedelic," but the most common ones in popular discourse are:

Shrooms	DMT	MDMA
LSD	Ayahuasca	Ketamine

So, with all these options (and the countless other plant and chemical compounds with psychedelic effects, some of which we'll explore in chapter 11), the first question is: *How do you choose which psychedelic substance is right for you?*

Before we get into how you might answer that question, a disclaimer: We're not doctors; we're journalists. And we don't know you or your situation—everyone's needs and psychological and physical health are different. So please don't take anything in this book as medical advice. We'll provide you with a lot of information to help you start assessing the right path for you, but it's still always good to consult with a psychedelic integration therapist, trusted facilitator, or doctor before embarking on a psychedelic journey.

Regardless of who is helping you prepare for your journey, you'll want to understand some basics around potential contraindications. We get into this in each psychedelic-specific chapter, but we'd also point you to Spirit Pharmacist, an online resource intended to help people understand the risks of psychedelics, as a starting point.

Beyond that, there is no right way to answer the question of what substance to choose and there, indeed, may not be just one answer. As you'll see, many of the most common psychedelics are showing promise for the same conditions. Many people, for example, look to tripping to improve their day-to-day mood, but ketamine, shrooms, LSD, and ayahuasca have all shown promise in rigorous scientific studies for depression. So while we'll cover the basics, and we always encourage folks to do their homework (you're in the right place!), there's also an element of intuition involved in the decision-making process. Is there a particular experience, based on what you learn, that you just feel drawn to? That's as important as understanding fundamentals such as dosage and duration. Typically, when people consider tripping, they first consider one of the "classic psychedelics," such as shrooms or LSD, so we'll begin there.

The Classic Psychedelics: Shrooms, LSD, and DMT

When you think of the stereotypical "psychedelic experience"—the grass beneath your feet swirling into patterns, the flowers and clouds assuming personalities as seen in *Alice in Wonderland*—then you're most likely thinking of the effects associated with "classic" psychedelics: LSD (a.k.a. acid), psilocybin (or magic mushrooms), and DMT (and substances that contain DMT, such as ayahuasca).

These psychedelics activate the brain's serotonin 5-HT2A receptors, which play a role in learning, memory, and other fundamental cognitive processes as well as mental health conditions, like depression, anxiety, substance dependence, and eating disorders. No one knows exactly *how* psychedelics work, but one thing is for sure: Generally speaking, these substances increase and decrease activity in various regions throughout the brain. Notably, they decrease activity in the default mode network (or DMN).

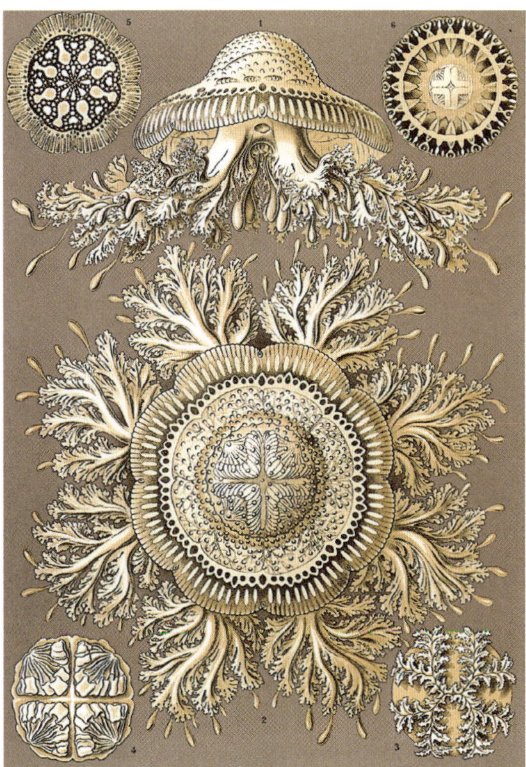

It's in the DMN where core parts of who a person perceives themself to be, sometimes referred to as "the ego," live. The DMN is a large-scale neural network that is most active when a person is not focused on the outside world and the brain is at a wakeful rest, such as during daydreaming and mind-wandering. This is also the region where the brain processes identity; perceives time in the past, present, and future; and stores memories.

During a psychedelic experience, when activity in the DMN decreases, a person might experience what scientists call "ego death" or "ego dissolution." That's why it's not uncommon, when under the influence of a substance like psilocybin, to, for instance, lose one's sense of time or regular sense of identity.

A temporary quieting of the DMN has been linked to therapeutic outcomes, such as helping a person release addictive behaviors or thought patterns that no longer serve them. It also allows for greater activity in other parts of the brain that don't normally communicate with each other—which could lead to a phenomenon called synesthesia, where one of the senses, like sight, stimulates a usually unrelated sense, like hearing. Yes, this means you can actually hear colors or see sounds.

And that is only one of the many trippy, disorienting, far-out sensations that can occur during a psychedelic experience. You might see the Divine, feel like you're dying and being reborn, be surrounded by love, or just spend many hours feeling slightly uncomfortable. It's impossible to predict what a trip will be like until you're in it—which is why so much of the psychedelic experience, no matter which substance you use, is founded upon 1) trusting the process and 2) ensuring that the set and setting—your internal state of mind and body and your external surroundings—going into a trip are the best they can be (we'll cover more on this in chapter 2).

What About MDMA and Ketamine?

Distinct from the classic psychedelics are MDMA and ketamine.

MDMA is methylenedioxymethamphetamine—otherwise known by its street names *molly* (which mostly refers to a pure version of MDMA) and *ecstasy/E* (which sometimes refers to a less pure version of MDMA, cut with other substances). MDMA has a variety of connotations, but in today's scientific community, it's best known as a PTSD treatment. This is why many people seek it out these days for therapeutic reasons, although it's also commonly used among partners, friends, and families for resolving interpersonal conflicts. It's also used for, well, having a good time—at festivals, clubs, and even just among romantic partners looking to connect. If you ever find yourself pooping out on the dance floor but want to shake it all night long, MDMA just might be your psychedelic of choice.

MDMA is special because, rather than ushering the user into another world, the experience is grounded in this reality—from a place of compassion and empathy. Its primary mechanism of action is through the release of serotonin, dopamine, and norepinephrine in the brain, giving it its unique pharmacology. It also triggers the release of oxytocin, which popular science refers to as the "love hormone"; the warm, fuzzy feelings a person may have while on MDMA are often attributed to oxytocin, though its role in human behavior isn't actually well understood. Additionally, functional MRI studies have shown that MDMA reduces activity in the amygdala, a part of the brain that plays a crucial role in activating the "fight or flight" response, which appears to help people experience their memories, including traumatic ones, with reduced fear.

A person with PTSD often experiences flashbacks. Internal or external triggers, such as a sudden loud noise, can cause them to reexperience a traumatic event, like an assault, and this happens over and over again. It's thought that PTSD arises from the inability to fully process trauma because it is, well, too traumatic to think about intentionally. But MDMA helps ease the overwhelm, so that a person who has experienced trauma can process their past and move on. All that said, before you rush to roll on MDMA to address trauma, remember that the promising results of the research reflect specific protocols in a controlled environment; that isn't to say that doing it on your own will not be therapeutic, but there are no guarantees (not even if you're doing it clinically).

Like MDMA, ketamine is known for being a gentler psychedelic and, for some who are afraid of tripping, perhaps an easier way into these consciousness-shifting experiences. It's also currently taking the place of cocaine in a lot of party settings. You'll find people snorting lines of it or spritzing it up their noses in DIY nasal sprays everywhere from warehouse parties to Burning Man. In small doses, it's a social lubricant and energizing.

Unlike MDMA and classic psychedelics, ketamine is technically legal for use in clinics around the United States and globally for the treatment of depression, trauma, and other conditions. Indeed, many think this trendy treatment is paving the way for legal psychedelic clinics that will eventually serve an entire menu of substances in conjunction with therapy. For now, however, generic ketamine is prescribed "off label," which means that it hasn't actually been approved by the FDA for mental health. As of this writing, only one company has secured FDA approval for a ketamine product for depression. It's called Spravato, and it is a ketamine nasal spray that is administered under medical supervision at clinics.

Ketamine is considered a dissociative psychedelic because it can induce feelings of detachment from one's surroundings and from one's own body (this especially comes in contrast to MDMA, which might engender feelings of connectedness and increased embodiment). Ketamine's dissociative

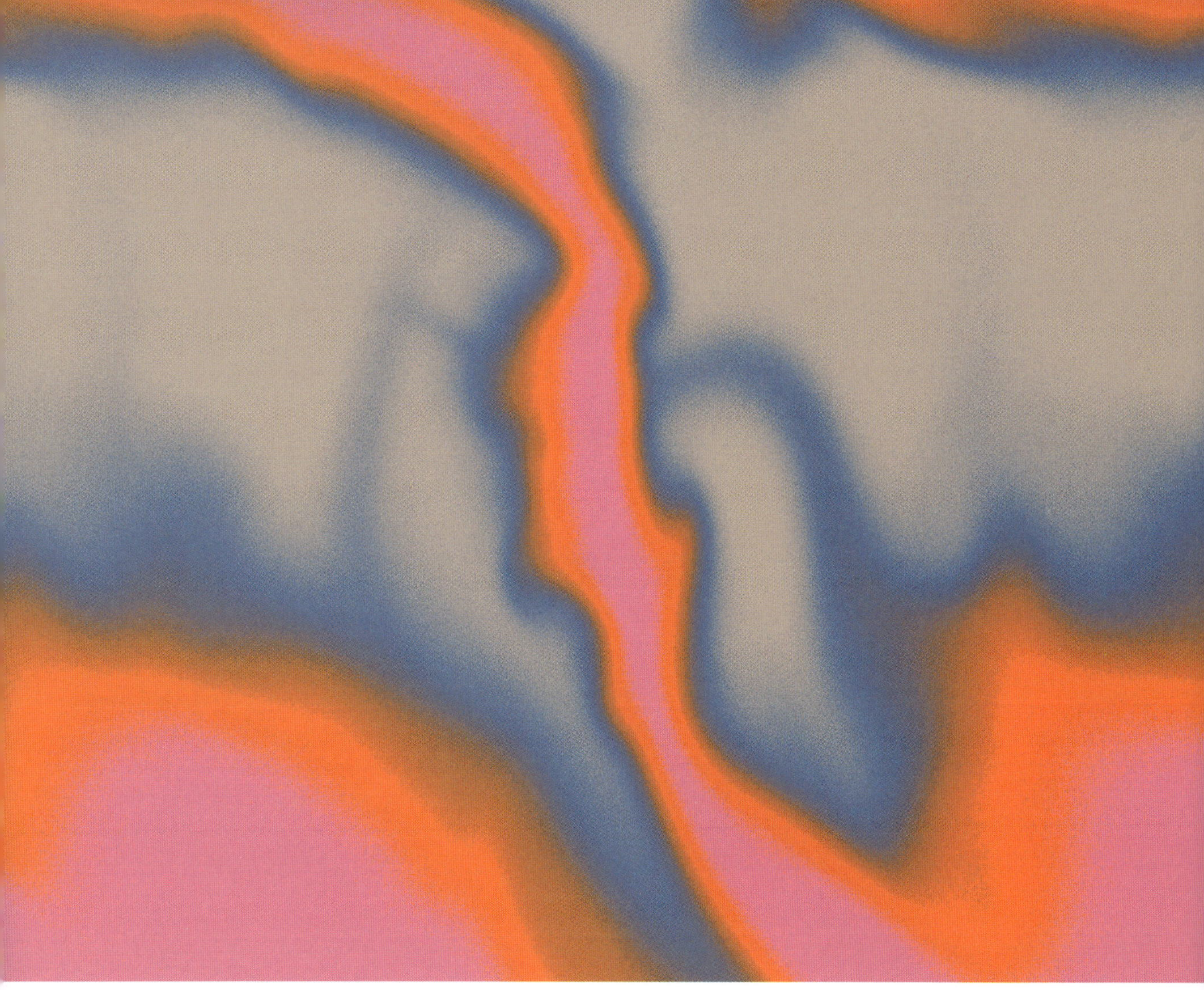

effect comes as a result of its ability to block the brain's N-methyl-D-aspartate (NMDA) receptors, which are involved in sensory processing, perception, and other critical brain functions.

Although dissociative effects may sound negative, they can actually be therapeutic in certain contexts. With ketamine, they may help break the cycle of negative thought patterns and rumination that can contribute to depression and other mental health conditions. By creating a temporary detachment from one's thoughts and emotions, ketamine can offer new perspective or reprieve. In some cases, the dissociative effects may also help in the treatment of chronic pain, as it can help interrupt the pain signals that are sent to the brain and reduce the perception of pain.

---

flip
verb

to combine drugs

In the world of psychedelics, popular drug combinations include MDMA and shrooms (hippie flipping); MDMA and LSD (candy flipping); and shrooms, LSD, and MDMA (Jedi flipping). One small study found that combining MDMA with LSD might induce a more positive mood. That said, flipping is not recommended for psychedelic newbies, as it can be more intense than doing a drug on its own and there's no rigorous research on this practice.

"Natural" vs. Synthetic Psychedelics

corporadelic
adjective

corporation + psychedelic = corporadelic

Corporadelic describes organizations and people who prioritize profit over purpose in their psychedelic industry pursuits. The term is most often used to describe stakeholders who are putting psychedelics through the drug development process with the intention of getting them on the market as prescription medications. Most of these entities are researching drugs under a for-profit model and taking millions of dollars in investment from venture capital funds using a big pharma model that has been criticized for inflating prices at the expense of patients. In the case of psychedelics, there's been criticism, in particular, of companies that are tweaking psychedelic compounds so that they are eligible for patent. Psilocybin, for example, is in the public domain and can't be patented, but a unique delivery system, such as a psilocybin nasal spray, would be eligible for patent and grant the developer exclusivity on sales for a period of time as well as control over pricing.

In addition to considering the effects and duration of a psychedelic (which we'll cover for each substance in its dedicated chapter), some people make their choice based upon whether a psychedelic is natural (i.e., grows in the ground) or synthetic (i.e., is made in a lab). This is a philosophical choice as much as a pragmatic one. Much like there are people who want to eat only organic foods that are not genetically modified, there's a contingent in the psychedelic community who prefer "plant medicines." In this category we find a number of substances derived from plants and fungi (e.g., psilocybin mushrooms, ayahuasca, wachuma/San Pedro cactus), as well as, in some cases, substances from living animals (e.g., 5-MeO-DMT from the venom of the Sonoran desert toad). For some people, this preference for plant medicines arises from Indigenous cosmologies, which, throughout the world, are infused with the philosophy of animism, the idea that there are spirits in all living beings, including plants, and that when we take plant medicines, we can commune with these spirits.

From a scientific perspective, it may be easiest to understand the choice between natural and synthetic substances through the example of cannabis. Some argue in favor of utilizing the whole plant (or, more accurately, the whole plant part) because the full package and variety of the plant's natural compounds work in harmony with each other, according to a synergy known as the "entourage effect." That is to say, even if a person is seeking the effects of just one of the cannabis plant's compounds, like THC (its main psychoactive element) or CBD (among its most popular, highly therapeutic nonpsychoactive compounds), some researchers hypothesize that THC or CBD work better in the presence of other compounds that occur naturally within the whole plant. The same has been hypothesized of psychedelic mushrooms, which contain a variety of alkaloids beyond psilocybin that differ depending upon the species.

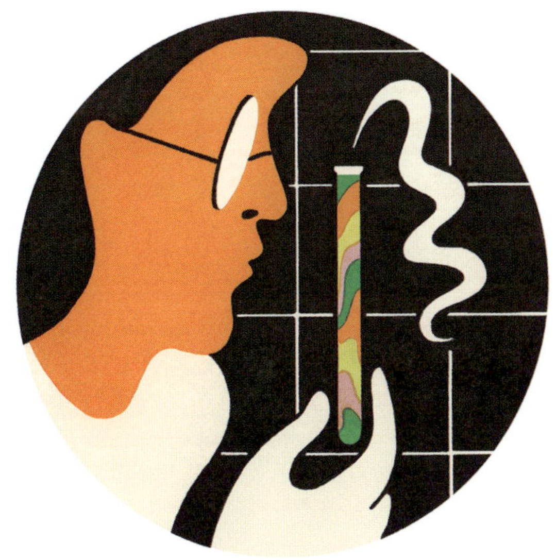

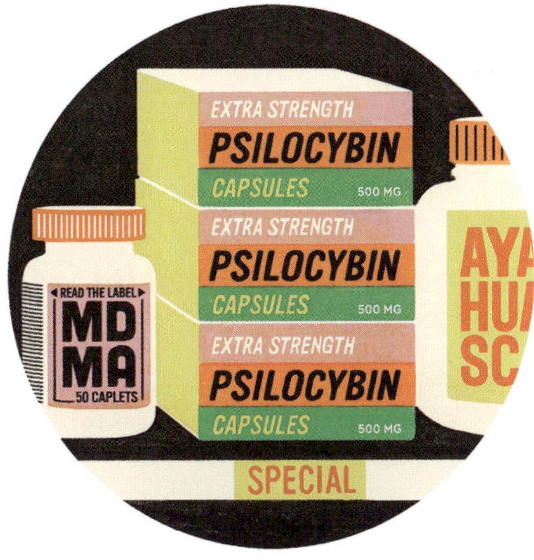

Synthetics, some hypothesize, just may not be as therapeutically effective because you're getting the benefit of only one compound, as opposed to many working together. That said, there's been hardly any rigorous research done on whole psilocybin mushrooms.

An arguable downside of working with natural material, however, is that there is not a clear delineation of just how much of a substance's active compound is present or exactly how potent it is. A gram of cannabis bud doesn't indicate exactly how much THC it contains; in the same vein, a gram of magic mushrooms doesn't indicate how intense the experience of the psilocybin may be, especially since its chemical profile may vary from species to species and strain to strain, or even batch to batch, depending on the growing conditions. It's just harder to standardize dosages of material that comes from the earth. In the case of a plant, it's also sometimes difficult to determine the grower's methodology with regard to using pesticides or other sustainability practices.

That is, in part, why some people prefer isolated chemical compounds, which are easier to measure and guaranteed to be pure. Thus, for instance, in FDA-approved clinical trials exploring the therapeutic potential of psychedelics, scientists at institutions like Johns Hopkins are using synthetic, lab-made psilocybin, which is subject to fewer variables than a comparable amount of psilocybin contained within actual mushrooms grown within a facility or in nature.

Legality

Before you dive into your journey, it's essential to consider the laws around the psychedelic you're considering using. Psychedelics in general are not legal, but we are fast on our way to a post-prohibition world. That's all to say, through government-sanctioned research at the federal level and local grassroots initiatives, psychedelic plant medicines and synthetic compounds are becoming decriminalized or legal—in the context of therapy—throughout a perpetually increasing number of jurisdictions. Psychedelic laws are changing or may change in the future in a number of ways, from rescheduling to decriminalization, and they all may affect the risks you incur when you decide to journey.

RESCHEDULING

First, you probably know about the possibility of certain psychedelics becoming legalized as FDA-approved medicines. At the time of this writing, both psilocybin (in synthetic form) and MDMA are in the final stages of research to be approved in what's called "psychedelic-assisted psychotherapy" to treat depression and PTSD, respectively. As of now, it's unclear whether psilocybin and MDMA, on their own, or just the specific formulations used by the companies doing this research will become rescheduled (meaning they will no longer be categorized as Schedule I controlled substances, which is the most highly restricted category, by the US government). However, even if psilocybin- and MDMA-assisted psychotherapy become legal for the treatment of depression and trauma, outside of this context, these two compounds would remain illegal substances at the heart of thriving underground, unregulated markets. It's also important to note that even if these forms of psychedelic-assisted psychotherapy become legalized through the FDA, not everyone will qualify for them. We say this because we've heard some folks say they want to wait for federal legalization, but, at this moment, it's likely not going to happen soon—and it won't change things for most people in the United States.

DECRIMINALIZATION AND STATEWIDE LEGALIZATION

As of this writing, your best shot at having a legal psychedelic experience in the United States (unless you've been prescribed ketamine for the treatment of depression or certain other disorders) might be at a state-approved clinic. Two states—Oregon and Colorado—have legalized facilitated psilocybin experiences. These experiences are being licensed and approved at the state level, and they are distinct from the clinical trials, which are seeking to legalize psychedelic therapy federally. Basically, any adult—whether they're a resident or not—can have a supported psychedelic journey in these states at approved locations under the supervision of professionals licensed by the state. Please note, though, that at this time these experiences usually run in the thousands of dollars.

Alongside this, in an ever-growing list of localities that began with Denver, Colorado, and Oakland, California, and has since expanded to places like Ann Arbor, Michigan, and Somerville, Massachusetts, adults can possess, grow, gather, and gift mushrooms and other natural psychedelics under local decriminalization bills that have been passed by city councils or at the ballot box.

For the layman, the distinction between legalization and decriminalization can be a bit hazy. Decriminalization typically involves reducing or eliminating criminal penalties for drug possession or use, while often still maintaining some level of regulation or control for larger quantities. Under decriminalization, drug-related offenses may be subject to civil penalties like fines or set as law enforcement's lowest priority. Decriminalization is often seen as a more lenient approach to drug policy, with a focus on reducing the harm associated with drug use and addressing drug addiction as a public health issue. It basically means you can possess and gift these substances without risk of incarceration by local law enforcement, but you can't sell them.

Legalization, on the other hand, makes the possession and sale of a substance legal, though it may still be subject to restrictions like age and possession limits, and in some cases licensing may be required for certain retail or production purposes (such as what we've seen with the legal cannabis industry). Typically, legalization comes with some kind of regulated marketplace that involves sales. And whether we're talking about legalization or decriminalization, it's important to note that these measures apply only at state and municipal levels, while federal prohibition is still in effect.

As it stands today, a number of grassroots activist organizations are leading the charge to end psychedelic prohibition. One such group is Decriminalize Nature, a collection of independent chapters throughout the United States that have launched successful efforts to decriminalize naturally occurring psychedelics (other than, for the most part, peyote, at the request of the Native American Church, which is concerned about the cactus's risk of endangerment). Other efforts have originated within state legislatures (such as in the states of California and New York) and through ballot initiatives (such as in the case of Oregon's full-scale drug decriminalization policy and legal psilocybin therapy program). If you're passionate about psychedelic reform or want to meet other psychonauts in your town, a great way to do it is by becoming involved in a local decrim initiative.

RELIGIOUS EXEMPTION

Aside from medicalization and decriminalization, another route to a post-prohibition world exists through protections that afford religious organizations the right to use psychedelics as a sacrament, so long as they can prove their sincerity. This policy exists in part thanks to the Religious Freedom Restoration Act (RFRA) of 1993, which has enabled churches like the União do Vegetal (UDV), for instance, to use ayahuasca (which contains DMT) and the Native American

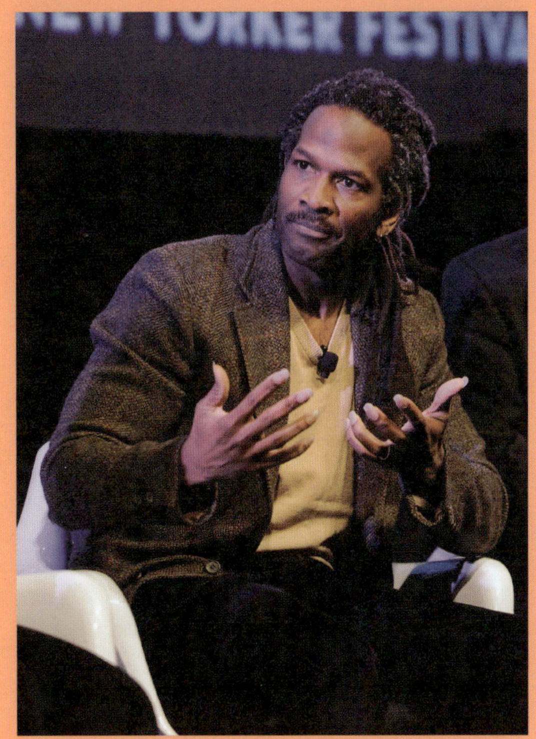

BEYOND THE JOURNEY

THE "PSYCHEDELIC EXCEPTIONALISM" DEBATE

In 2021, as psychedelic decriminalization bills were sweeping the nation, Columbia University professor and neuroscientist Carl Hart came out with a widely covered book, *Drug Use for Grown-Ups*, advocating for the legalization of all drugs. He popularized the term *psychedelic exceptionalism*, which refers to the idea that some drugs that are believed to have therapeutic potential (i.e., psychedelics) are "good" and others that are believed to cause harm (i.e., heroin) are "bad." This ideology is problematic, he and other drug policy advocates argue, because it justifies removing criminal penalties for some drug users while continuing to incarcerate others. If we're going to decriminalize any drugs, they say, we should decriminalize them all.

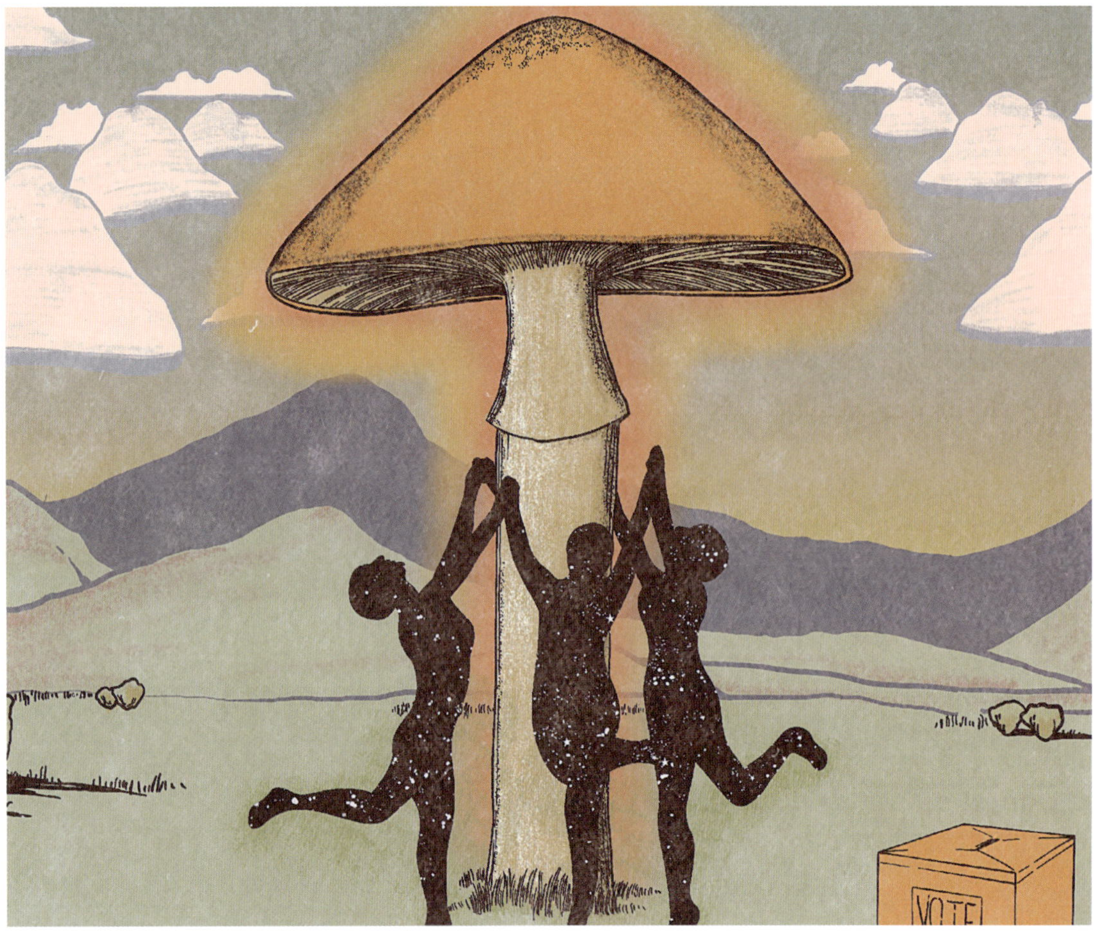

Church to use peyote (which contains mescaline). Here, we'd like to place emphasis on the word *sincerity*. There are dozens of groups out there now claiming that they're legally serving psychedelics through their "church" and that they're protected by religious freedom, but they have not been officially granted exemption from federal laws restricting psychedelic use. It remains controversial as to whether or not the federal government should be able to determine the sincerity of someone's psychedelic use.

PSYCHEDELIC RETREATS ABROAD

A handful of countries have a booming psychedelic retreat center industry. The legal situation varies in these countries, but over the past decade, people who either feel called to sit in Indigenous-led ceremonies or do not want to wait for their home country to approve psychedelic therapy have begun going to places such as Mexico, Costa Rica, or Jamaica for mushroom retreats; Peru, Colombia, or Brazil to do ayahuasca; Gabon to try iboga; and beyond.

It's worth noting that even in countries where psychedelics are legal or decriminalized, there may still be risks associated with their use, and it's important to research the safety and legitimacy of any retreats or ceremonies before participating. Additionally, it's important to approach these substances with respect and caution, and to participate in ceremonies or retreats only under the guidance of experienced and qualified practitioners who have an understanding of their traditional use. You can find more information on how to vet a retreat center on page 146.

Stewardship and Reciprocity

Increasingly, we're seeing discourse within the psychedelic industry on the importance of supporting and giving voice to Indigenous communities that have long preserved the knowledge around psychedelic plants and fungi. As millions of dollars began to pour into pharmaceutical companies looking to develop psychedelics into FDA-approved medicines, reciprocity efforts among organizations, led by and working closely with Indigenous groups, grew, too. They've put out a call to the psychedelic field to acknowledge Indigenous people as the stewards or protectors of traditional plant knowledge and requested that people without ancestral ties to these medicines prioritize biocultural preservation. Ongoing reciprocity efforts within the field include psychedelic conferences allocating money to fly Indigenous healers from their territories to speak alongside researchers and therapists; nonprofits raising money for Indigenous communities; and dialogue about the ethics of taking a sacred plant or fungus from its place of origin and trying to patent a synthetic version of it for profit.

There's also been a rising conversation around how individuals who are taking psychedelics can engage in reciprocity with Indigenous stewards. At DoubleBlind, efforts to give back to and include Indigenous voices in our work is central to our values. Yet it can be complicated to figure out what that actually looks like.

Indigenous people are not a monolith. There are an estimated 476 million Indigenous people across ninety countries, and while there's no definitive data, many of them have deep-rooted traditions involving the use of psychoactive plants. Some of these communities, such as the Native American Church, have requested that non-Natives do not participate in their ceremonies at all. Other communities, such as the Shipibo-Conibo (often referred to as the Shipibo for short) in the Amazon, hold ceremonies for foreigners who have brought invaluable financial resources into their territories. In this book, we highlight just some of these voices.

There's also ongoing debate about the degree to which someone who is taking a psychedelic that does not have Indigenous roots, such as LSD or MDMA, should be responsible for engaging in reciprocity. We believe that all journeyers should make an effort to give back to Indigenous stewards, because while certain substances may not have direct ties to a specific ancestral tradition, the broader psychedelic movement is deeply rooted in Indigenous knowledge and practices. By supporting Indigenous communities, we honor the cultural and historical foundations that paved the way for contemporary understandings of altered states of consciousness, ritual, mysticism, and plants and fungi as beings with a spirit, as opposed to inanimate objects that we consume for our own benefit.

So, if you want to engage in reciprocity, how might you do that? It might sound obvious, but a good way to begin is by learning about the history of psychedelic plants and fungi, including the communities they come from and the contemporary challenges they're facing. While Indigenous communities hold a wide variety of cosmologies, all maintain a deep connection to the earth and a significant majority have fought for the right to stay on their land. This is relevant to psychedelic users because, for these communities, sacred plants and fungi cannot be protected separately from their territories and all the other living beings contained within them. Traditional medicines such as peyote and ayahuasca live within ecosystems that need protecting as a whole, and many of them today are still actively under threat by corporate interests, such as industrial farming and oil and mining extraction.

At the end of the book, we include a list of organizations that host ongoing talks, papers, and conferences with Indigenous people. Generally, learning about the traditional use of plant medicines will help you approach your journey with respect.

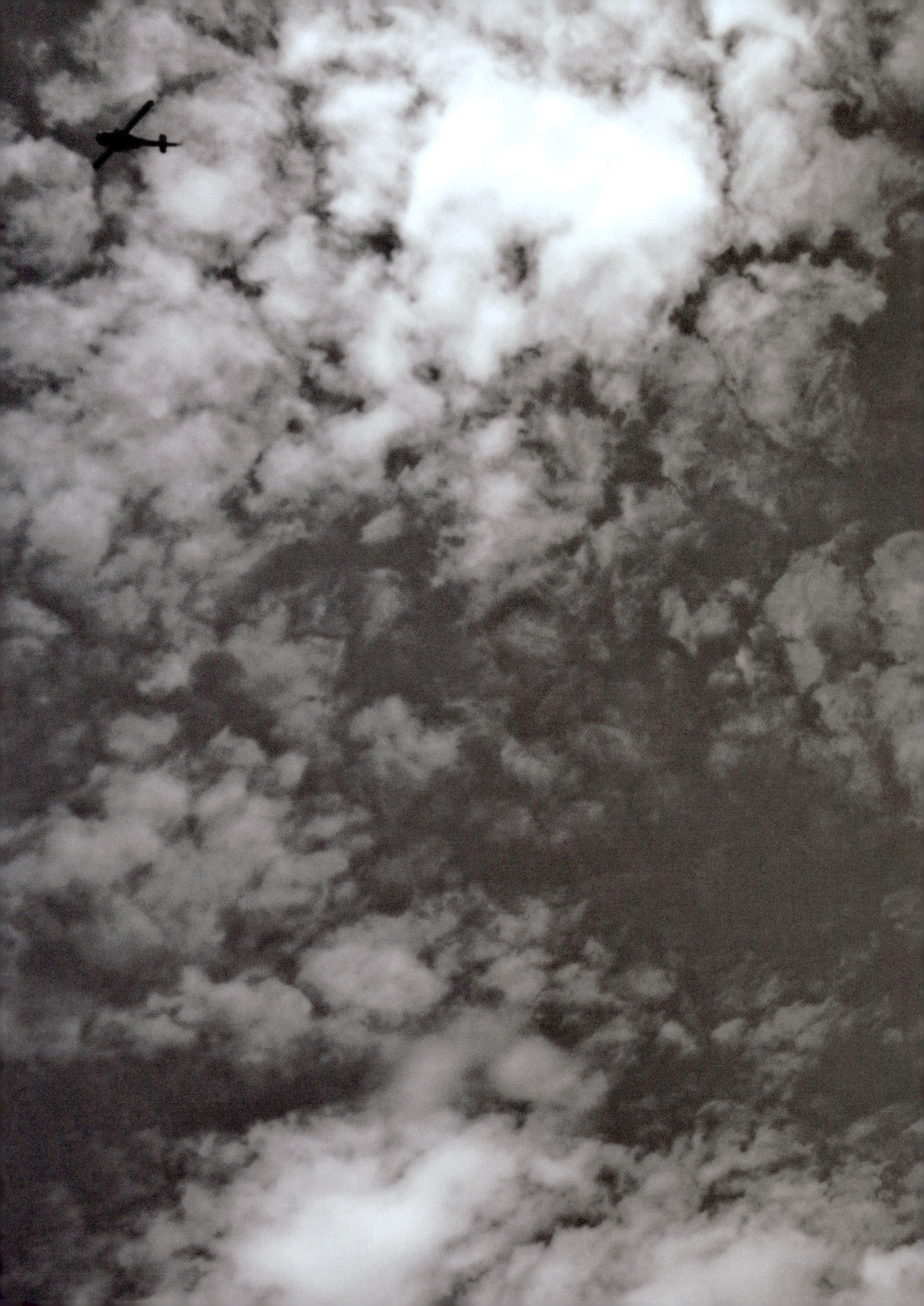

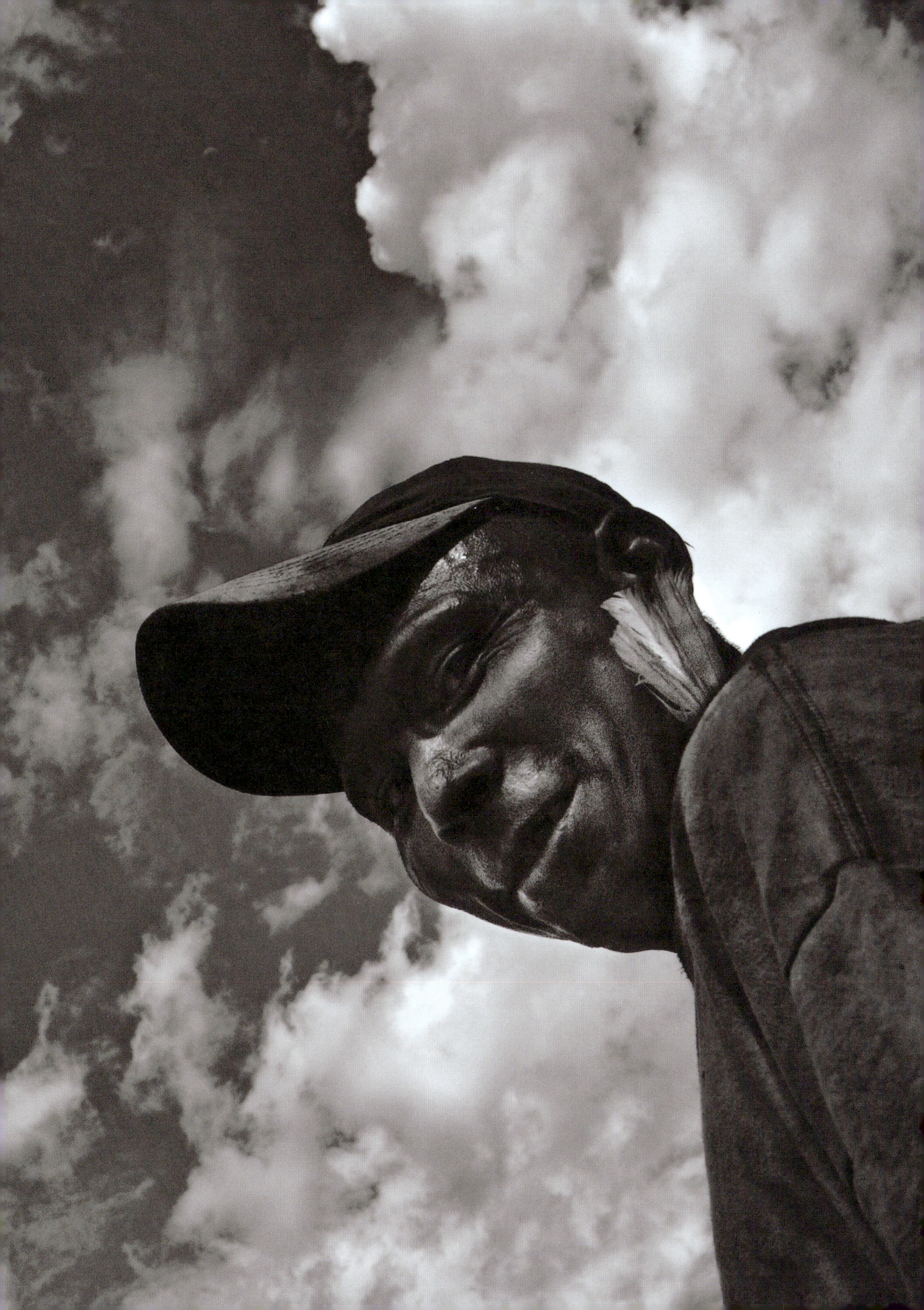

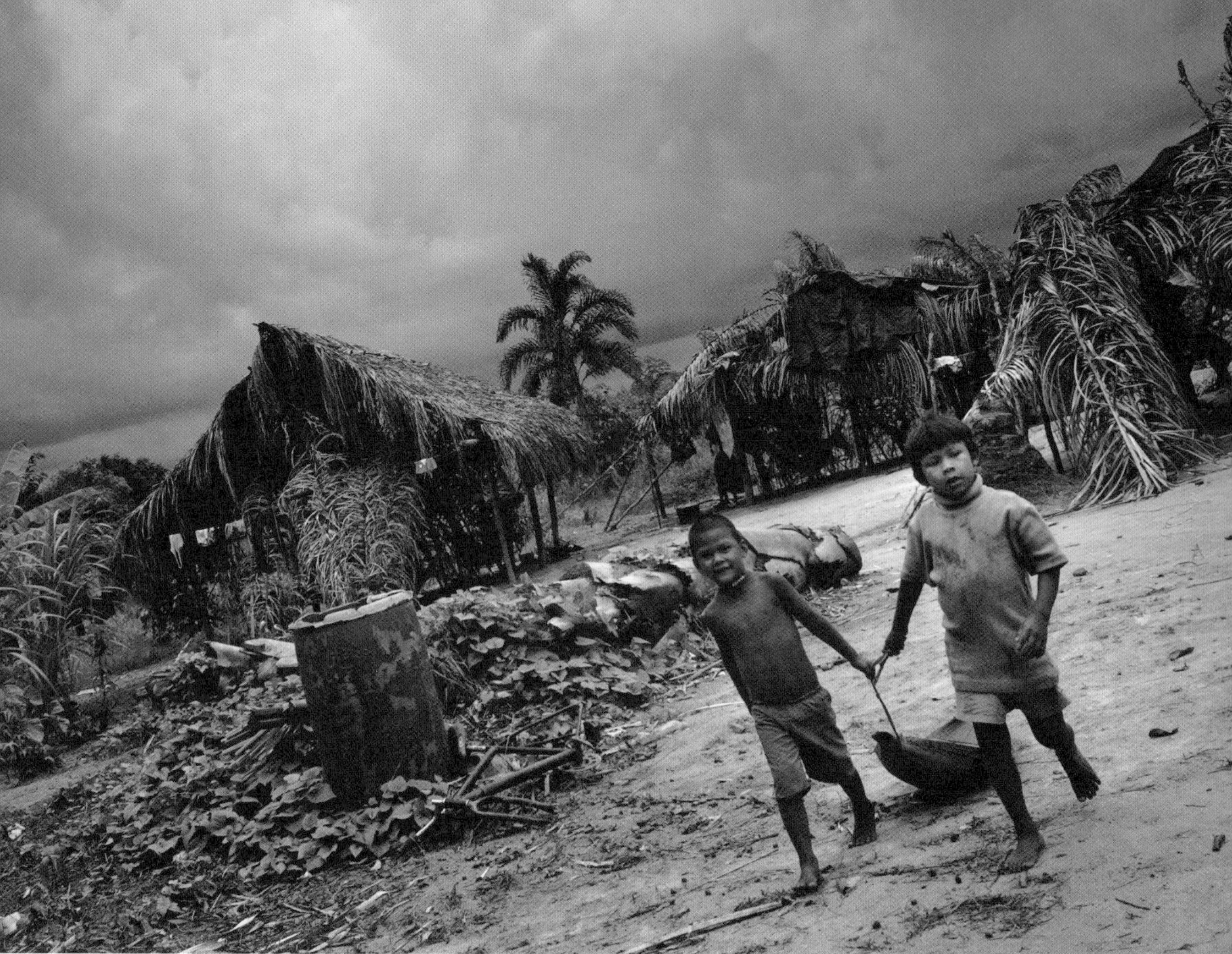

The Nukak Maku people, nomadic hunter-gatherers violently driven out of their jungle territories in Amazonia by Colombian guerrilla and paramilitary squads, are seen here living in a refugee camp close to San José del Guaviare, Colombia, September 4, 2009.

Previous pages: **A Nukak man watches a Colombian police helicopter flying over the Nukak settlement.**

One of the first steps toward reciprocity is not creating a hierarchy of wisdom (i.e., assuming that scientific data is a more legitimate way of knowing than Indigenous traditions of learning through prayer, ritual, and communing directly with the spirits of these plants and fungi). Other ways to practice reciprocity include donating to nonprofits working with Indigenous communities (see page 218 for a list); ensuring that the psychedelics you're taking are sourced sustainably, especially plants with a history of being poached, such as iboga and peyote; and attending a retreat that is directly engaging in reciprocity through equitably compensating Indigenous healers.

Last, we'll just say that reciprocity doesn't always have to be tied specifically to giving back to Indigenous communities (although we encourage this) but can also look like taking care of your own community. Within the Indigenous framework, we are all connected, and thus any form of giving back is reciprocity in action. This can take the shape of volunteering, trip sitting for someone, helping raise awareness about ways to avoid harm when taking a psychedelic—really all types of altruism.

Stewardship and reciprocity is a complicated topic, and one that is, frankly, worthy of its own book, but all of these steps are a great starting point.

CHAPTER 2

PREPARATION

Before embarking on a psychedelic experience, whether you're a newbie or a seasoned psychonaut, it's essential to prepare to maximize its potential benefits. Taking a psychedelic is not just about getting the right dose or finding the perfect setting; it's about creating a "container" for the experience, a space where you can safely explore your inner world, spiritual connection, relationships, and whatever else you put into your intention.

Set and Setting

The concept of set and setting was first popularized by Harvard psychologist Timothy Leary and his colleagues and laid out in their 1964 psychedelic guidebook, *The Psychedelic Experience: A Manual Based on the Tibetan Book of the Dead*. *Set* refers to your mental and emotional state. It's about how you're feeling, your intentions, your expectations, and your overall mindset going into a psychedelic experience. *Setting* is the physical environment in which you're taking the psychedelic. It's about the space, the atmosphere, the current events, the season, the music, the people around you, and other external factors. Every aspect of your space is going to shape how you feel, so take care in arranging it. Clean ahead of time, from removing clutter to dusting to washing your sheets. Make sure the lighting is not grating by turning on lamps as opposed to overhead fixtures. Place anything you want out so that it's easily accessible: extra blankets and pillows, an essential oil, incense. Perhaps most important, make sure that any potential disruptions are taken care of. This includes roommates coming home and people stopping by unexpectedly. If possible, it's great to have private indoor and outdoor areas available so that if you're wanting a change in scenery, you can access it easily.

Both set and setting are critical for shaping your psychedelic experience. They can create a safe and supportive environment that allow you to explore your inner world with openness and curiosity. On the other hand, a negative frame of mind and disruptive environment can create a challenging experience, leading to feelings of anxiety, fear, or even paranoia. Just know that whatever you are exposed to before and during your psychedelic experience can cognitively prime you and influence what comes up during the journey.

Who Should I Trip With?

If you're new to psychedelics, first things first: Don't go it alone. While it's important to prepare for your experience and curate your set and setting to maximize the best possible outcome, it's also nearly impossible to predict exactly how it will go. That said, if you are unfamiliar with psychedelics, having someone else present can help foster feelings of safety and therefore enable you to go deeper into the experience.

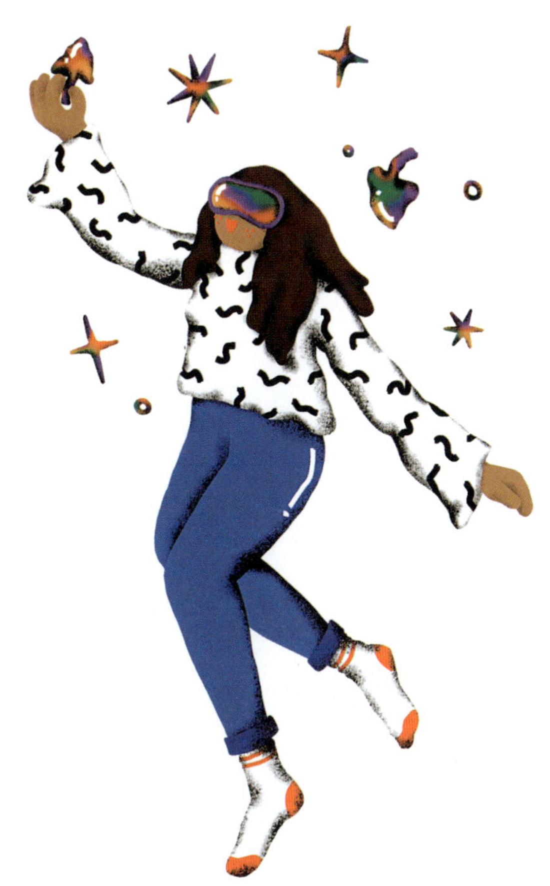

On the other hand, if you're a seasoned psychonaut, solo journeying can offer a profound opportunity for self-insight and self-exploration.

Beyond tripping with someone who is there to support you or tripping solo, there are a number of options. You can trip with a group of friends, you can trip with one other person who is also on psychedelics (as opposed to being sober and present just to support you), you can have a private trip with a professional guide, or you can trip in a ceremony. There are pros and cons to each, and ultimately, as with every other aspect of your journey, you have to decide what feels right for you.

TRIPPING SOLO

Taking a psychedelic by yourself allows you to connect with your inner world without distractions. However, it can also be isolating and challenging, especially if you hit some bumps along the road. While there are resources, such as the Fireside Project, which offers a hotline for anyone having a challenging psychedelic experience, using your phone can be tricky, exposing you to messages or notifications that you may not want to see when you're tripping.

TRIPPING WITH LOVED ONES

Tripping with friends, family, or a romantic partner can provide a sense of safety, support, and connection, while fostering a more playful and fun experience. However, it's important to be sure that you are comfortable with the present company, as any unresolved or latent relational issues can compromise feelings of emotional safety and potentially lead to a challenging experience. If you want to focus on your own healing, journeying with someone who needs your support might distract you from addressing your own feelings. A journey done with a loved one can end up becoming about your relationship with that person; you both may want to talk about past or current issues that exist between you or you may just want to have fun together. That's okay, but just understand that tripping with other people adds variables that may not be conducive to you focusing on yourself, if that's what you want.

JOURNEYING WITH A GUIDE

A one-on-one, personalized experience may be ideal for a first-timer looking to focus on a specific issue. The best way to figure out whether you want this level of attention and care is to get clear on your intention. (Learn more about setting your intention on page 49.)

If you feel called to employ a guide, it's important, first, to explore the different types that exist. Do you want a licensed therapist who is working underground? This may be ideal if you're dealing with a formal mental health diagnosis such as post-traumatic stress disorder. If you're someone without a formal diagnosis, depending on the level of your psychological distress, a trained guide who is not licensed as a therapist or even a friend or family member who offers to be by your side may be sufficient. You'll want to vet any person serving you medicine, but once you find the right fit, a trained guide can help you prepare for and navigate the experience. They may also be able to help you process or integrate your experience afterward (see chapter 4 for more information on that). In essence, it is like having a babysitter while you're tripping. The downside here is that, at least in the United States, Canada, and much of Europe, unless you're enrolled in a clinical trial, you will be working with someone who is operating "underground," which means it may be trickier to find them. It can also be expensive, with many guides asking for $1,000 or more for a single session.

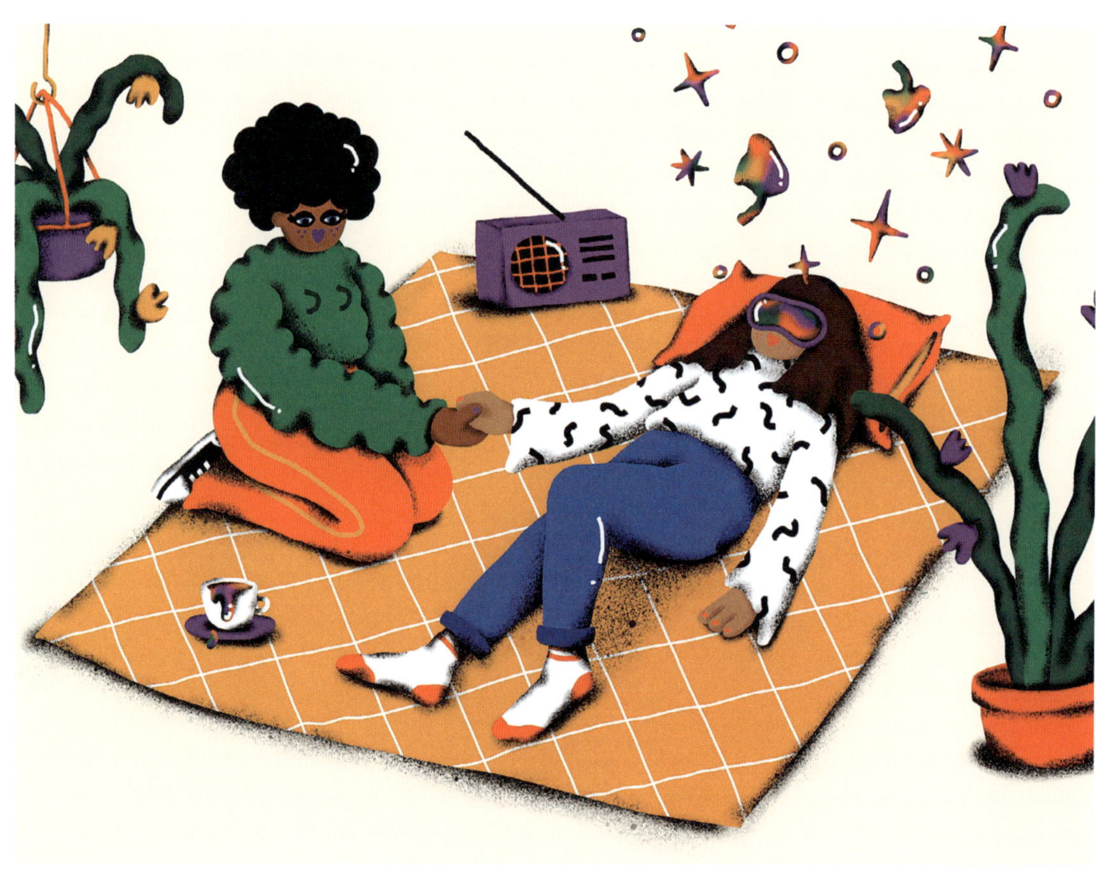

JOURNEYING IN A CEREMONY

All the psychedelics we discuss in this book are offered in group settings. More and more, clinics and facilitators are exploring group journeys, particularly for MDMA and ketamine, because they can bring the cost down for each participant. That said, typically when someone talks about a "ceremony," they're referring to a psychedelic being administered in a ritualistic setting, at night, with songs, incense, and other aspects influenced by Indigenous traditions.

The most common psychedelics offered in a ceremonial environment include ayahuasca, peyote, and mushrooms. Wachuma is also offered in ceremony, but traditionally during the day rather than at night. Ceremonies provide a structured and guided environment for exploring psychedelic consciousness, often offering a sense of community, ritual, sacredness, and spiritual connection as well. Regardless of what type of ceremony you're sitting in, it's important to vet your facilitator to make sure that they are trustworthy (unfortunately, issues like sexual assault or even just chaotic environments in ceremony are not uncommon and can be psychologically, if not also physically, dangerous). It's also important to ask critical questions about ceremony scholarships, Indigenous reciprocity, and other ethical practices to ensure they align with your values. (You can find more information on how to vet a retreat center in chapter 8.)

Journeying with others in a ceremonial context can be an incredibly profound experience, but for some people, it also may lead to a feeling of restriction, as there will be rules about what is and isn't permitted in the space. Depending on the ceremony and the facilitator, you may be asked to stay in a spot that's been designated to you, likely around the size of a yoga mat, and to not talk with others. Varying levels of noise are permitted: It's normal to laugh, cry, and even let out sighs and grunts when deep in a psychedelic experience, but you might be asked to quiet down if you're too loud or disruptive. Some people would rather be in a space—with friends, alone, or in a one-on-one session—where anything goes.

BEYOND THE JOURNEY

HOLOTROPIC BREATHWORK

Did you know you can trip with just your breath? We're not talking light visuals here. We're talking full-blown revelations and emotional releases. In the 1970s, after Richard Nixon outlawed classic psychedelics such as shrooms and LSD, psychiatrist Stanislav Grof developed a method for inducing altered states of consciousness just by manipulating the breath. The technique, called holotropic breathwork, uses accelerated breathing, evocative music, and bodywork to induce deep psychological and emotional experiences. It aims to facilitate self-exploration and personal growth without the need for, well, the drugs.

Holotropic breathwork is a great way to prepare for a journey (and to integrate a journey once it's over), because if it gets too intense at any time, you can just stop. So if you're nervous about what might come up for you during a psychedelic experience, breathwork can help you begin looking at what's living below the surface of your day-to-day mind, with an added sense of control. You might start to feel an uncomfortable tingling sensation in your body, sadness, or frustration. In these moments, you can practice embracing what's coming up so that when you're tripping you feel more confident that you have the inner resilience to do the same.

Types of Space Holders

There are many different types of trip sitting. There's the close friend who's just there to be a warm, safe body in the room, the shaman trained by a lineage or lineages of medicine servers, and many roles in between. There is no "right choice" when it comes to which modality to go with, but the choice you make will shape your journey profoundly, so be sure to weigh your options and wait for a space holder you feel good about. Here are a few broad categories.

TRIP SITTER

A trip sitter is someone you know who does not necessarily have professional training in space holding. This could be a friend, family member, or partner. For someone without a severe mental health condition, a trip sitter may be sufficient—and most convenient. Note, however, that just because you love someone doesn't mean they're the best trip sitter for you. If you have a complex interpersonal history with someone, you may feel more comfortable being supported by someone else.

Note that no friend or family member should trip-sit for someone who has a history of trauma or severe mental health issues. In this case, a professional space holder who is trauma informed is recommended.

PROFESSIONAL SPACE HOLDER

This is someone who has experience holding space for others but doesn't have a degree in therapy. There are many qualified professional space holders, from people who have supported facilitators for many years in ayahuasca ceremonies to folks who have some kind of training or certificate that isn't accredited or doesn't license them to do therapy through the state. It can be tricky to vet these types of space holders, so be sure you're getting a recommendation you trust—and see "Questions to Ask a Psychedelic Guide" on page 48. They can also be expensive and hard to find if they're working underground. That said, a professional space holder may be necessary if you don't have a trusted friend or family member to sit with you or if you're concerned that you'll need more qualified support to get through the experience.

THERAPIST

From principal investigators in FDA-approved clinical trials to licensed therapists who are offering psychedelic sessions underground, many people with training in mental health offer psychedelic space holding. If you'd like to enroll in a clinical trial, you can see if there's one in your area at clinicaltrials.gov. If you're looking for a licensed therapist who is offering psychedelic work underground, finding one can be tricky, as they risk losing their license if they get caught. Start by cultivating a relationship with a psychedelic integration therapist who is offering legal preparation sessions and take it from there.

SHAMAN

Shaman is a tricky word. Indigenous communities all have their own words for healer. There's also a fast-growing number of people from the Global North learning with Indigenous people to lead ceremony, all with widely varying degrees of training, dedication, and integrity. That said, this category broadly refers to people who are supporting others through plant medicine journeys in a ritualistic context. When it comes to Indigenous healers from a specific lineage, some serve medicine only to their communities and remain quiet about it. Others serve to foreigners who have come to work with them in the shamans' home countries, or they travel abroad and serve medicine underground in places like the United States and Canada. Again, vetting is incredibly important here, as there's been a rising number of phony shamans taking advantage of foreigners—see "Questions to Ask a Psychedelic Guide" on page 48 and "How to Find a Vetted Retreat Center" on page 146.

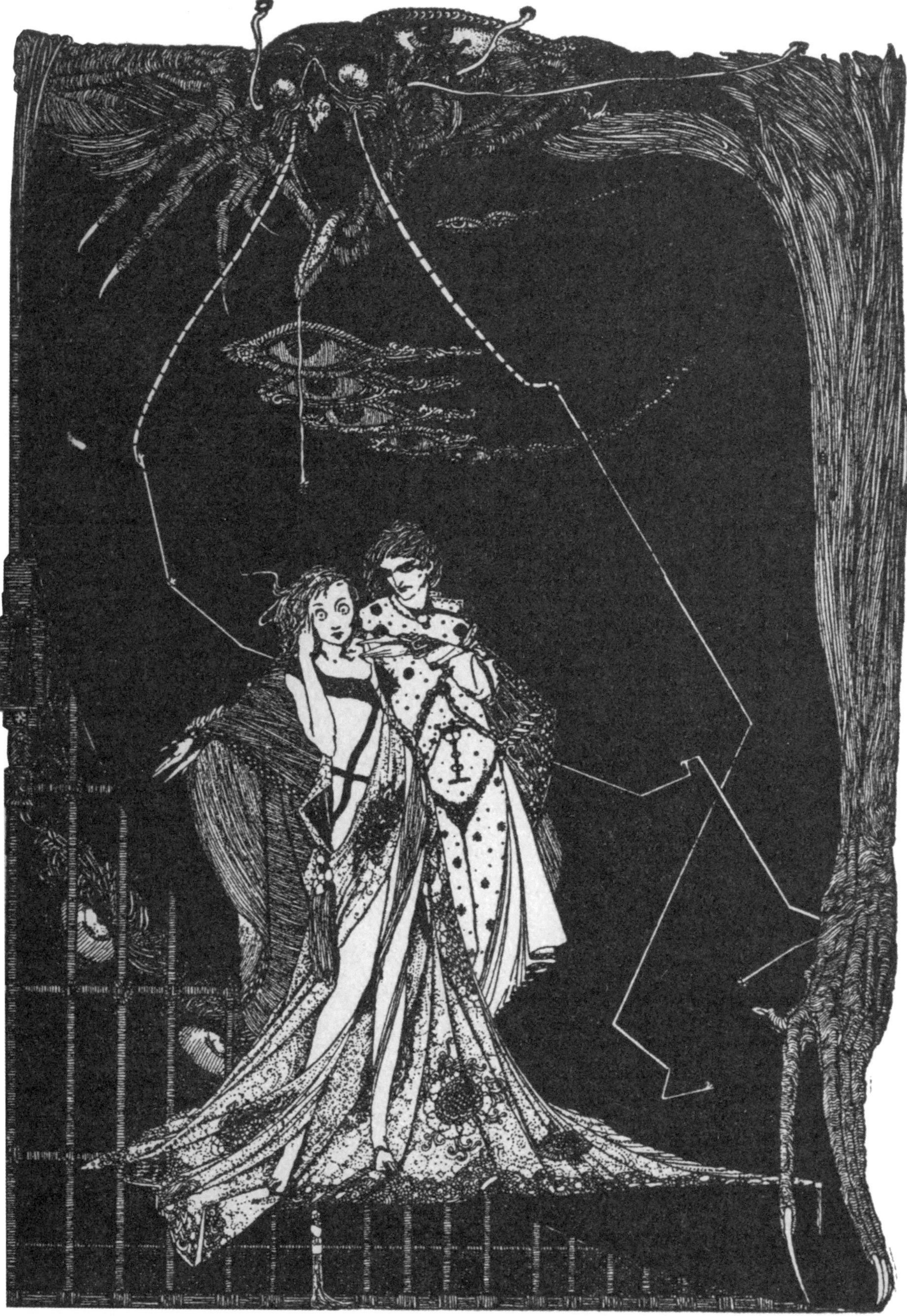

QUESTIONS TO ASK A PSYCHEDELIC GUIDE

If you're considering working with a guide, it's important to do your research and make sure that you are comfortable with their approach, background, and experience. It's best to have an in-person meeting with a potential guide to get a sense of their personality and to ask any specific questions you might have. If they are unable to meet in person with you, they should at least be willing to talk on the phone. Either way, to ensure they are the right fit, start with these questions:

- What is their personal experience with psychedelics? How long have they been working with the medicine? People have varying opinions on whether it's important for a guide to have journeyed on the psychedelics they are serving. Some think that it's sufficient for a guide to have gone through training on how to support others on psychedelics, regardless of the guide's personal experience. Others feel strongly that guides can't properly support others unless they've been through the experience themselves. You have to decide what makes you most comfortable.

- What is their training and background?

- What is their commitment to social justice? Do they prioritize the safety and well-being of their clients? Do they uphold ethical guidelines and respect diverse perspectives?

- What is their philosophy of psychedelic use? What are their views on the potential benefits and risks of psychedelics?

- How do they approach guiding others through their experiences? What are their methods for setting intentions, creating safe spaces, and supporting integration?

- What kinds of stories can they share with you about outcomes achieved by people they've supported through a psychedelic experience? Can they provide you with references?

- What would they do in the event of an emergency? Are they trained in CPR?

- Are they doing their own inner journey work?

- Do they offer preparation? Integration? Many guides create safe environments for the journey but do not have the capacity to provide support before or after the experience.

- Are their prices comparable to market rate? If not, why not?

- What kinds of clients do they work with? Are they trauma informed? This is a good question for everyone to ask, but it's particularly important if you are dealing with acute psychological distress or have traumatic experiences in your past.

- What are their boundaries with regard to factors like touch, time parameters, sharing about their own lives, and so forth?

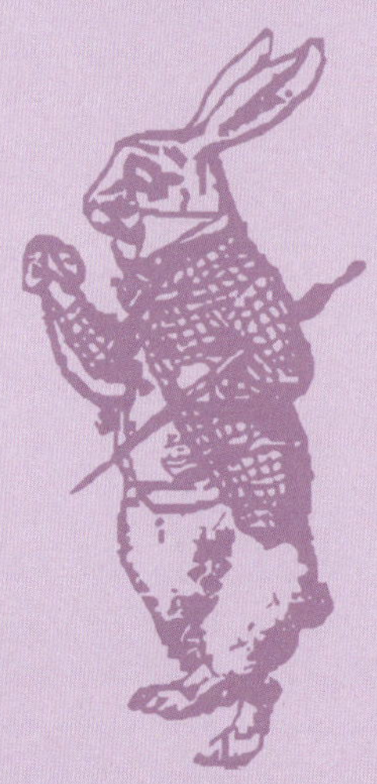

Setting an Intention

An intention is a clear, focused statement of what you hope to achieve or focus on during your psychedelic experience. It could be a word or phrase, like *self-love* or *boundaries*, or it could be centered on a more specific outcome, like "I will nurture my inner child" or "I will explore my relationship with [person]." Here are some questions, written with the help of DoubleBlind facilitators and teachers Skye Weaver, Tony Moss, Ido Cohen, and Deanna Rogers, to help you set your intention:

- What is the most alive thing for me (in the present), both energetically and emotionally?
- What do I want to get from this experience?
- Why am I doing this?
- What do I want to work on?
- What kind of joy do I want to experience?
- What is blocking my joy?
- What's holding me back?
- What pieces of myself or my life need some love or improvement?
- What do I want to cultivate?

Once you've set an intention, it's important to write it down or say it out loud. This helps solidify your intention and make it a part of your conscious awareness. Especially if you hit rocky waters or lose sight of why you decided to trip, the intention can offer a grounding anchor, bringing you back to focus. While it may provide a sense of purpose, however, it is not an expectation; you may have a certain intention and end up nonetheless exploring something else. (Perhaps you'll come to see how your experience connects back to your original intention in the integration phase; see chapter 4.)

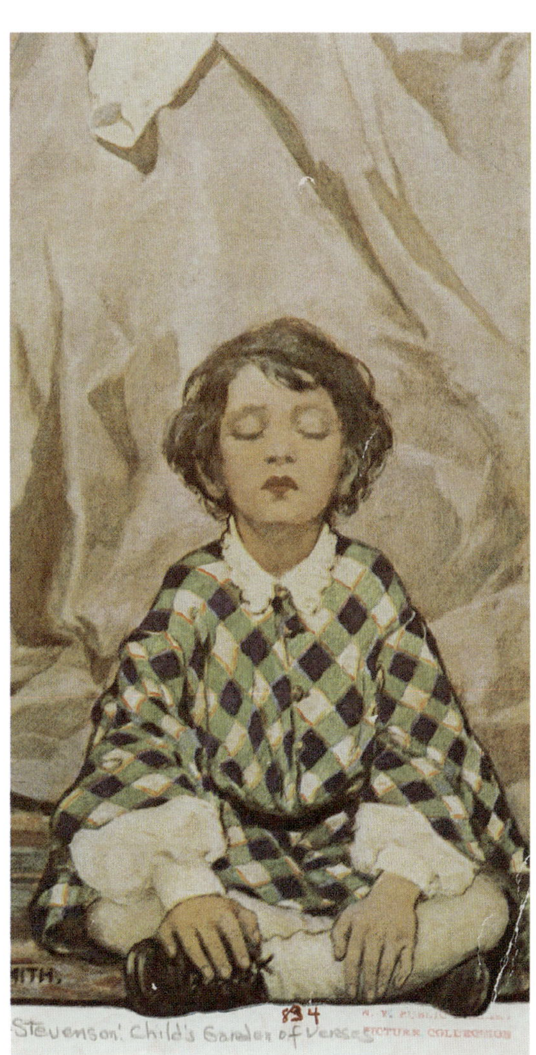

Making a Playlist

The importance of music during a psychedelic experience cannot be overemphasized. Music can greatly impact your mood, associated thoughts, feelings of connection, and so forth. It can soothe the experience or make it feel more challenging. There are tons of existing playlists for tripping out there (including on DoubleBlind's Spotify—scan the QR code below for one of these), but the most important thing is to just choose music that you enjoy and that resonates with you. Consider the setting and the mood you want to create. If you're tripping in a quiet space, you might want mellow and ambient music. If you're tripping with friends, you might opt for more upbeat and danceable music. You may wish to choose music without lyrics, so you're not influenced by messages that can distract from the journey, or songs with specific lyrics to influence the experience.

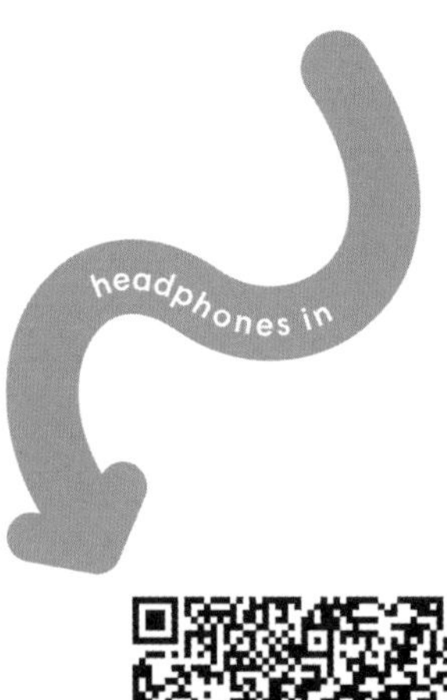

In addition to the songs themselves, it's important to consider the length of your playlist as it compares to the duration of effects for the psychedelic you're taking. There's nothing worse than having to fidget with technology while you're on a psychedelic, especially if you're playing music from your phone, in which case you may then suddenly get bombarded with notifications. So make sure you have plenty of songs to last the entirety of the journey. With shrooms, that's going to be about six hours. With LSD, it will be about twelve. (Each substance's typical duration is addressed in the relevant chapter.)

It's also worth thinking about curating the songs to mirror the arc of the journey. During the come-up (the first third of the journey), you might like calmer music without lyrics. During the peak (the middle third), sometimes it's helpful to have music that's more activating, with drums. During the come-down (the final third), it can be cathartic to have music that speaks to themes of love and peace or sentimental songs from your past—really anything that you find comforting. There are also albums that have been composed specifically for psychedelic journeying. Jon Hopkins's album *Music for Psychedelic Therapy* is intended to be listened to while on ketamine, for example, mirroring how the experience grows in intensity and then declines over about an hour. East Forest has an album titled *Music for Mushrooms: A Soundtrack for the Psychedelic Practitioner*, which lasts an ideal four hours and fifty-nine minutes to listen to while on psilocybin. If you're unsure of what kind of music to play while tripping, we recommend not overthinking it and just going with one of these albums or a playlist that's already been curated. Most important, don't forget to download your playlist in advance and make sure all your devices, including your speakers or headphones, are charged.

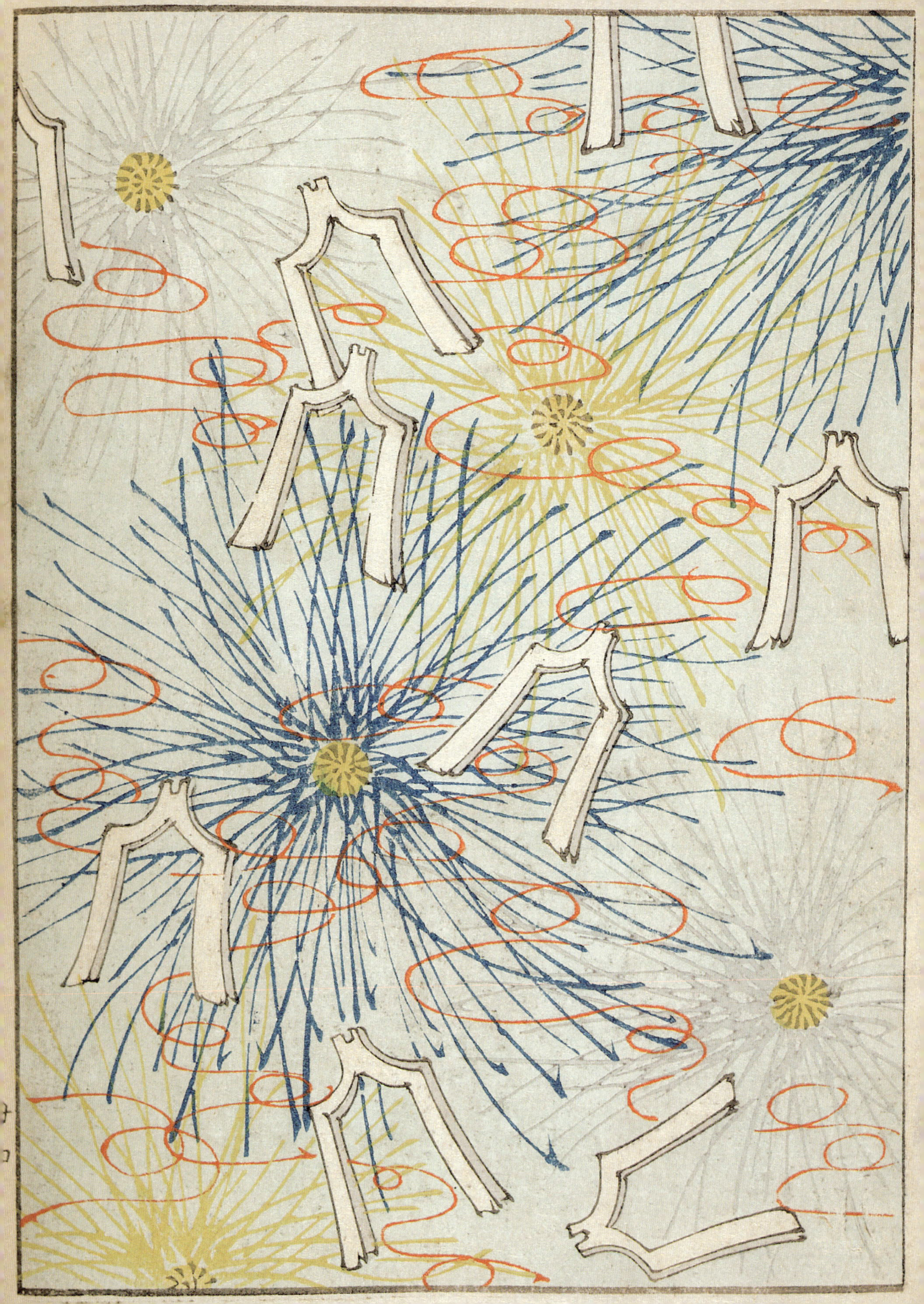

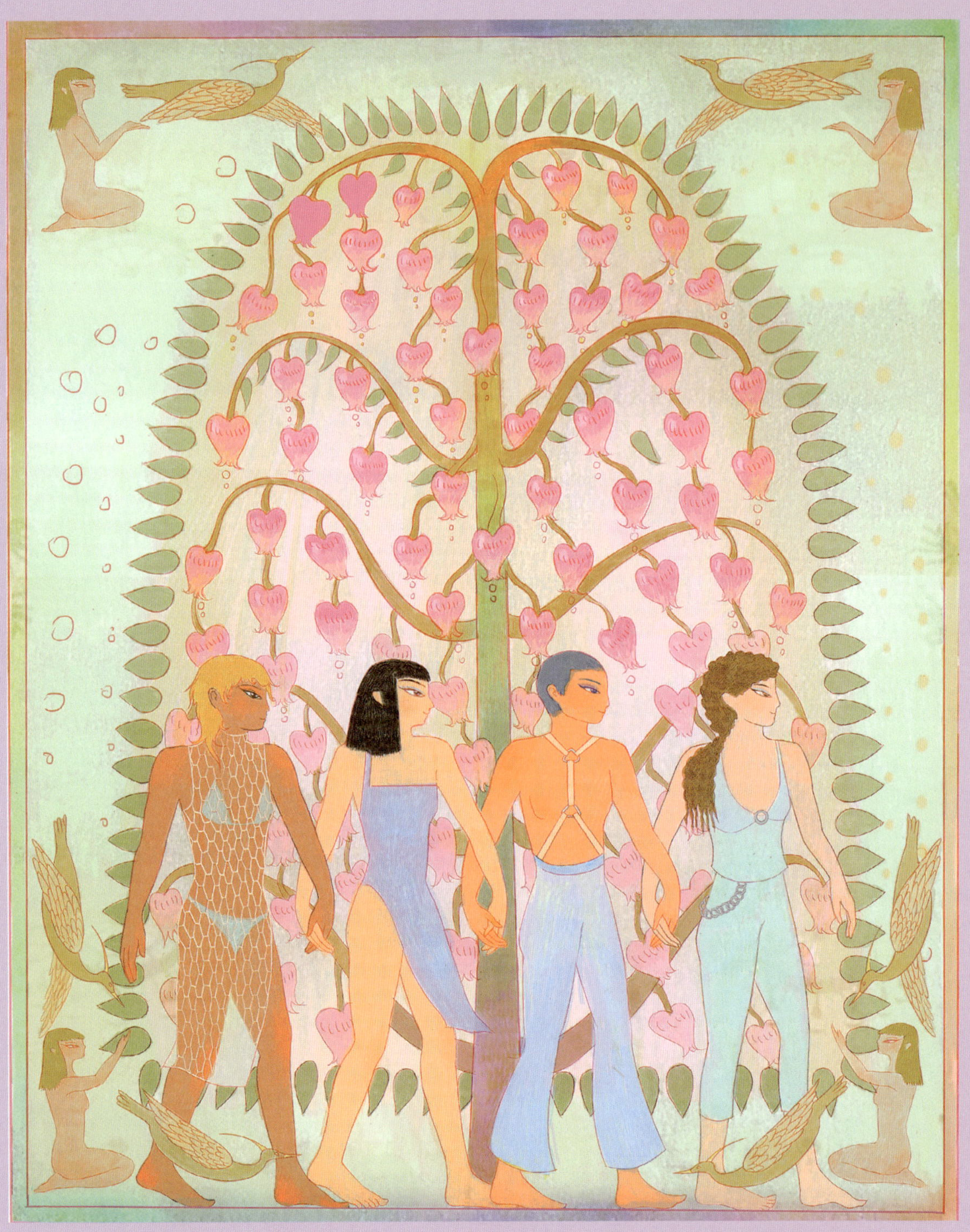

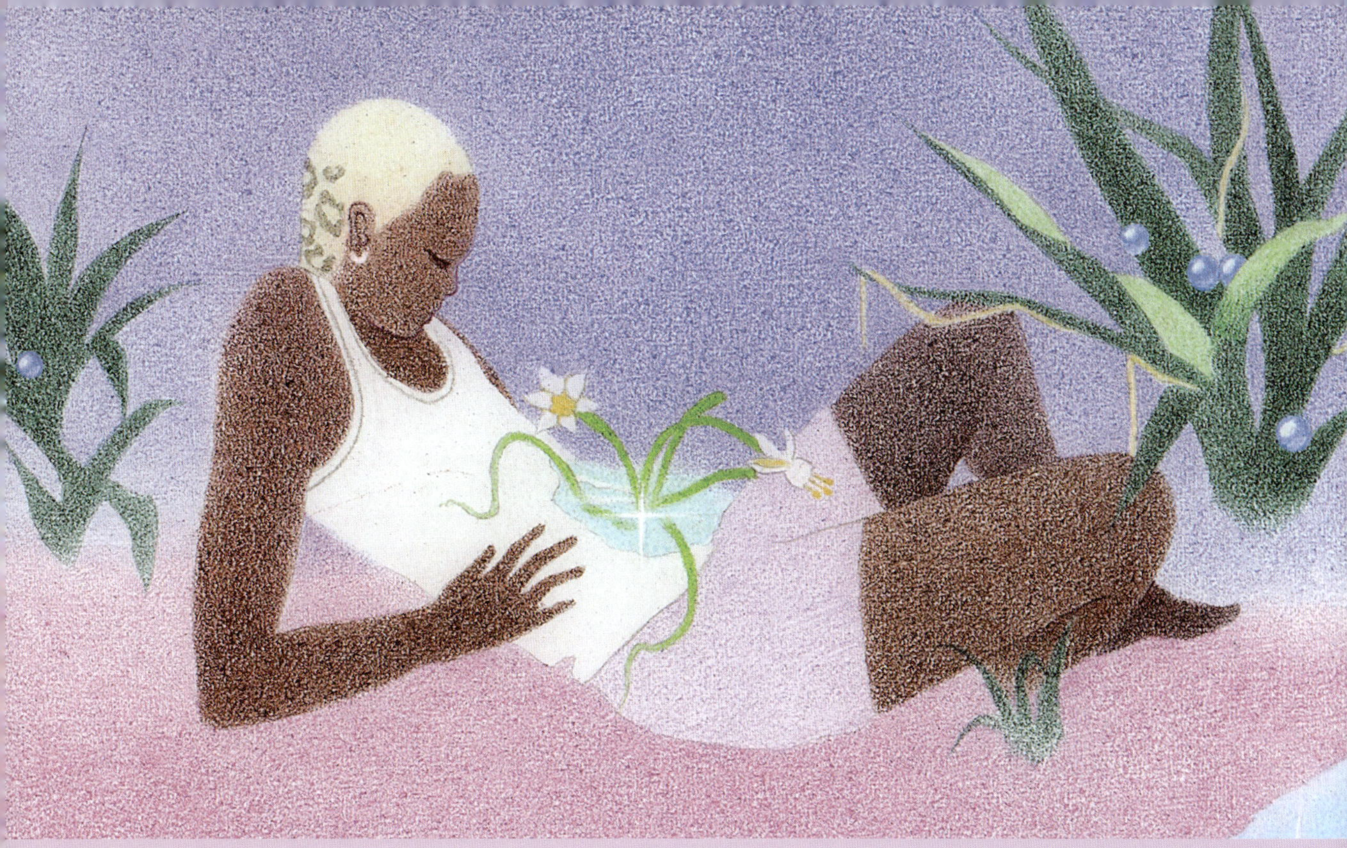

QUEERING PSYCHEDELICS

Queering psychedelics is a growing movement to foreground and uplift the experiences of LGBTQIA+ people who are working with psychedelics. The term—and the dialogue that has followed—was spurred by a conference series hosted by Chacruna, a nonprofit devoted to highlighting marginalized voices within plant medicines, and their subsequent book by the same name. Since then, the movement has inspired the creation of ceremonial spaces, clinical trials, and even psychedelic parties with queer and trans experiences in mind.

While popular understanding used to be that ingesting these perception-shifting substances has the effect of making us more compassionate beings with broader, wilder, more inclusive mindsets—more sexually free, honoring of diverse identities, and perhaps even more queer ourselves—we've seen a rising understanding of psychedelics as "non-specific amplifiers," something that reinforces preconceived biases, as opposed to challenging them.

If we flip through the pages of psychedelic history, we find now-famous figures like Richard Alpert (Ram Dass), Timothy Leary, and Stan Grof endorsing the notion that psychedelics can cure a person of homosexuality and, in some cases, conducting gay conversion therapy—the attempt to change someone's sexual or gender identity in a formal therapeutic setting.

If our "set and setting" no longer presumes that gender is binary and that everyone is straight, we can break the molds that limit our compassion and discover a vast, shimmering liberation that magnifies our capacity for joy. When we queer psychedelics, we find ourselves in a time where queer and trans ceremonialists, researchers, and edgewalkers are present, brilliant, and speaking for themselves. We might find our own voice there, too, distinct and interconnected, rising up.

This excerpt comes from a story reported for DoubleBlind's print magazine by Noelle Armstrong.

Preparing Your Physical Vessel

Your body is the vessel that carries you through your journey, so you'll want to make sure you're feeling strong enough and well enough to handle it (especially if the psychedelic substance itself brings on physical sensations like nausea, weakness, or intensity). Here are some tips:

- Eat a healthy diet in the days leading up to your journey. Focus on whole, unprocessed foods that are rich in nutrients. Avoid foods that may make you feel sluggish or uncomfortable. (Note that if you are doing ayahuasca, your server may recommend you follow a specific "dieta," which you can read about in chapter 8.)

- Hydrate! Hydrate! Hydrate! Especially on the day of the event. But do not overhydrate. You don't need to overthink this. Generally, about 8 fluid ounces per hour keeps a person hydrated, unless it's very hot. Just try to stay in that range. Some facilitators may have specific recommendations regarding water intake.

- Get enough sleep. This will ensure you're refreshed and energized for your trip.

- Engage in regular exercise or movement, which can help you get out of your head and into your body, improve your mood, reduce stress, and increase present moment awareness.

- Practice mindfulness. Whether it's meditation, breathwork, yoga, walks in nature, or something else, having a mindfulness practice in place before the experience will make it easier to engage with the psychedelic consciousness and integrate it afterward. When it comes to breathwork and meditation, in general, there's a seemingly infinite number of modalities you can try. Holotropic breathwork (see page 45) is great but can be fairly intense. You can use meditation apps, like Insight Timer, to try different mindfulness practices and see what works for you. You can also just practice observing your diaphragm expand and contract with your breath naturally, with your eyes closed.

Building Community

The final piece of advice we'll give you about preparation is to be sure to let others in your life know that you are doing this so you can feel held in the aftermath. It can be isolating to have a transformative psychedelic experience and then to return home to find that friends and family don't understand the weight of what you went through—or, worse, that they're judging you. Providing partners, parents, and others you're close to with some literature (or even this book) ahead of time can help. If you don't know anyone you can talk to about it, consider joining a local psychedelic community (which you can find through the Global Psychedelic Society's database) and/or finding a psychedelic integration therapist who is available after the journey to help you process what happened. If you can establish care with a community or therapist before you journey, you'll feel more comfortable reaching out for help with integration afterward. Following a profound experience, it can be incredibly validating (and important) to be able to speak to others who understand what you have gone through.

CHAPTER 3

NAVIGATION

The psychedelic journey is a voyage into the unknown. It's an exploration of your inner landscape, a process of self-discovery, an opportunity to confront your fears, embrace your shadows, and awaken to a deeper level of awareness. In order to help foster a feeling of safety during the experience, it's helpful to understand the arc of the journey: how long it's going to last and the phases it will pass through. Typically, we think of these phases as taking place in three parts: the come-up, the peak, and the come-down.

The Come-Up

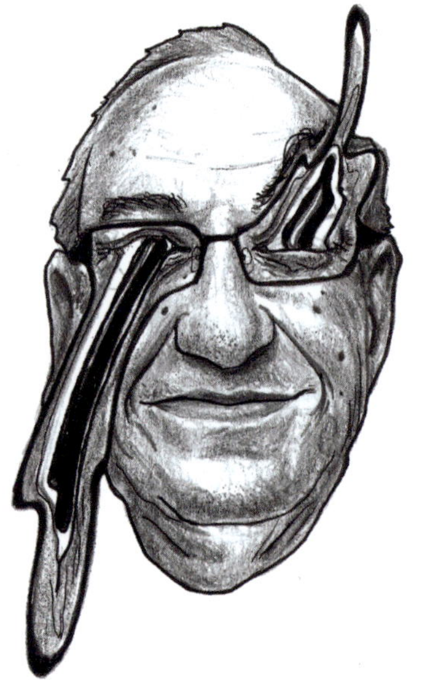

After you first dose, and especially with classic psychedelics like LSD or mushrooms, the come-up can feel like a slow-motion dance, a waiting game where you're anticipating what's to come and may or may not begin to notice subtle shifts of perception. You might feel a gentle tingling in your limbs, a heightened awareness of your breath, butterflies or nausea in your stomach, or a sense of warmth and expansion. The world might seem a little brighter, a little more alive, and your senses might be a little sharper.

The best thing you can do during this time is to just relax and observe what's happening with curiosity as opposed to judgment. Many facilitators recommend starting the journey in silence so you can be especially attuned to what's happening as the psychedelic begins to take effect. Get as comfortable as you can; you might try lying down with an eye mask on or meditating in a seated position. You may find it supportive to focus on the simple in and out of your breath. Exhaling for longer than you inhale may help your nervous system relax. You might also find it supportive to melt into some yoga postures. Think of the come-up like a prelude, a soft invitation to the adventure that awaits.

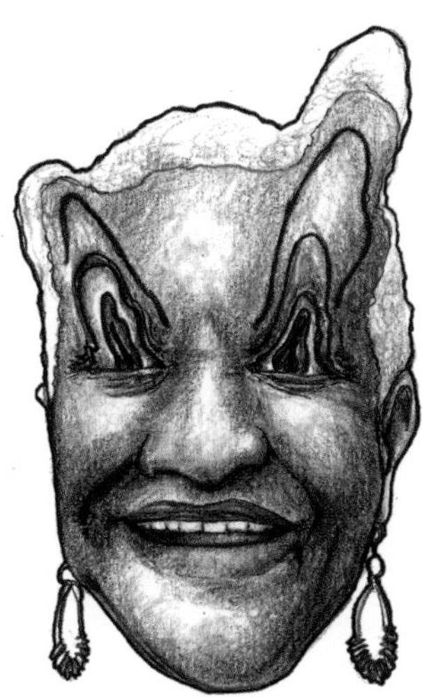

The Peak

The peak is the most intense part of the experience, when the psychedelic effects are strongest. Since every journey is different, it's impossible to say how the peak is going to feel for you and when it will happen, but oftentimes it will be defined by powerful emotions, visuals, sensations in the body, and/or an active mind.

Typically, you can anticipate that you will peak around one-third to half of the way into the experience. The length of the journey will vary each time, but you can use rough predictions based upon the average durations provided in this book for each substance. We don't recommend paying close attention to the clock or spending too much time wondering whether you've reached the peak while journeying, as these thoughts can take you out of the present moment. That said, we do recommend that you take a look at the clock before you take a psychedelic and know roughly how long it's supposed to last. If and when the experience starts to feel intense, these details allow you to identify, based on how much time has passed, whether you are in the peak window and how much longer your journey is likely to last. This can help calm you if you start to lose your perception of time and feel like the trip is never going to end. (Don't worry—it happens to the best of us!)

The Come-Down

Sweet relief! At least, that's how we feel as we approach the come-down. You often don't recognize that you're in the come-down right away, as the intensity of the journey is not always perfectly linear. Generally, when you're on shrooms, LSD, or DMT, you can expect the intensity to grow and then fade. But within that trajectory, there will be swells of emotions and visions. Some people don't realize they're coming down until, well, the experience is basically completely over. But it's generally pretty safe to assume that if you're more than two-thirds of the way through the typical duration of the journey, you'll be coming in for a landing soon. During this time, just try to get the most you can out of the remaining moments of your experience. Breathe. Stretch. Drink some tea. It can be tempting, especially if you're with friends or in ceremony, to start talking about your trip in the past tense with others before it's really over or to just chatter and hang out. But taking this time instead to journal, play an instrument, or perhaps engage in other calming activities can be deeply healing.

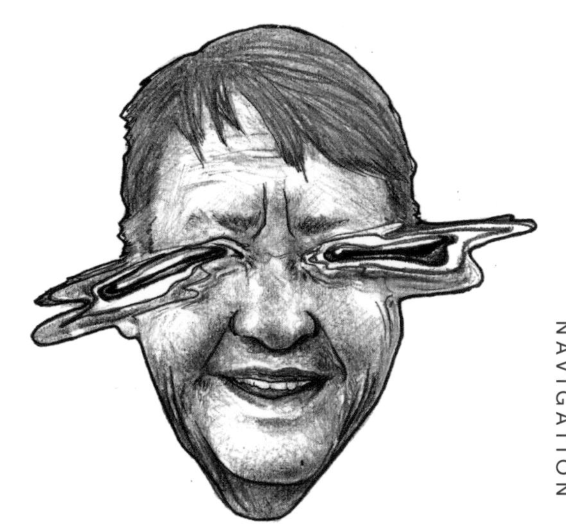

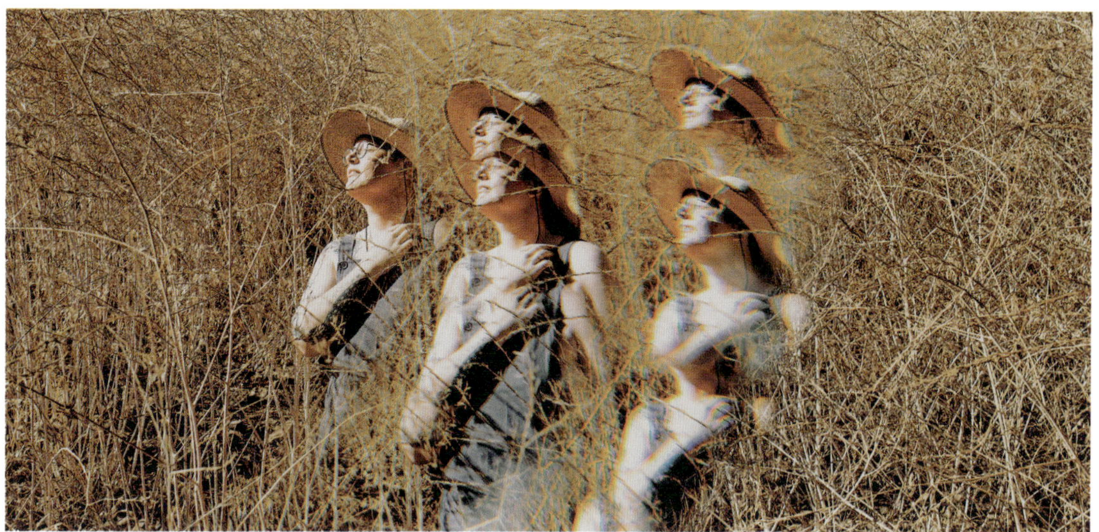

Boosters

A booster is a dose that you take after your initial dose. People can take boosters when tripping on all the most common psychedelics, including MDMA, psilocybin, and LSD. Your window of opportunity to take a booster dose typically extends to about two and a half hours after the first dose when the intention is to deepen the experience rather than elongate it. For all common psychedelics, it's not recommended to take a booster more than halfway into the experience, unless you're okay with the journey lasting longer than initially anticipated.

A booster is generally about one-quarter to half the original dose. We recommend having this dose prepared ahead of time and easily accessible so you're not trying to weigh it out or fumble through things while you're coming up.

Whether or not to take a booster dose is a delicate decision. There are those who take a booster because they aren't feeling the original dose, and those who simply want to have a stronger experience. If you're thinking about taking a booster, we recommend first removing distractions and going inward by meditating or lying down with your eyes closed. Observe what's happening for you, and then ask yourself whether you feel you need more of the substance in order to achieve the shift in consciousness you were hoping for. Remember: You're not always going to get exactly what you want out of a psychedelic experience. We've heard stories of people who took extremely high doses and felt nothing at all. While it's hard to explain to a newbie, if you haven't taken a high enough dose for you, you might experience what feels like a struggle to go into the psychedelic realms, as though a part of you is operating in the same way it normally does and another part of you is being pulled into a different way of perceiving or feeling. You might experience this situation as an uncomfortable limbo between tripping and normality. If that's where you are and you feel safe to do so, better to take the plunge and go for a booster. You've gotten this far; you might as well go all in.

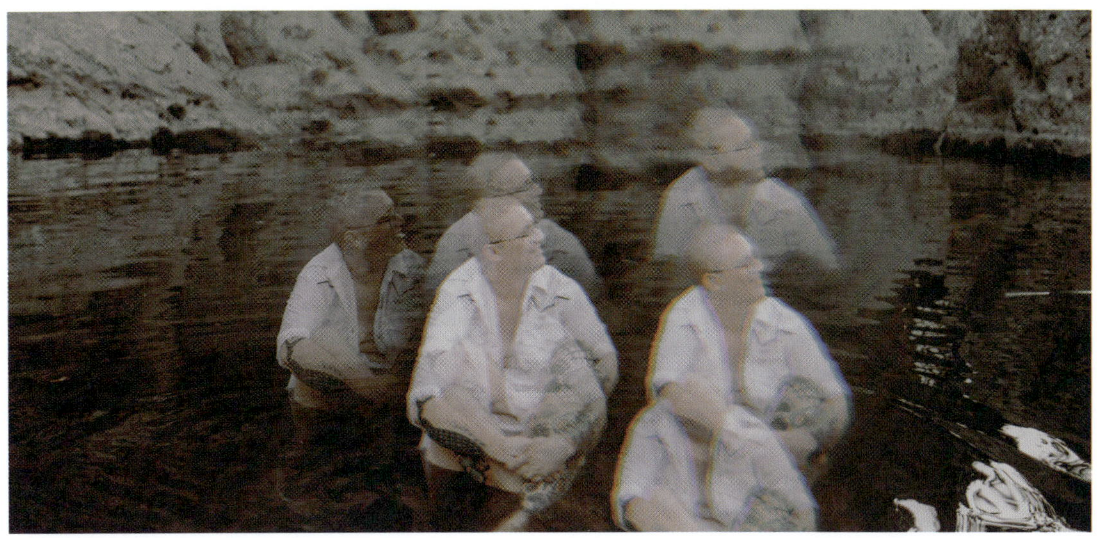

Asking for Help vs. Going Inward

Psychedelics can sometimes trigger challenging emotions and experiences. It's important to remember that you're not alone—even if you are *physically* alone. If you're feeling overwhelmed or scared, reach out to your trip sitter, a friend, the Fireside Project (which offers a free psychedelic support hotline), or, if you believe in a higher power, a supportive divine entity. Don't be afraid to ask for help. It's a sign of strength, not weakness.

If you're experiencing a medical emergency or have any doubt about your safety, the best thing to do is to call 911. However, please be aware that most hospitals do not have a competency in psychedelics and being in a medical environment while tripping can be deeply uncomfortable. That's why, if you have any health concerns, you should make sure you're safe to journey before you do so by meeting with a psychedelic integration therapist to discuss your medical history and any medications you may be taking. Generally, psilocybin, MDMA, and LSD have all been shown to be safe for healthy adults in clinical trials. But if you're feeling unsure about the experience, it's best to journey in a ceremony or with a trained therapist so they can assess whether physical symptoms you're experiencing actually need to be addressed by a doctor or you're just processing emotions that will pass on their own.

Embarking on a journey with psychedelics necessarily involves learning to distinguish between those times when you should seek out help and those times when you should turn inward and face your discomforts or fears. For a tripping beginner, this can be challenging. Sometimes the most helpful thing you can do is to lean into an uncomfortable experience, treat it with curiosity, gracefully and humbly accept the feelings that are coming up, and trust that you have the inner strength to navigate them.

In the psychedelic community, many facilitators talk about the concept of the "inner healer," meaning the idea that we all have within us a wisdom that can be a powerful source of healing. Some challenge this notion, saying it overemphasizes the need for self-reliance when oftentimes healing also happens in relationship and in community, but it's generally accepted among experts across ideologies that your body is a strong source of intuition and guidance, and that the psychedelic experience may, in fact, help you get in touch with it. This is all to say that it can be incredibly powerful to talk to someone or even have someone hold your hand during a journey, but it's also incredibly powerful to let go and explore what's emerging within.

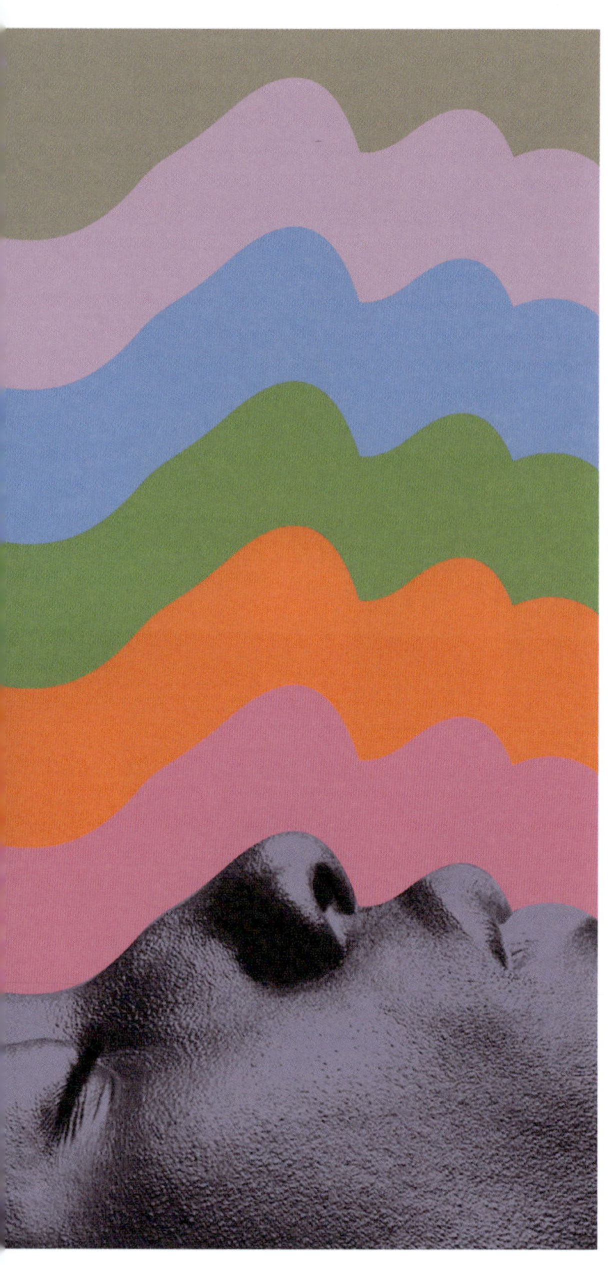

4-7-8: A SIMPLE GROUNDING TECHNIQUE

The 4-7-8 breathing technique, developed by Dr. Andrew Weil, pioneering author, physician, and psychedelic advocate, is a simple yet powerful method for reducing stress, promoting relaxation, and improving sleep. This practice is rooted in ancient yogic traditions and is known for its calming effects on the nervous system.

It involves inhaling for a count of four, holding your breath for a count of seven, and exhaling for a count of eight. The speed of counting (and breathing) will vary by the individual; just do it at a pace that feels slow enough to be calming but not so slow that you have difficulty maintaining the cadence. You'll get the hang of it as you practice.

This technique is a tool you can use anywhere to quickly induce calm and restore balance—and it can be particularly useful during a psychedelic trip if you need to slip out of your mind and into your body. You can also try adding an affirmation, such as "I am safe" or "It is okay," or perhaps a phrase centered on the intention you set prior to your journey.

DROP IN WITH THESE FIVE SIMPLE STEPS:

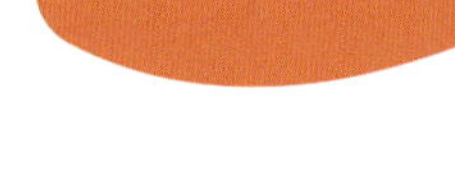

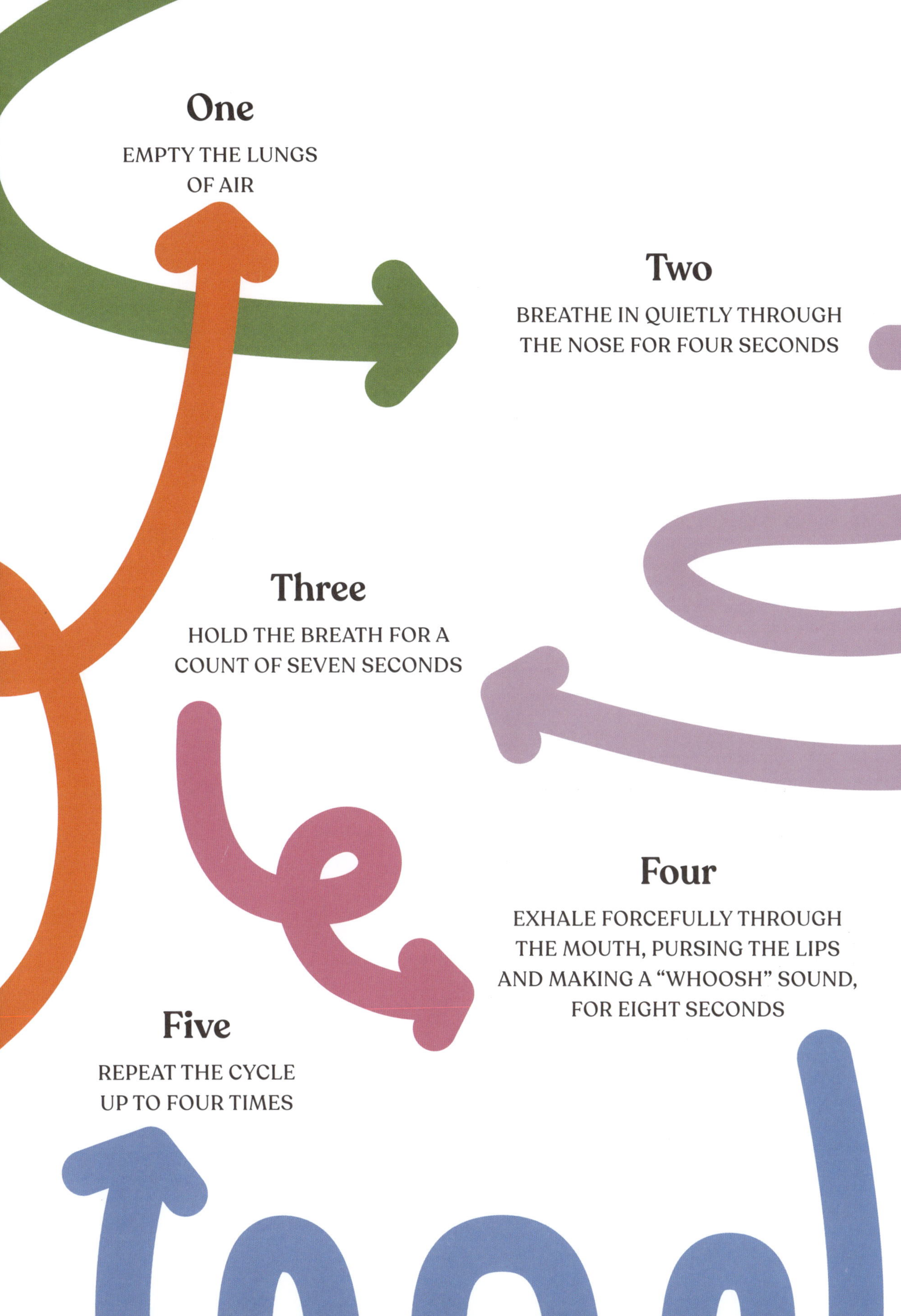

One

EMPTY THE LUNGS
OF AIR

Two

BREATHE IN QUIETLY THROUGH
THE NOSE FOR FOUR SECONDS

Three

HOLD THE BREATH FOR A
COUNT OF SEVEN SECONDS

Four

EXHALE FORCEFULLY THROUGH
THE MOUTH, PURSING THE LIPS
AND MAKING A "WHOOSH" SOUND,
FOR EIGHT SECONDS

Five

REPEAT THE CYCLE
UP TO FOUR TIMES

Navigating a "Bad Trip" (Rule #1: Don't Call It a "Bad Trip")

No one, even the most seasoned psychonaut, is immune to challenging psychedelic moments. But they don't have to define the entire experience.

Challenging experiences can involve intense emotions like fear, anxiety, paranoia, disorientation, dissociation, or confusion. Typically, as is the case for journeys in general, the recommended way to approach these emotions is with curiosity. Sometimes you may be experiencing discomfort simply because you're, well, uncomfortable—you're with people who aren't making you feel safe or in an environment where you're struggling to relax. But if there's nothing obvious that can or needs to be shifted externally, then the best next step, if you can, is just to close your eyes, breathe, and remind yourself of your intention. Focus on your body, on the air coming in and out of your lungs. You can try putting one hand on your heart and one hand on your stomach to ground yourself, humming, or any other practices that you know help regulate your nervous system.

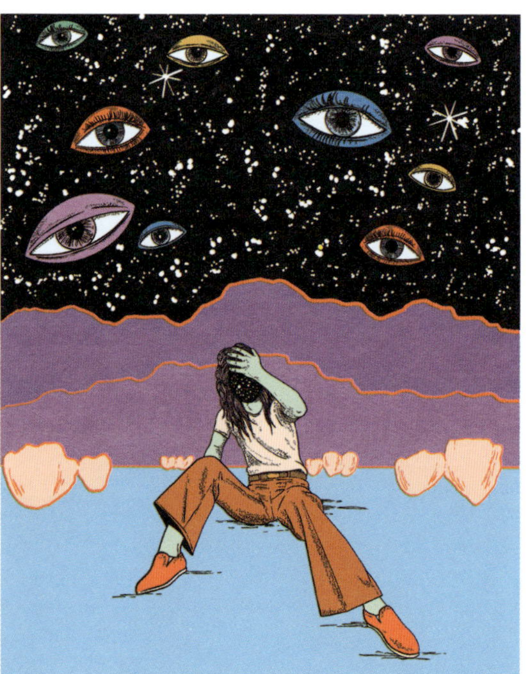

If this doesn't work, you can try to:

- Change your environment. If you're outside, go inside; if you're inside, go outside. Go for a walk, adjust the lighting, go to a different room.

- Engage in physical activity. Movement can be helpful for grounding you in the present moment, releasing tension, and getting you out of your head and into your body. Try dancing, yoga, or simply walking around.

- Listen to music or change what's playing. Or better yet, pick up an instrument and sing or play something yourself.

- Engage in sensory activities. Pick up a crystal, drum, chant, draw, or look at an art book.

Remember: The key to navigating a "bad trip" is to stay grounded, to focus on the present moment, and to trust that you will eventually come back to a place of balance and peace. Oftentimes, when we go into those challenging feelings, as opposed to resisting them, they shift and transmute—and there's something beautiful on the other side.

---

surrender
verb

to relinquish control and relax into the psychedelic experience with trust and curiosity

People in the psychedelic community often say that you must "surrender" to the medicine, but that's easier said than done and can take practice. Breathing, stretching, and any activities that help you get out of your mind and into your body can help.

CHAPTER 4

INTEGRATION

The psychedelic experience can be transformative, insightful, healing, spiritual, and even life-changing. It can also be just for fun—and that's okay! But know that the real benefits of the experience only really begin to take shape after it's over; that is, the more you invest in the integration phase, the more you have the potential to grow from it.

Integration is the process of making sense of your psychedelic experience and incorporating the insights and lessons that come from it into your daily life. The integration phase, which could last from days to years afterward, is about taking the time to reflect on the experience, explore the meaning behind it, and apply it to your thoughts, beliefs, and behaviors.

Integration is essential for making the most of your psychedelic experience and using it to create positive change in your life. Without integration, the insights and realizations you gain during a psychedelic experience can feel fleeting and ephemeral, like a dream you can't grasp once you wake up. Integration helps you ground those insights in your mind and body, allowing them to become part of your waking life.

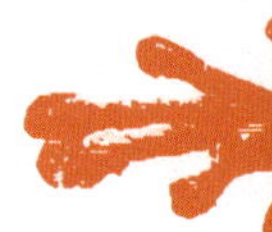

The Phases of Integration

Integration is not a singular event. It's an ongoing process that unfolds over an extended, undefined period that differs for each person. The first phase of integration happens in the days and weeks after the experience. This is when the insights and realizations you gained during your trip are most fresh and vivid. It's also a time of heightened awareness and sensitivity. People often report a "sparkle" or "afterglow" effect; they feel lighter and more joyous. Be sure, however, that you do not make any major decisions in the first three weeks following a journey (unless your trip has led you to decide to leave an abusive or dangerous situation, in which case, if you can, consult with a therapist or trusted resource to help you make swift, well-thought-out plans).

The second phase of integration happens over the months and years following the journey. It's a time of deeper processing and reflection. In this phase, you may look back on the experience and continue to draw fresh or deeper insights. You may also by this point have put into practice some of the lessons you learned from the journey.

Note that there are different levels of integration. There's the degree of integration that occurs within the scope of the mind and cognition—reflecting on various insights; treating your memories of the psychedelic experience with curiosity; noticing the joy, pain, and other thoughts and feelings that came up. And then there's the type of integration that happens through the body—not only thinking about the experience, but doing something about it, taking action, whether it's adopting a practice like meditation, getting a new job, or engaging in a cause like environmental activism.

Integration can also be sensory. You might take souvenirs of the psychedelic experience and engage with them in the aftermath, such as listening to the music that played during the experience, speaking regularly to people from the community you journeyed with, practicing the same yoga postures that you did under the influence, smelling the same scents that were present during the experience (incense, essential oils, sage), and so forth.

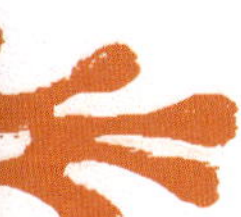

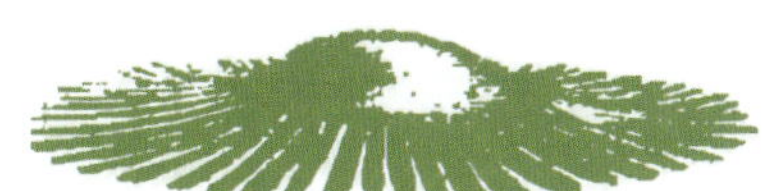

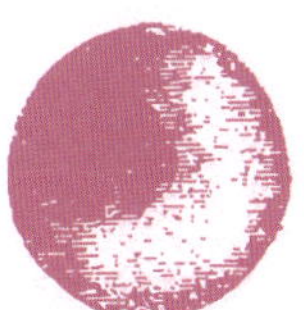

Tools for Integration

You can use a variety of tools to support your integration process, and we describe the more common ones here. But the process is uniquely personal. There is no right or wrong way to do it—and no right or wrong order in which to partake in these activities. Be patient, be kind to yourself, and trust the process.

BREATHWORK. Deep breathing exercises like box breathing or holotropic breathwork (see page 45) can allow you to release tension and connect with your body. Dedicating a few minutes daily to intentional breathing can help keep your nervous system regulated so that you can continue to face any lingering thoughts and emotions that may be stuck or challenging. You can find instructions for many forms of breathwork on YouTube and free apps like Insight Timer.

JOURNALING. Write about your experiences, thoughts, and feelings in a notebook or digital journal. Focus on key insights, emotions, or recurring patterns that arise post-journey to deepen your understanding. Oftentimes, images, thoughts, and feelings that we don't comprehend emerge during the journey, and through journaling, we begin to make sense of them.

MOVEMENT. Engage in physical activities like stretching, tai chi, or even gentle walks. It might seem obvious, but it's incredible how physical movement can help bits of the journey come to the fore in ways that talking and writing cannot. And don't neglect the power of dance! Put on that favorite record or the playlist from your journey and move intuitively. Shake it out, sway, whatever feels good.

PRAYER. Use prayer as a way to express gratitude, ask for guidance, or find peace. You can create your own affirmations or use traditional prayers that feel meaningful to you. Not everyone is comfortable with praying, and that's okay! But whether you have a prayer practice or not, it might be worth giving it a try.

CONNECT WITH NATURE. Spend time outdoors, whether in a park, in a forest, or at the beach. Ground yourself by walking barefoot on the earth, hugging a tree, or simply observing natural beauty around you. Profound psychedelic experiences can help us feel connected to a force greater than ourselves, and nature can put us back into that frame of mind. (Yes, we just told you to hug a tree.)

AROMATHERAPY. Slowing down and engaging in simple acts of self-care that you normally wouldn't make time for can be a part of the integration process. Diffuse essential oils in your space or apply them to your wrists and temples; try essential oils like lavender for relaxation or peppermint for clarity.

MEDITATION. Practice mindfulness or guided meditations. There's an infinite number of meditation techniques, so use apps like Insight Timer to find what resonates with you. It's amazing how supportive five minutes with your eyes closed in the morning can be.

OTHER MINDFULNESS PRACTICES. Mindfulness is really just about taking your time as you move throughout your day and checking in with yourself to see how you're feeling. Practices like eating slowly and savoring your food, writing a list of things you're grateful for, or scanning your body from your head to your toes to see how each part is feeling can help with that. Even just pausing for thirty seconds in between activities to become aware of how you're feeling can make a profound difference.

Integration Therapy

If you're struggling to understand a psychedelic experience or navigate the emotional shifts that have come up in the aftermath, if the experience left you feeling destabilized, or even if you're feeling great about your journey but want to get more out of it, an integration therapist might be worth seeking out. (Note that if you're experiencing acute distress during or after a trip, the Fireside Project has a hotline you can call for free integration support.)

An integration therapist is a mental health professional who specializes in assisting you in making sense of your psychedelic experience. They can provide support, guidance, and therapeutic techniques for processing your experience and applying it to your life. An integration therapist can guide you as you explore the emotions, insights, and realizations that came up during your journey, address any challenges in the aftermath, set goals and intentions for the changes you want to make moving forward, and continue to reap what you can from the journey. You can work with a therapist to integrate a journey you just had or even one from years ago.

If you're already working with a mental health professional but they don't have a background in psychedelics, they may be able to help you with integration, but you may find it supportive to have a couple of sessions with an integration therapist, too.

It's also incredibly valuable to integrate in community. Most major cities have psychedelic societies that hold meetups. They can be found through Facebook, websites such as meetup.com, or the Global Psychedelic Society's database. Many of them offer "integration circles" (get-togethers where people talk about and process their psychedelic experiences) virtually and in person. A benefit to these, in addition to being able to meet fellow psychonauts, is that they're much more financially accessible than a therapist. There are also integration circles specifically for marginalized groups, including BIPOC and queer folks, that can be especially helpful for anyone who feels safest processing their psychedelic experiences with people of a similar background.

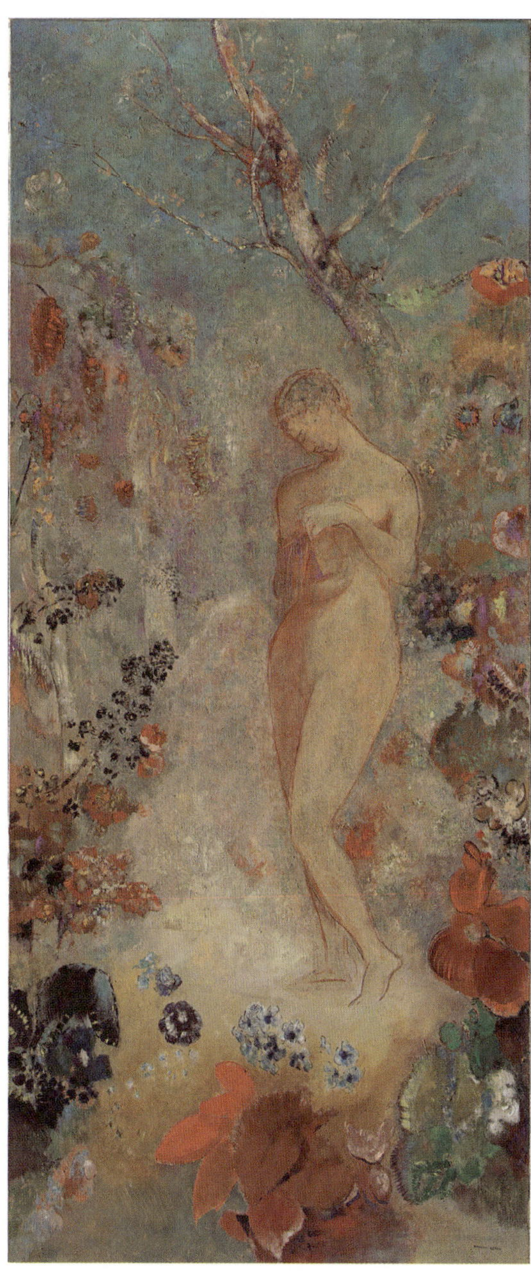

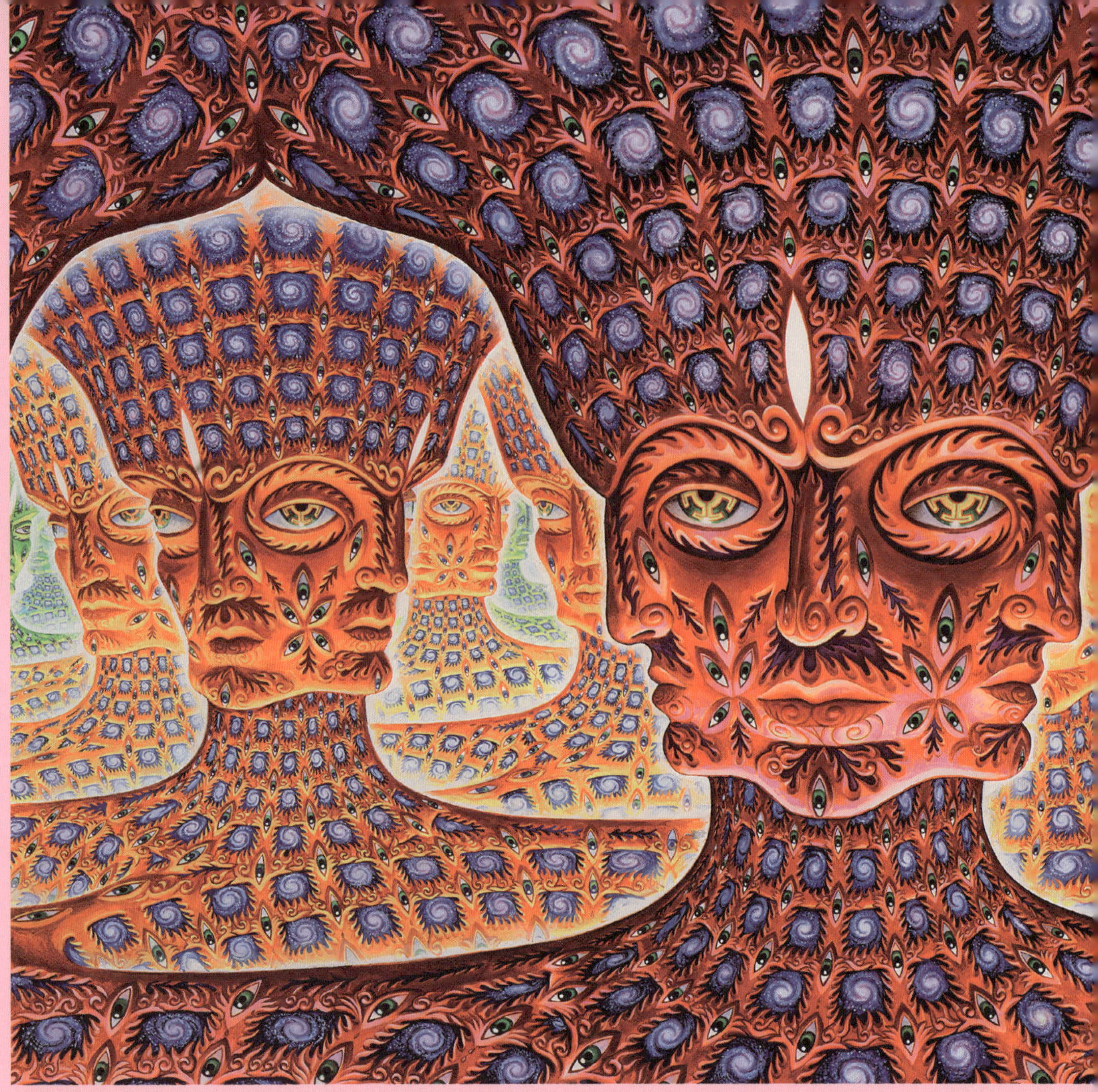

BEYOND THE JOURNEY

VISIONARY ART

Perhaps one of the most challenging parts of integrating a psychedelic experience is how elusive it can be. How can you possibly make sense of something that you can't describe? Since time immemorial, art has filled the void when words have failed us—and the psychedelic experience is no exception. Making art can be a cathartic practice in the weeks following a journey; so can looking at it. From the intricate and stunning paintings of Peruvian shaman Pablo Amaringo to the trippy, fractal-like works of Alex Grey, there's no shortage of visionary art to meditate on. And as Grey told us, it's one of the best ways for people to recognize the universality of their experience. "I can culturally pave the way for people to not be frightened of the visionary state with my art, and that validates people," Grey says. "When they see my art, they say, 'Oh my God, okay, I'm not crazy.'"

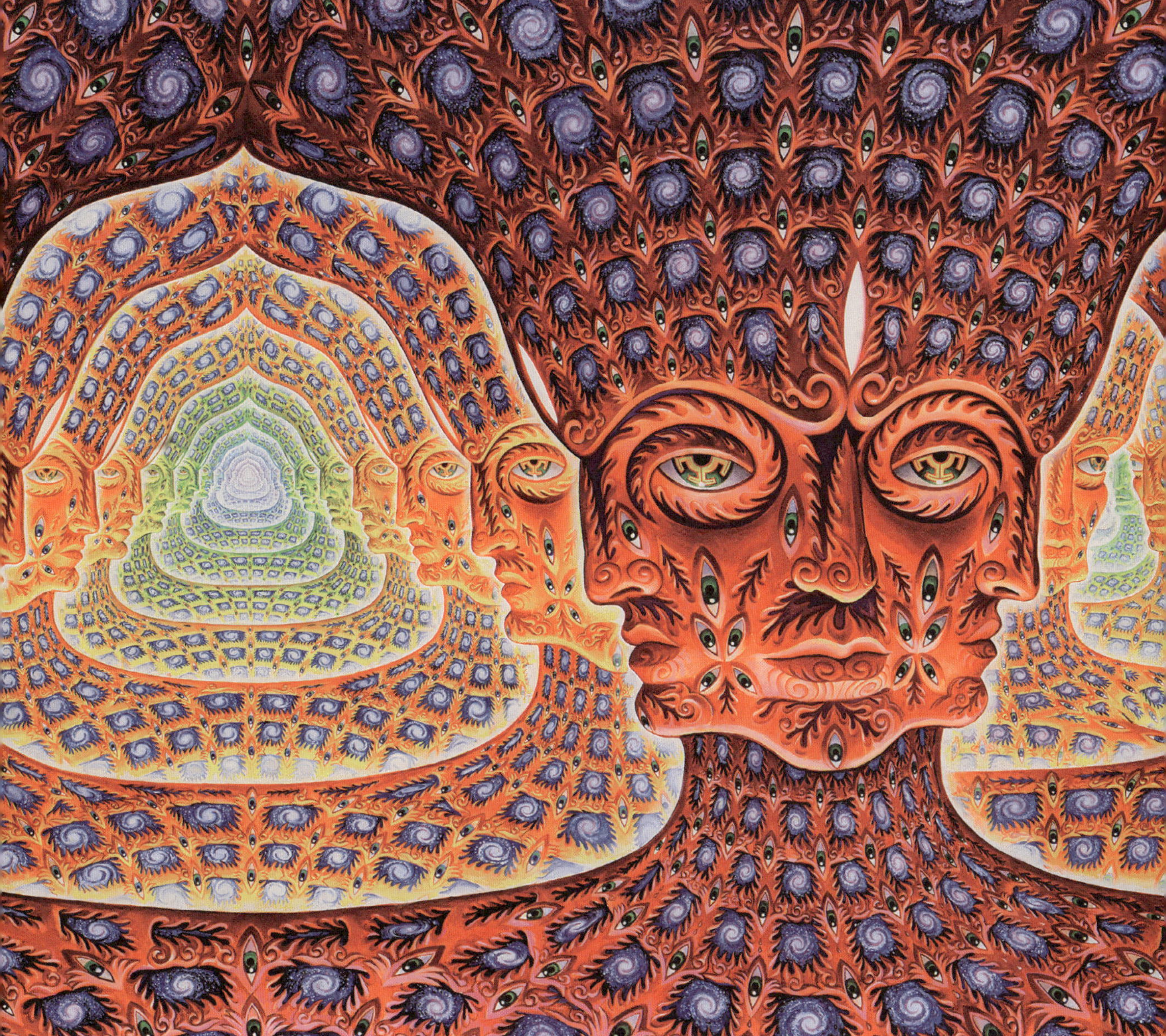

Above: Net of Being by Alex Grey

Page 70: El Encanto de las Piedras by Pablo Amaringo

Page 71: Huasi Yachana (Templo del Saber) by Pablo Amaringo

Page 72: Moon Womb by Mariela de la Paz

Page 73: Flower of Fire "Kodkille Rayen" by Mariela de la Paz

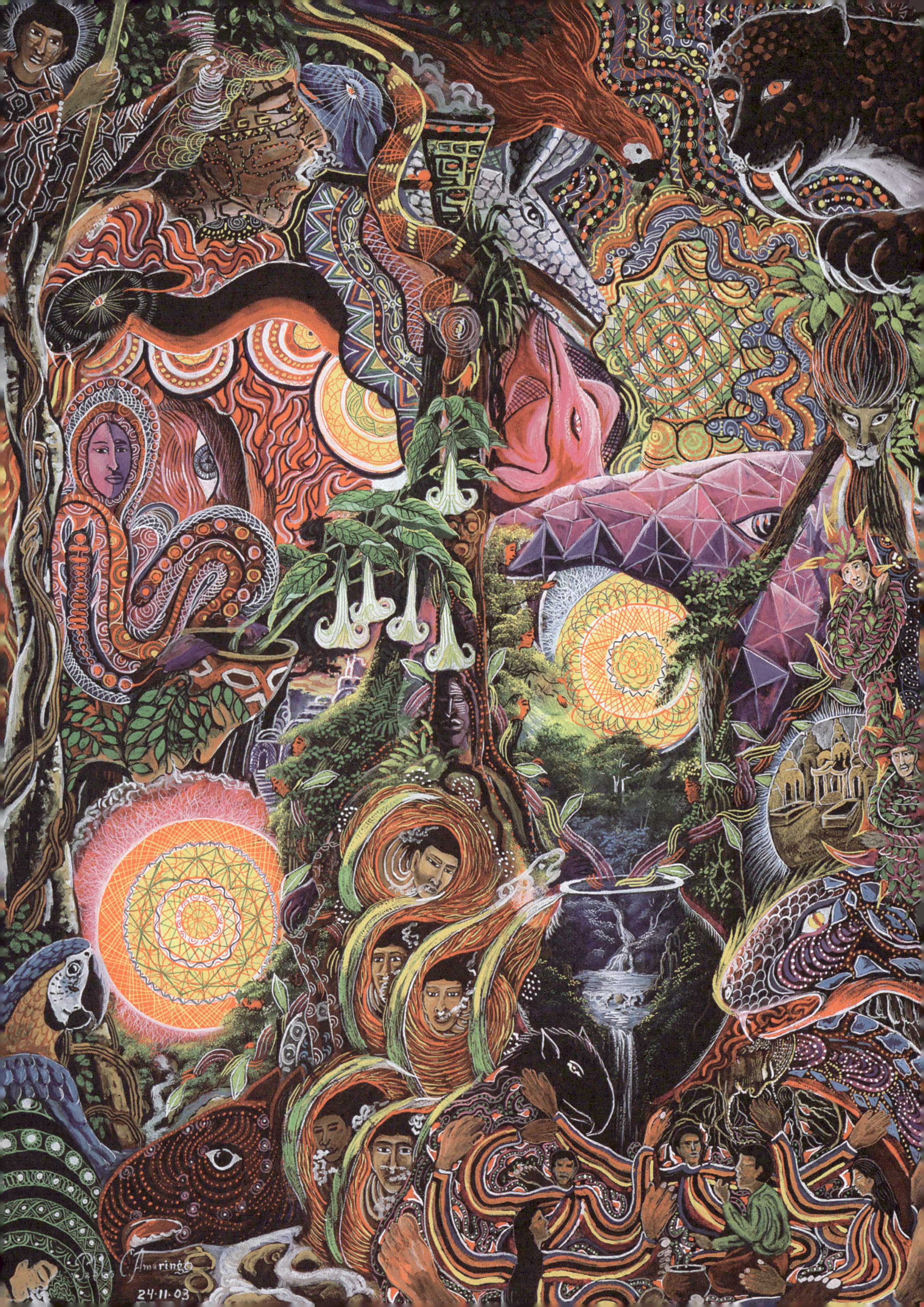
Amaringo
24·11·03

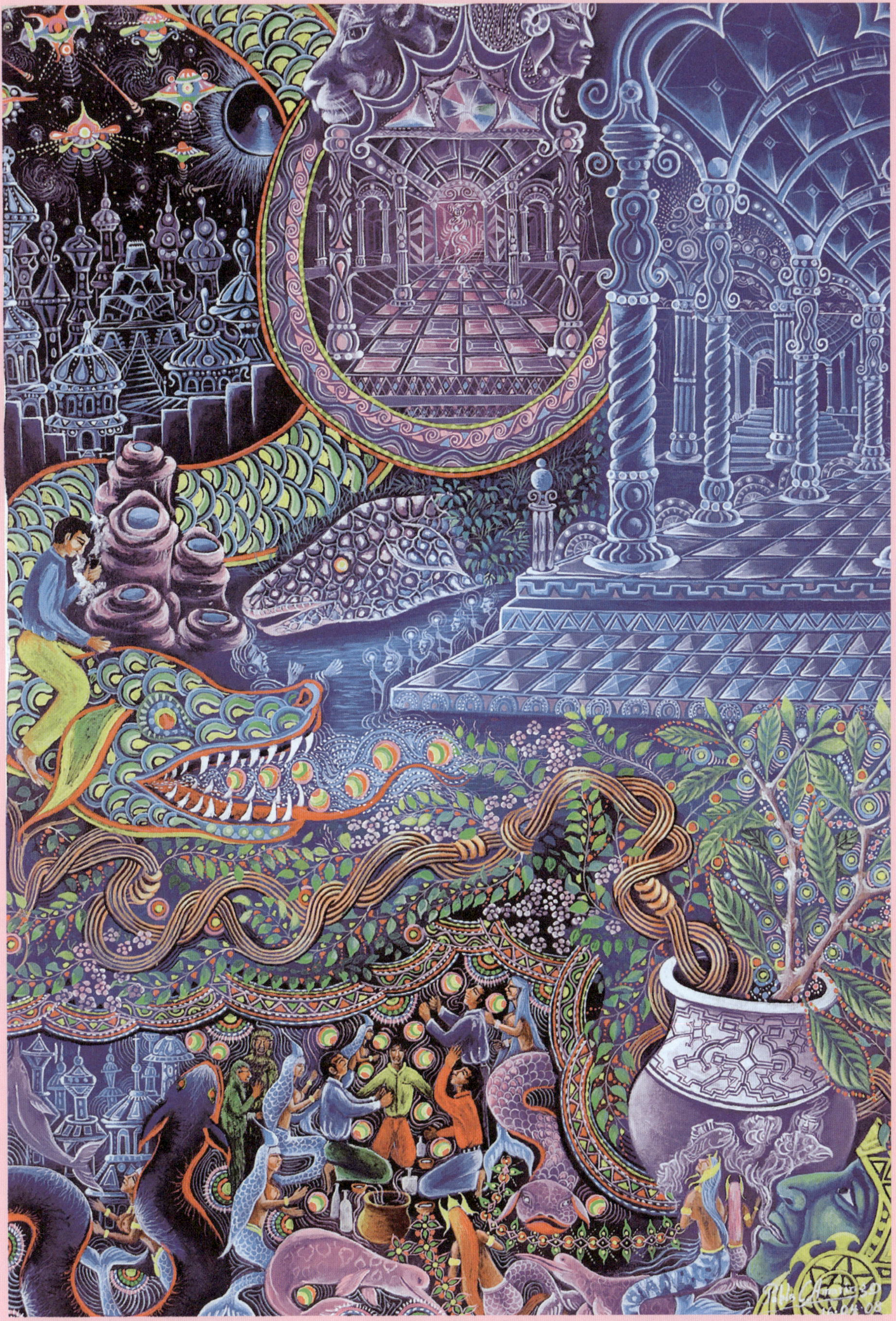

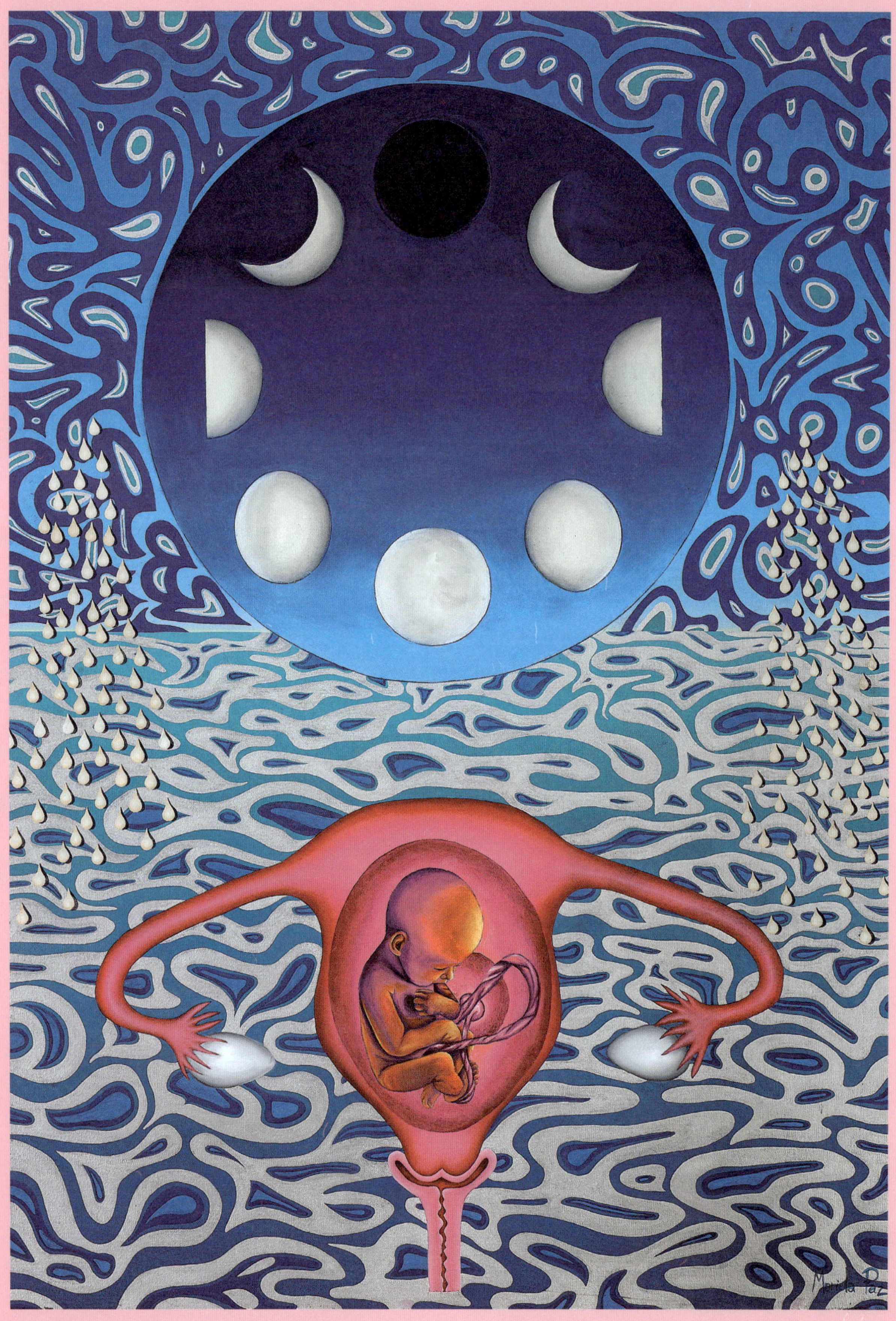

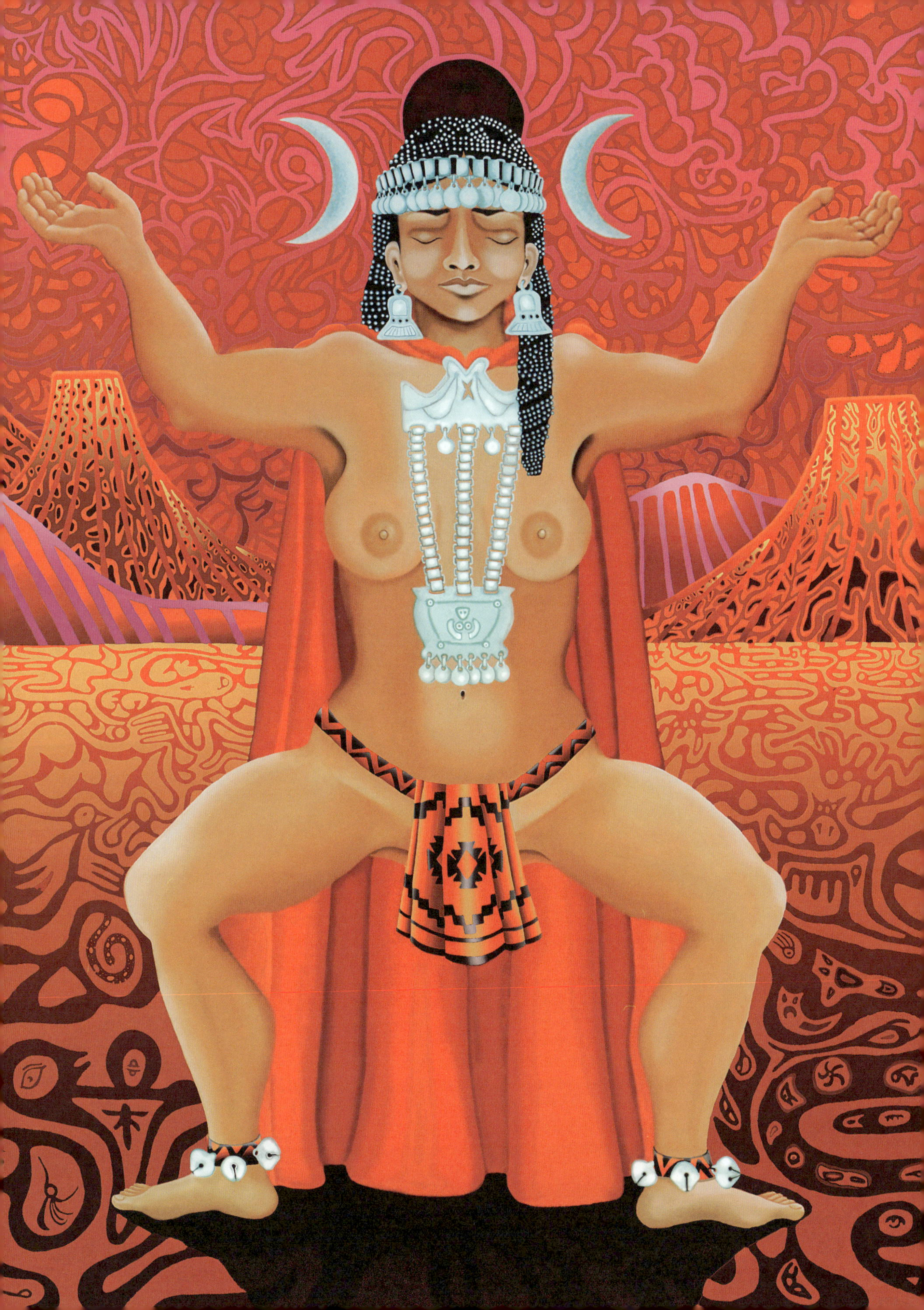

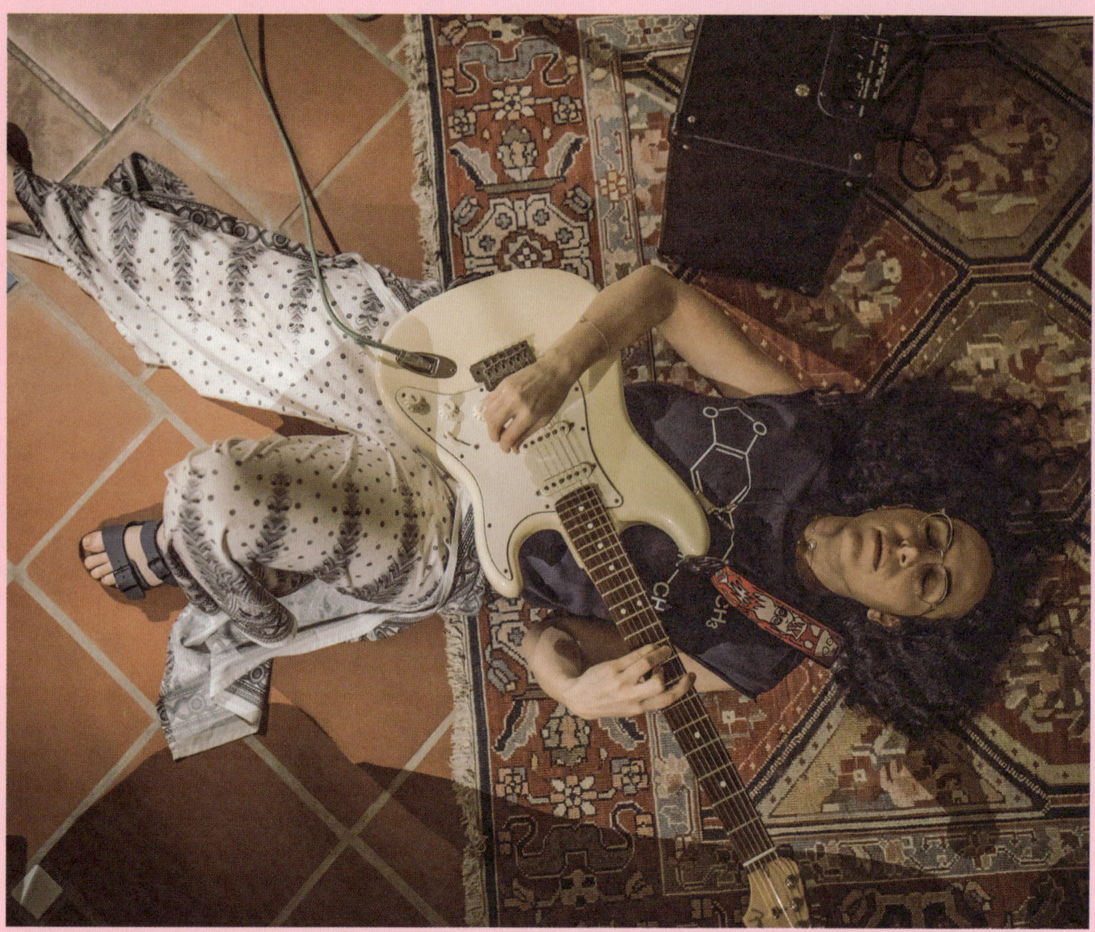

Haya Al-Hejailan plays guitar in her family home in Riyadh, Saudi Arabia

BEYOND THE JOURNEY

ARAB PSYCHEDELIC SOCIETY

Haya Al-Hejailan never anticipated her interview on psychedelics in *Arab News* would receive such overwhelmingly positive responses. But, after it did, she knew there was a need for a community in the Arab world devoted to reframing substances such as psilocybin and MDMA as potential tools for healing. So Al-Hejailan, who is from Saudi Arabia and has trained in harm reduction and ketamine therapy, started the Arab Psychedelic Society (at first, as an Instagram page). She highlights that her efforts aren't actually introducing psychedelics to the region, but reviving ancient, regionally rooted practices—such as the use of acacia and Syrian rue, and Sufi rituals—through a scientific lens. Since its inception, APS has led a fundraiser to train Arab mental health practitioners in MDMA-assisted psychotherapy; facilitated online integration circles; and hosted in-person gatherings. Future plans include mentorship, scholarships, translations of educational texts on psychedelics (like Michael Pollan's *How to Change Your Mind*), and, ultimately, culturally tailored clinical trials investigating the potential of psychedelics for health issues facing the Arab world such as obesity, depression, and smoking cessation.

Spiritual Emergence vs. Spiritual Emergency

Think of a spiritual emergence as a blossoming open of the soul. It can happen as a result of many intense experiences, such as a deep meditation practice, a profound personal crisis, or a peak psychedelic event. It can feel like a gentle awakening to your true nature, a shedding of the false or limiting beliefs of the ego as you step into a more expansive, integrated understanding of who you are. In brief, it's a spiritual awakening that can be accompanied by an expanded sense of creativity, alignment, compassion, and more.

A spiritual *emergency* is similar in that it can be experienced as a powerful shift in consciousness, but in this case it is amplified and at times overwhelming or chaotic. A spiritual emergency can present like a wave or a storm, leaving you feeling confused, lost, or perhaps out of touch with or detached from reality. It's not uncommon for someone undergoing a spiritual emergency to have psychosis or delusions of identity, such as believing they are the Messiah. If you or someone you know is undergoing a spiritual emergency, it's best to seek out psychedelic integration support or psychiatric care. It might even be necessary to seek hospitalization if a person having a spiritual emergency is a danger to themself or others.

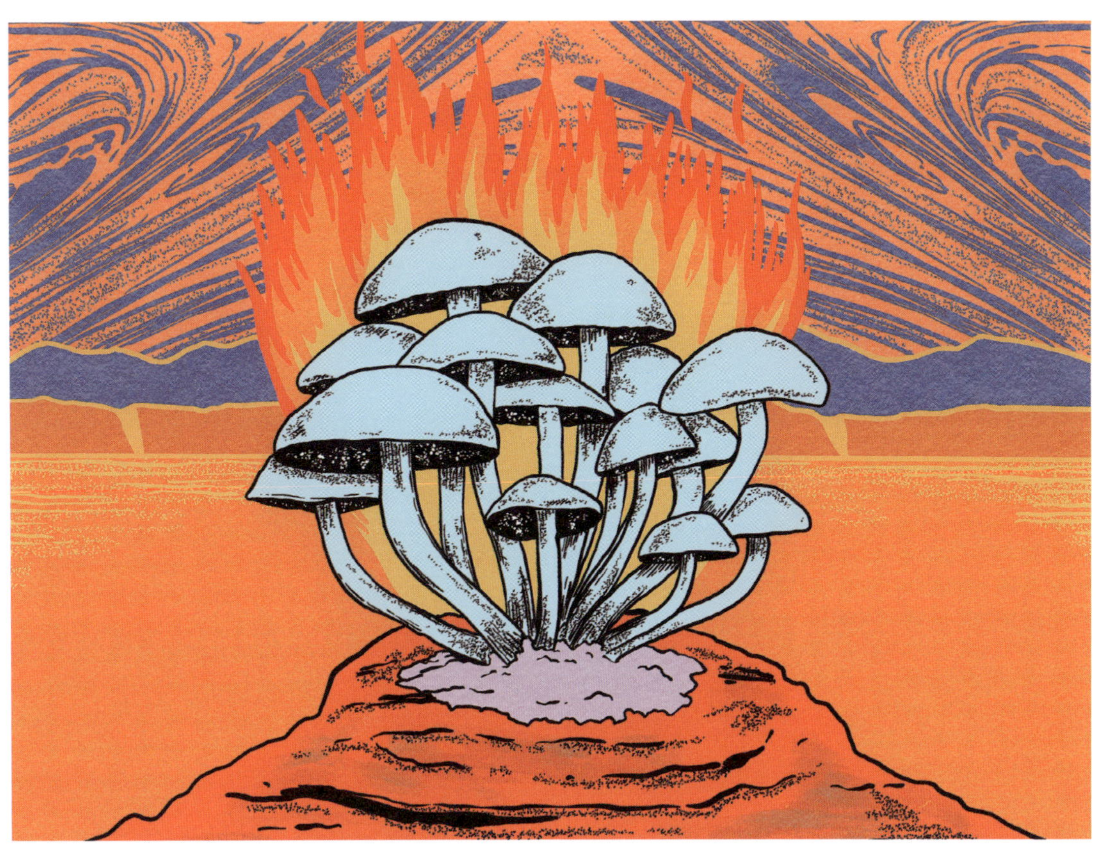

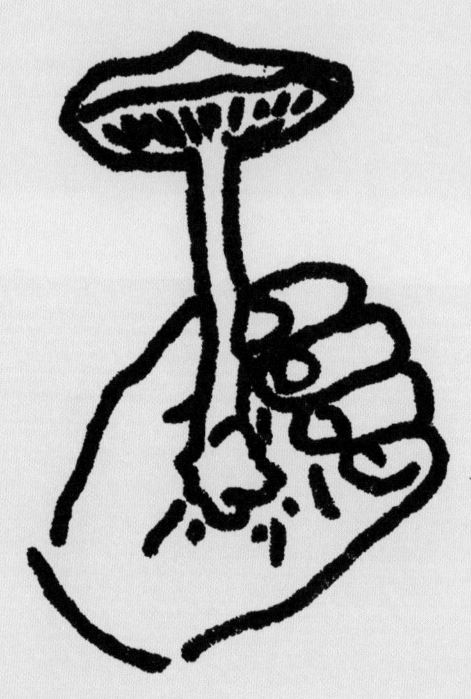

CHAPTER 5

SHROOMS

There's no one right way to do shrooms—and, even if you've decided there is, trips always have an element of unpredictability. People have transformative experiences on shrooms at festivals, in their homes, frolicking in nature (we can attest to this one), in ceremonies around the world, and beyond. And while shrooms have shown promise for helping people experiencing serious distress, these magical fungi can also be just a great time; sometimes the healing is just in letting yourself laugh.

When people talk about "shrooms," they're talking about mushrooms that contain the psychoactive compound known as psilocybin (i.e., the thing, among other alkaloids, that makes you trip). Psilocybin mushrooms have been used for thousands of years—in fact, according to one hypothesis, called the stoned ape theory, put forth by ethnobotanist Terence McKenna, the consumption of psilocybin mushrooms by early humans contributed to the development of consciousness, language, and culture. The theory suggests that the effects of these psychoactive mushrooms (visual activity, pattern recognition, neurogenesis, and heightened awareness) enhanced human cognition and communication, leading to more complex social structures, mythologies, and religion. It might sound a bit lofty if you've never done shrooms before (and the theory continues to be highly speculative), but you'd be amazed by how many people, right after their first psychedelic experience, actually say things like, "I've discovered the answer to all the world's problems!" (This is before they come back down to earth, of course.)

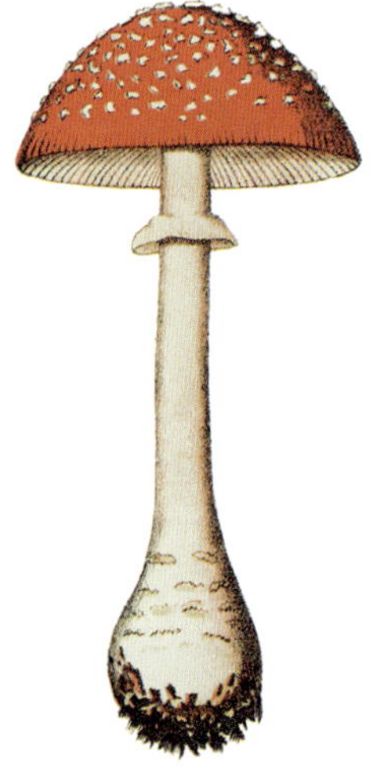

"Magic mushrooms," as they are sometimes called, were introduced to the West in the 1950s by ethnomycologist R. Gordon Wasson, who, along with his wife Valentina, participated in an Indigenous mushroom ceremony guided by the famed curandera (healer) María Sabina in Oaxaca, Mexico. Profoundly impacted by the ceremony, Wasson wrote about it for *Life* magazine in an article titled "Seeking the Magic Mushroom." He also sent some mushrooms to chemist Albert Hofmann, who is best known for synthesizing LSD but also, based on the specimens from Wasson, isolated and synthesized psilocybin for the first time.

It created a sensation. Inspired by Wasson's tale, many free spirits and seekers went down to Oaxaca to find Sabina and her famous mushroom. Tragically, their presence bred resentment among

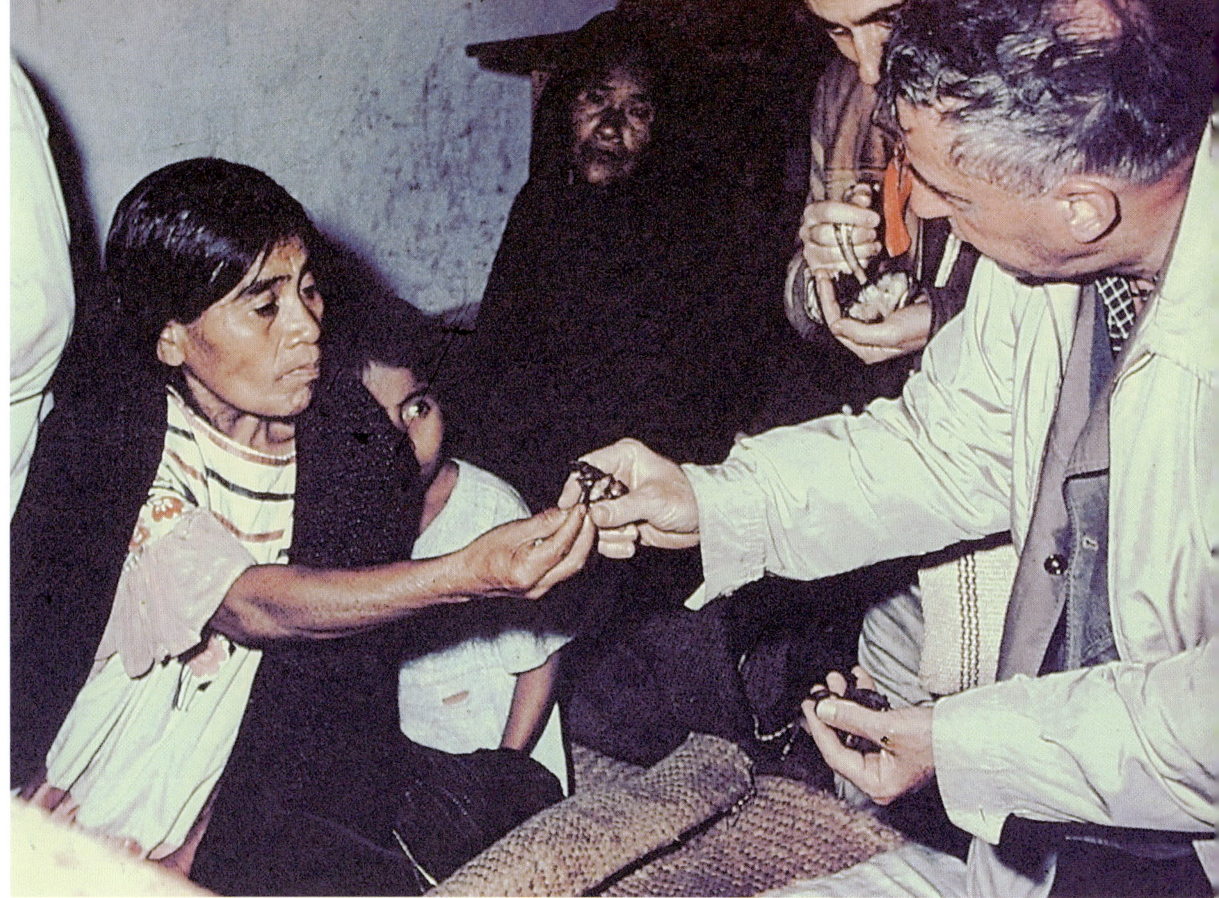

María Sabina hands a mushroom to R. Gordon Wasson before a ceremony, in the mid-1950s, in Huautla de Jiménez, Mexico.

Following pages: Sabina with her daughter Appolonia. During the ceremony, Appolonia often made sounds of birds, insects, and rain while her mother chanted.

locals, who felt their town had been overrun by tourists; they murdered Sabina's son and burned her house to the ground in retaliation. This incident, among others, adds layers of ethical considerations to conversations today about what it means to respectfully engage with Indigenous medicines by considering the needs and desires of their stewards. (In other words, do the people whose communities have traditionally taken certain medicines want outsiders taking them, too? If so, in what context?)

Meanwhile, in the United States, Europe, Canada, and beyond, the psychedelic revolution had begun. Research looking at the promise of psilocybin for mental health proliferated from the late 1950s into the early '70s. By the time Richard Nixon launched the War on Drugs in 1971, condemning psilocybin, along with substances like cannabis and heroin, to the category of Schedule I "drugs" (the most highly restricted category, making them generally prohibited), shrooms had already made their mark on the culture. Like acid, shrooms influenced some of the most iconic artists of the era; John Lennon, Bob Dylan, and Keith Richards are rumored to have been among the musical legends who visited María Sabina in Oaxaca. Lewis Carroll's 1865 *Alice's Adventures in Wonderland*—in which Alice stumbles upon a smoking caterpillar lounging on an *Amanita muscaria* shroom—took on a second life in this era, influencing hits like Jefferson Airplane's "White Rabbit."

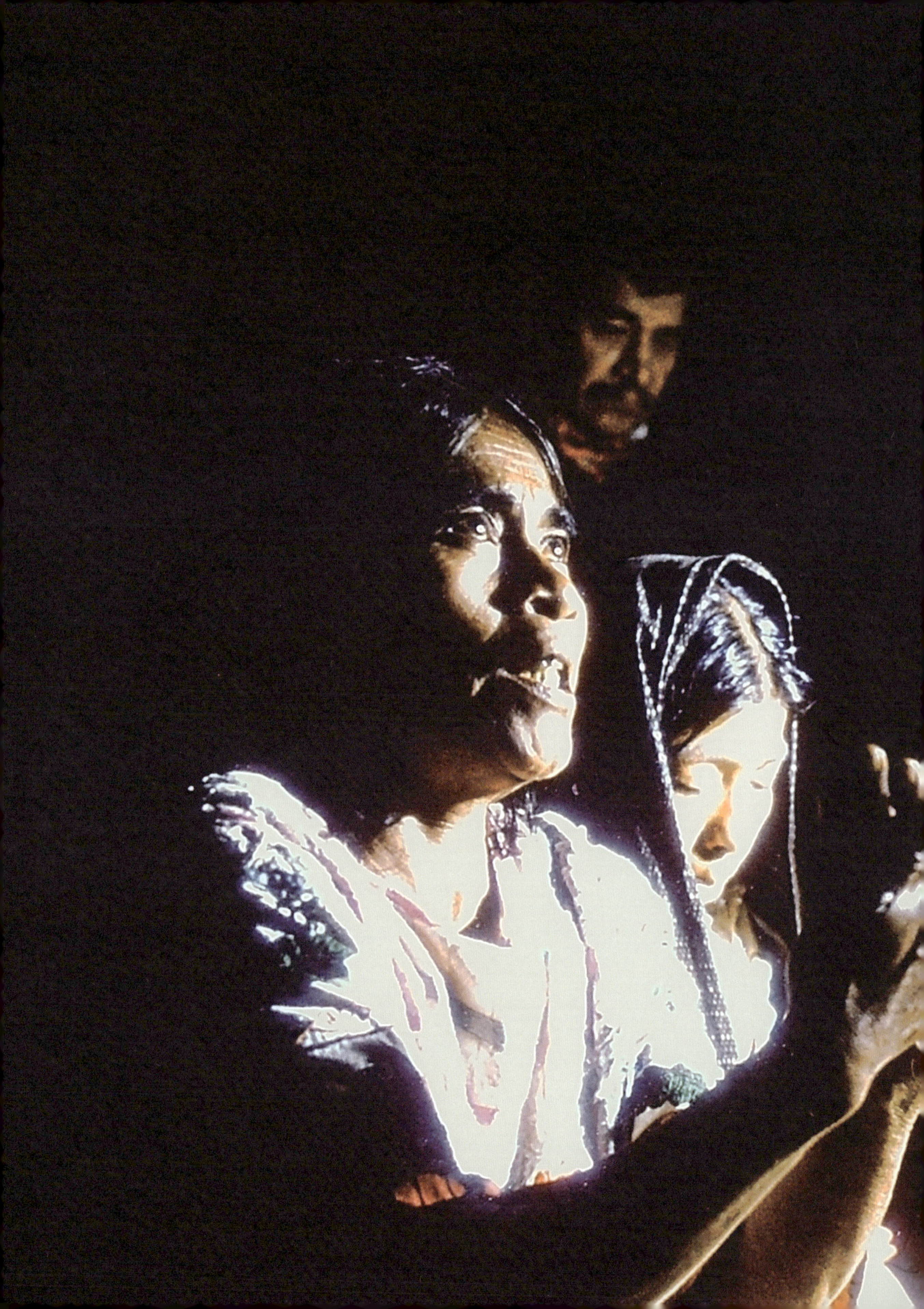

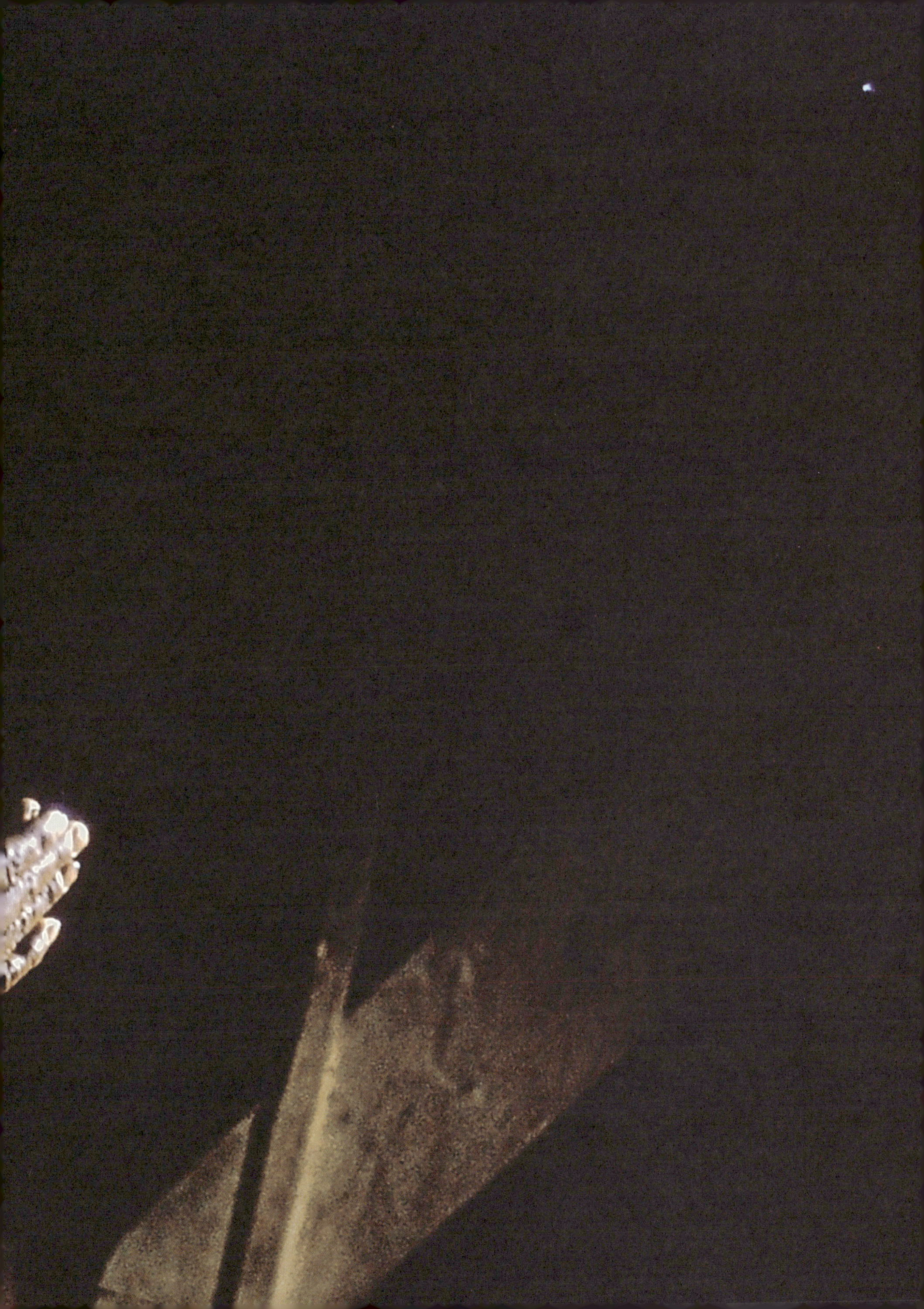

Meanwhile, for almost thirty years, psilocybin research largely went on hiatus. Today, a number of research institutions, as well as for-profit drug developers, have been granted FDA approval to study psilocybin for the use of conditions such as eating disorders, end-of-life anxiety in terminal patients, obsessive-compulsive disorder, Lyme disease, and more. This essentially means that officials at the FDA have recognized its promise as a treatment—and can help accelerate approval. In addition to medical conditions, clinical research has looked at psilocybin's potential to inspire mystical experiences and deepen meditation practices.

At the same time, a number of US cities have decriminalized psilocybin and other naturally occurring psychedelics with legislation geared toward making the growing, gifting, and gathering of these plants and fungi a low law enforcement priority. The movement to decriminalize psilocybin at the grassroots level began in Denver, which was soon followed by Oakland and then more than a dozen other jurisdictions. Many of the activists behind these campaigns see decriminalization—and a culture of growing your own fungi and gifting them to other people—as a grassroots alternative to legalization through the medical system or even the potential for recreational sales. They're passionate about making shrooms widely available so that people can use them in whatever manner they please (whether for therapy, for spiritual purposes, or simply to have fun). They're also invested in making sure that folks in marginalized communities with disproportionate rates of trauma are not prevented from having these healing experiences due to bureaucratic hurdles such as insurance coverage.

There's now a booming shrooms underground, with advocates and entrepreneurs around the world prepping for a lucrative, aboveground marketplace, but this time with much more sophisticated branding than we saw in the early days of weed. Think: artisanal shroom chocolates combined with maca and cayenne; lavender and shroom tea bags; shroom gummies; shroom capsules for microdosing, combined with lion's mane and other supplements. Aboveground, there are companies selling legal functional mushrooms (lion's mane, reishi, chaga) that are clearly readying themselves for a change of policy so they can sell psilocybin as soon as they're allowed to. It's a whole new world out there, folks, so take care as you navigate it.

Choosing Your Shroom

Though "shrooming" might sound as simple as getting your hands on some magic mushrooms and chomping away, there's much more to a psilocybin trip than meets the eye. For starters, there are more than 300 species of psychedelic mushrooms to choose from.

You're most likely to encounter *Psilocybe cubensis* mushrooms—sometimes referred to as cubes or (in reference to their golden caps) gold caps—because this species is one of the easiest to grow at home. You may come across a handful of other species (we'll describe some of them on pages 84–85), and there are hundreds more that are relatively obscure. Within each species, there are various strains or varieties with their own distinct genetic characteristics. Within the species of *P. cubensis*, for example, strains include B+, Penis Envy, and Golden Teacher. When people refer to different types of psychedelic mushrooms, they're oftentimes referring not to different species but to different strains of *Psilocybe cubensis*.

Until recently, hardly anything was known about the differences in potency between strains. In 2021, thanks to Oakland Hyphae, an organization that organizes psychedelic events and does potency testing, sixty strains were tested for their psilocybin and psilocin levels and *some*—albeit preliminary—trends began to emerge. The Penis Envy and Tidal Wave strains, generally, had higher psilocybin levels than other strains.

That said, these shroom strains mostly get their reputations from people's (unverifiable) tales of their trips (e.g., "Penis Envy is craaazzzyy" or "I really love Golden Teachers because they're much more spiritual"). The truth is, there are some psilocybin potency tests on the market, but for the most part, the only way to know what you've got is the old-fashioned way: to try 'em. That said, it is good to know the species and strain of any mushrooms you're considering, if you can, so you can see what people have to say about them online. Ask the person you're obtaining them from what their experience has been like—and then take their answer with a grain of salt.

As with any trip, but especially with shrooms, it is recommended to "start low" (as in a low dose) and "go slow" because there are so many unknowns. Bear in mind that, much like with weed, where people talk a lot about the percentage of THC (the molecule famous for getting people high), people who are into shrooms talk a lot about the psilocybin content, but mushrooms have many other alkaloids that work synergistically to create the effects, and we just don't have that much information about them yet.

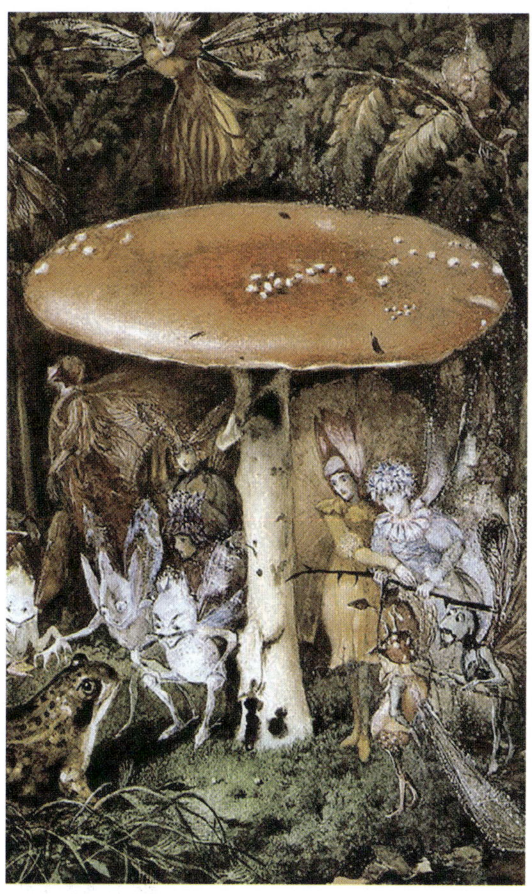

Types of Shrooms

There are more than 300 different species of psilocybin-containing mushrooms (holy cow!). Here are a few.

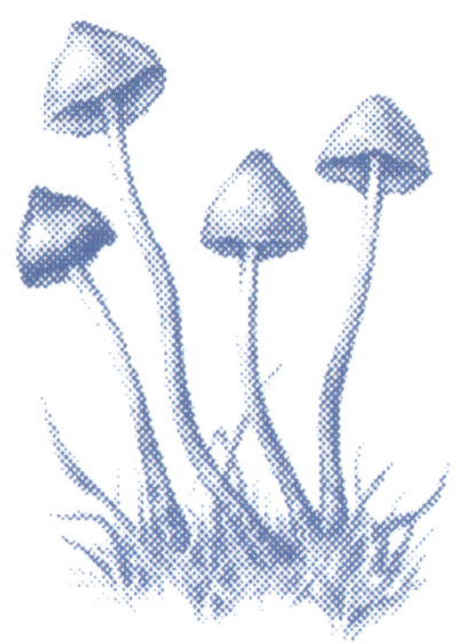

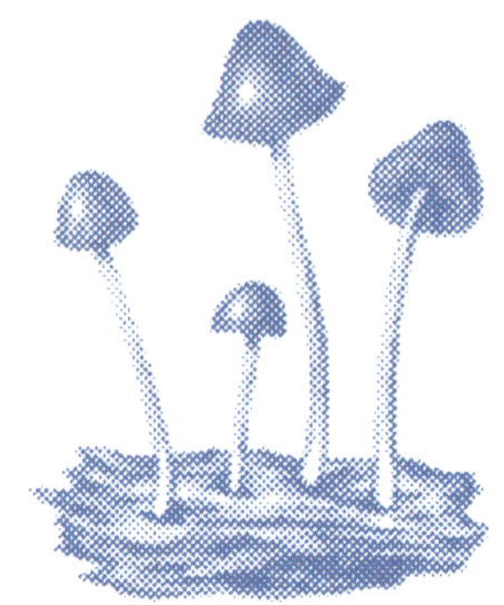

PANAEOLUS CYANESCENS

Panaeolus cyanescens (a.k.a. *Copelandia cyanescens*) mushrooms are sometimes referred to as blue meanies, which can be confusing because there is also a strain of *Psilocybe cubensis* called Blue Meanie.

PSILOCYBE AZURESCENS

P. azurescens—also known as flying saucers, blue runners, blue angels, or azzies—is considered one of the most potent wild-growing psilocybin mushrooms because of its high levels of psilocybin, though exact potency can vary and is influenced by additional psychoactive compounds and environmental factors.

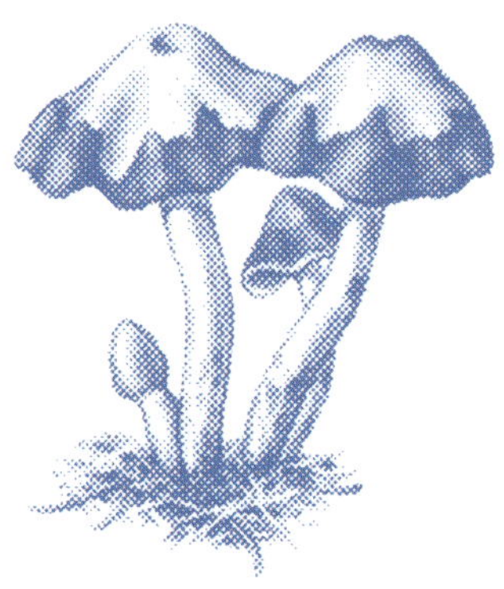

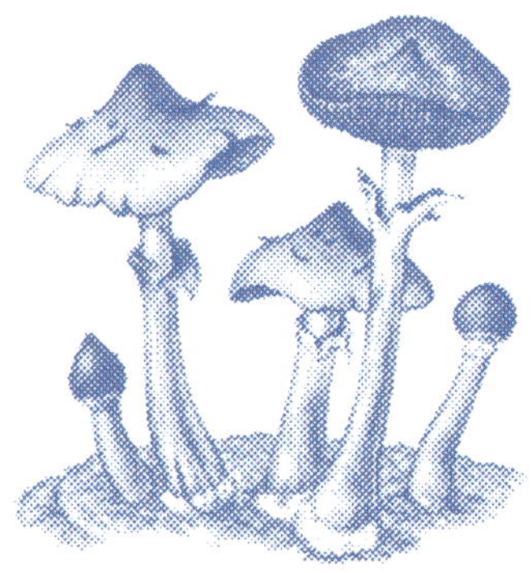

PSILOCYBE CAERULESCENS

Psilocybe caerulescens mushrooms are known as *derrumbes*, "landslides," in Mexico, where they grow naturally.

PSILOCYBE CUBENSIS

If you've eaten psilocybin mushrooms but had no idea what species they were, chances are they were a strain of *Psilocybe cubensis*.

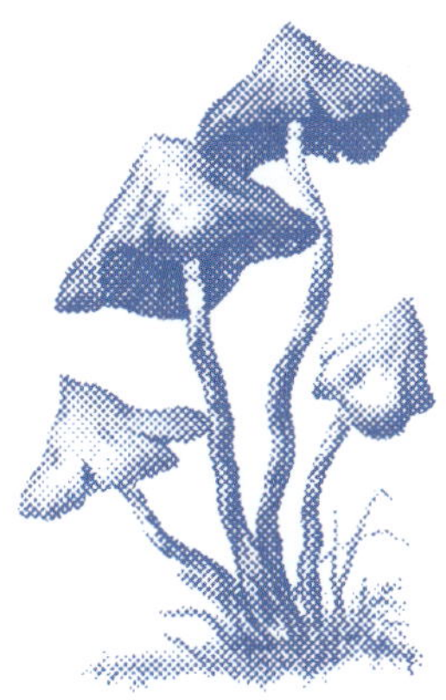

PSILOCYBE ZAPOTECORUM

Psilocybe zapotecorum is one of many species that grow in Mexico, producing some of the largest and most visually striking psychedelic mushrooms found in the Neotropics. The name "zapotecorum" was given in honor of the Zapotec community, an Indigenous group that uses and reveres this shroom.

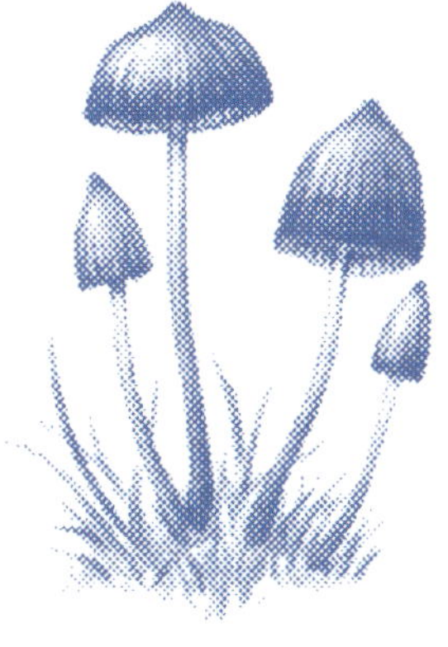

PSILOCYBE MEXICANA

Psilocybe mexicana has a rich history. It's believed that this is the species of mushroom that the Nahuatl or Aztec people used ceremonially.

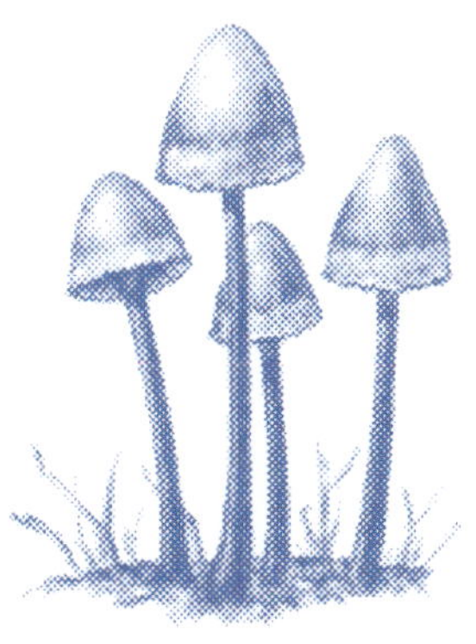

PSILOCYBE SEMILANCEATA

After *P. cubensis*, *P. semilanceata* is one of the most well-known species of psychedelic mushrooms, recognized by its small, bell-shaped cap with a pointed tip.

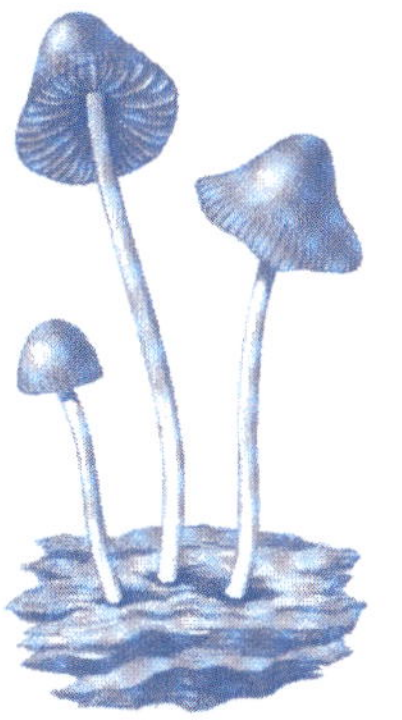

PSILOCYBE TAMPANENSIS

Psilocybe tampanensis is a rare species of psychedelic mushroom known for producing "magic truffles," or sclerotia.

What's a Mushroom Trip Like?

It's no mistake that psilocybin-containing fungi are called magic mushrooms—tripping on them can be straight up magical. But while the experience of shrooming can be euphoric, playful, spiritual, and introspective, it can also be frightening, anxiety-ridden, emotional, and heavy. The magic in the mushrooms contains multitudes of expressions, and it's nearly impossible to tell how it will go—as the common adage goes, "LSD puts you in the driver's seat; mushrooms take you for a ride." But you can do your best to have a safe, supportive, and nourishing trip by cultivating your set and setting (see chapter 2).

It's difficult to explain how tripping on shrooms will feel because the experience is so subjective and depends on not only the dose (see below) but also the individual and what they bring to the table in terms of their psychology, environment, and intentions. Psilocybin might cause you to feel your body in a different way; perhaps you will become more aware of your gut or your heart. On the flip side, it could cause you to feel totally light or even disembodied. It may cause hallucinations, like swirling patterns or auditory echoing, a brightened perception of color, or the illusion that inanimate objects are breathing or vibrating. During a mushroom trip, you might laugh or cry, or you might feel connected to the Divine or more in tune with your soul or with loved ones (living and deceased). The key, as with all psychedelics, is to remain as open and curious as you can.

The effects of psilocybin will begin to kick in about twenty minutes to an hour after ingestion, and they will last for roughly six to eight hours. The peak occurs about two to three hours in. The effects plateau for about another two hours and then start to wear off.

Shroom Dosage

So you've got a baggie of dried mushrooms—cracked white stems with some blue bruising, and amber caps. Or perhaps the shrooms came to you in the form of capsules filled with ground mushroom powder, or in an artisanal chocolate bar, with each square corresponding to a specific dose. Generally speaking, a "standard" dose of shrooms is said to be an eighth (of an ounce), or about 3.5 grams, but that's actually quite a lot and many folks prefer to do half an eighth, or about 1.25 grams, to start. A microdose is said to be between 0.1 and 0.5 gram (although 0.5 gram is more than a microdose for most); a low dose is 0.5 to 2 grams; a moderate dose is 2 to 3.5 grams; and anything above 3.5 grams is a high dose. The best way to figure out your dose is to get a small scale and weigh the dried shrooms. Also, please note that while potency does vary, even among the same species and strain, some shrooms are known for generally being stronger than others. Be especially mindful of your dosage if you're working with a shroom like that. DoubleBlind has more comprehensive strain and species guides on its website, but the most common potent shroom you're likely to encounter is the *Psilocybe cubensis* Penis Envy strain and varieties of it.

GROW YOUR OWN MAGIC!

Few things are more magical than growing your own food and medicine. Growing shrooms takes about six to eight weeks, from start to finish, and costs around $250 for all the supplies. It would be impossible to give a detailed-enough overview here to really get you started—there are whole books and classes devoted to growing shrooms, and everyone's environmental conditions and access to supplies are different. But to give you a window into the process, here are a few of the most important steps. If you can keep a plant alive, you can grow shrooms!

1. DECIDE ON YOUR TEK: *Tek* in the shroom-growing world means technique—that is, how you're going to grow your mushrooms. One of the most common methods for newbies, called the PF Tek, involves growing the mushroom mycelium on a substrate (kind of like soil for fungi) inside glass jars.

2. BUY YOUR SUPPLIES: Psilocybin spores are legal in all US states except California, Idaho, and Georgia. They also can be purchased in many other parts of the world. But beware: They're technically legal only for microscopy use in the United States, so once you start growing 'em, you're doing something federally illegal.

3. INOCULATE: This is basically when you inject your substrate with the spores.

4. WAIT: The hardest part of growing, honestly, may be having patience. If you did things right, within weeks you should start to see mycelium growing throughout the substrate (exciting!).

5. TRANSFER: The mycelium has colonized your substrate. It's white and gorgeous, with its tendrils reaching through the jar or bag. Now you'll dump them into a bigger bin of substrate.

6. MISTING AND FANNING: In this stage, you'll want to check in on your babies every so often, misting and fanning them to keep the temperature and humidity juuuuust right (the ideal temperature is around 75 to 80 degrees Fahrenheit, and the humidity should be around 85 percent). You can get a little temperature and humidity gauge to put inside the tub.

7. HARVESTING: Time to pick! Harvest your mushrooms right before the veil under the cap breaks. That's when they're at peak potency. Use clean hands or scissors to snip them at the base.

8. DRYING: To make mushrooms shelf-stable, you'll need to dry them completely. A food dehydrator works best, but a fan in a dry space can do the trick, too. You're aiming for a texture that's cracker-dry—no bendy mushrooms allowed.

9. STORING: Once they're dried, pop your shrooms into an airtight container with a little desiccant packet (like the ones that come in jerky bags). Keep them in a cool, dark place and they'll stay good for months—if you don't eat them all first.

And voilà! You've got yourself some shrooms—honestly, probably way more than you know what to do with. Interested in growing with DoubleBlind? Join our community of growers at doubleblindmag.com.

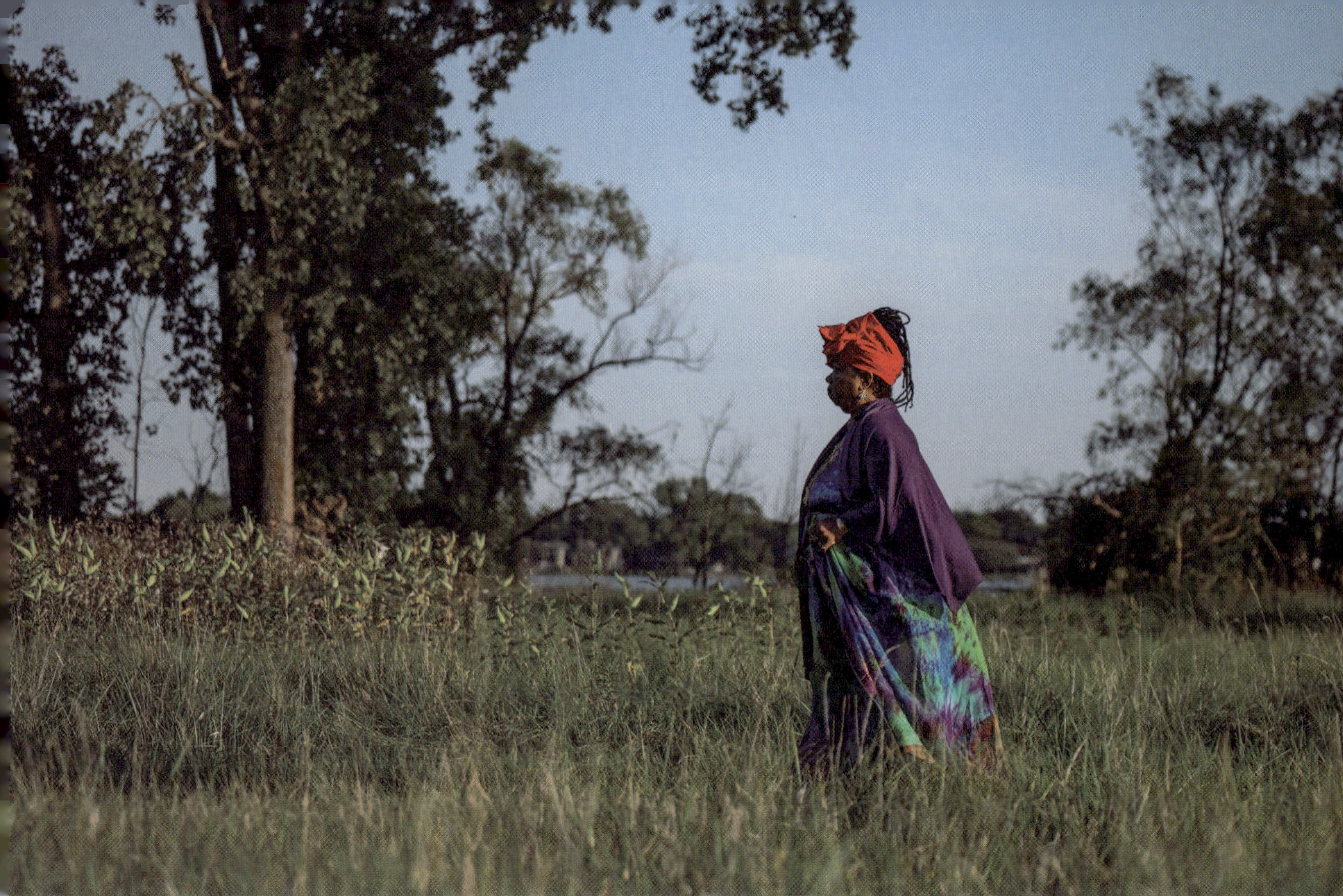

BEYOND THE JOURNEY

MAMA AYANA

While most may think of Berkeley or upstate New York as the origin points of the first psychedelic wave, Cleveland and Detroit are home to some of the most rooted mushroom cultures in America. And Ayana Iyi, lovingly known as Mama Ayana, is among a handful of practitioners who have been quietly serving these communities for decades, charting their own paths with high-dose journeys.

Two such practitioners were Kai Wingo—who was also a mushroom farmer and beloved among East Cleveland's local food community—and Baba Kilindi Iyi. Kilindi was Ayana's husband and a controversial, and also beloved, figure known for doing journeys of 30 to 50 grams (more than ten times what's considered "a high dose") and bringing back insights to his devotees.

Almost a decade has passed since Kai and Kilindi died. During his passing, Kilindi was surrounded by many powerful women who have carried his teachings into the world along with their own. Ayana—a legend in her own right within Detroit's psychedelic community—is holding down this local movement where it began, in the Rust Belt region, creating intergenerational spaces where healing can be done in community (as opposed to by individuals in psychedelic ceremonies or retreats far from home). She continues to host gatherings for women in psychedelics, including the Women and Entheogen conference in Cleveland, first hosted by Kai Wingo.

At a time when a growing number of people in their twenties and thirties—working outside the scientific and medical paradigms—are working to carve out a space for themselves within the psychedelic movement, she serves as a reminder that this work is not new.

This excerpt comes from a story reported for DoubleBlind's print magazine by Bett Williams.

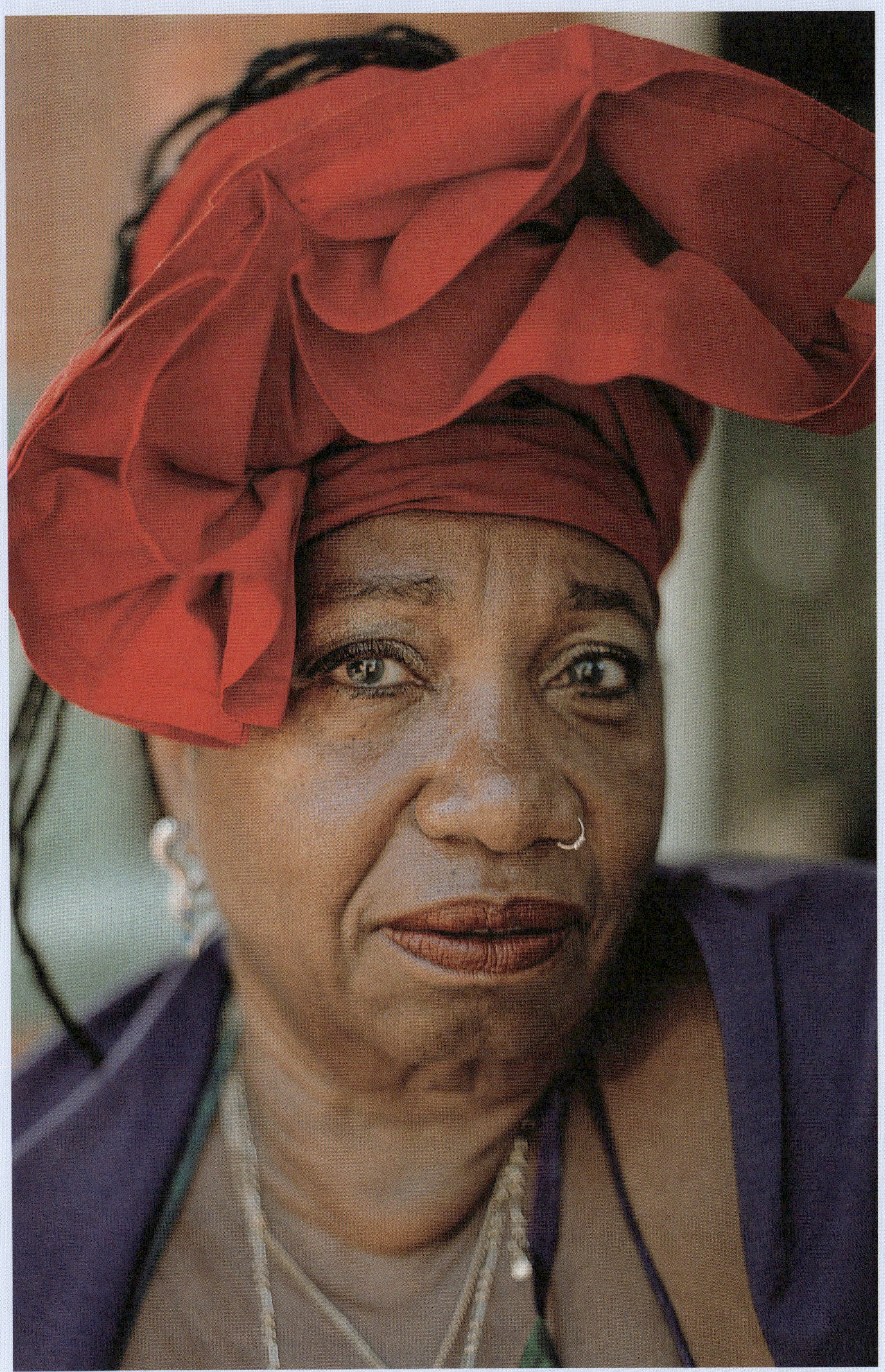

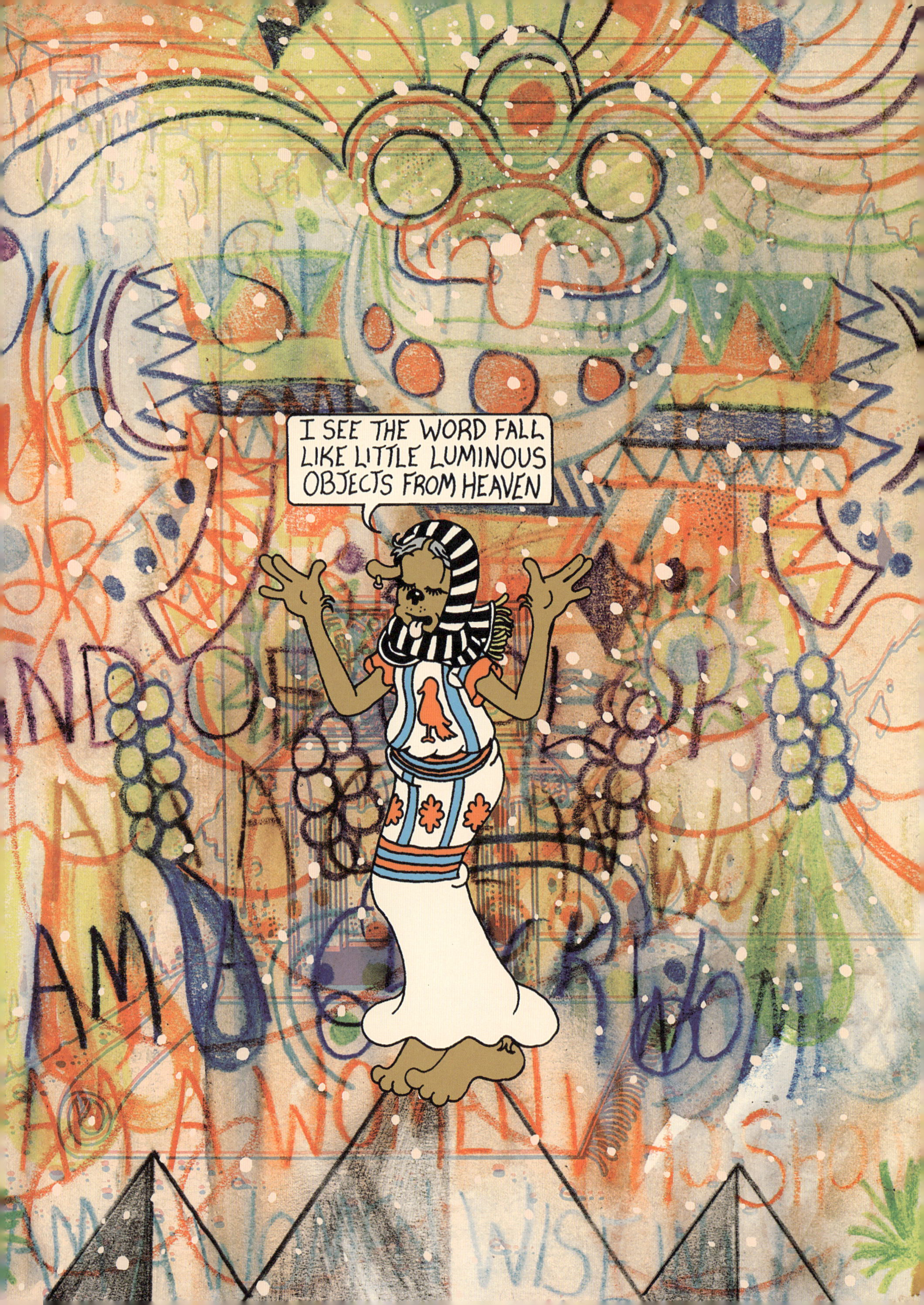
I SEE THE WORD FALL LIKE LITTLE LUMINOUS OBJECTS FROM HEAVEN

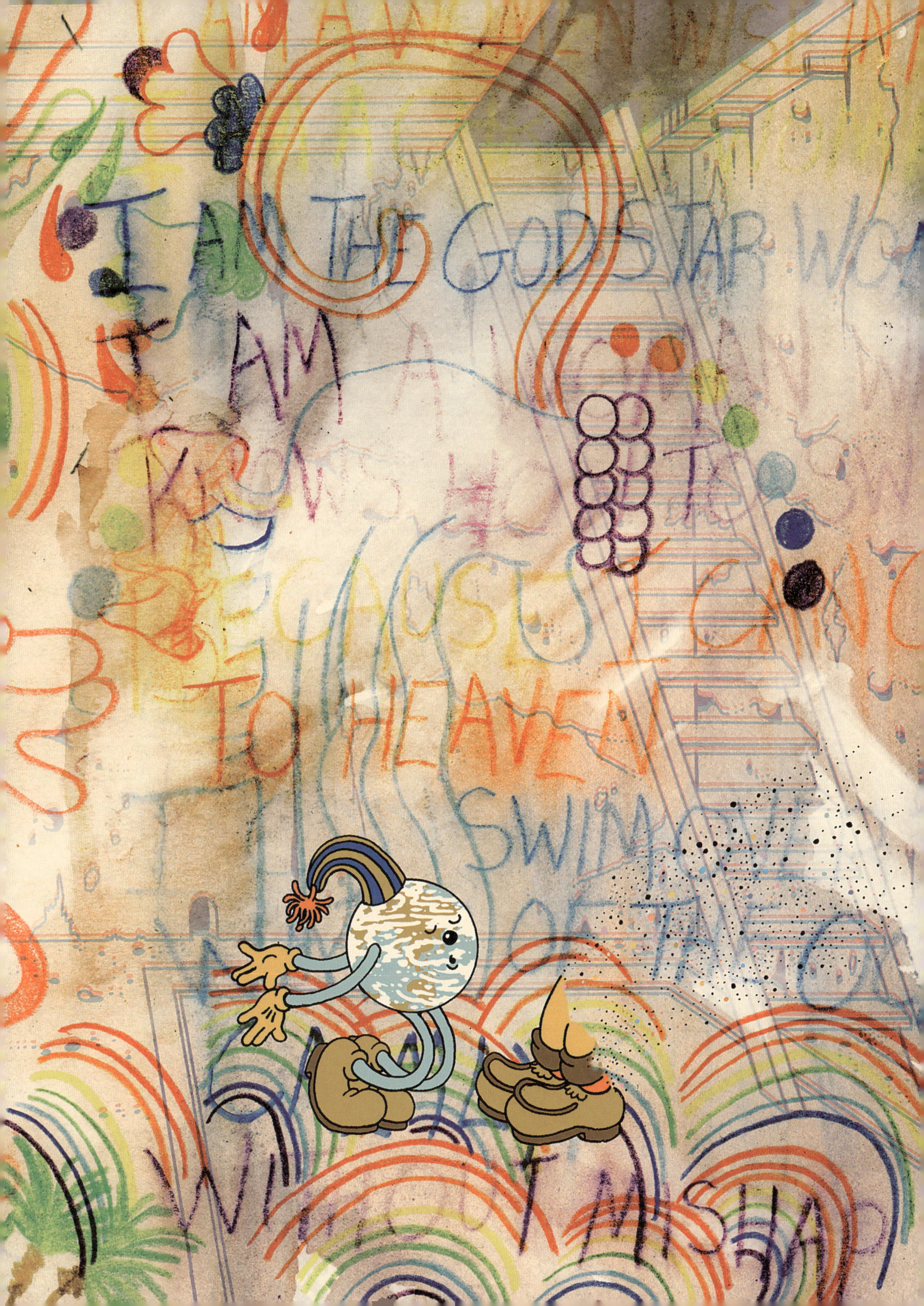

I AM THE GOD STAR
I AM
BECAUSE
TO HEAVEN
SWIM
WITHOUT MISHAP

SHROOM RECIPES

While some people choose to eat them on their own, mushrooms can admittedly smell like feet and taste like mud. There's actually a burgeoning field of shroom cooking (much like there was for cannabis cooking in the early days of legalization), which includes cookbooks and even a class taught by DoubleBlind. Slightly more appetizing options include the following:

LEMON TEKKING

This option entails soaking your shrooms in citrus juice prior to the trip. Start by grinding your dose of shrooms into a powder, using a coffee or cannabis grinder, and then transfer the powder to a shot glass. Squeeze lemon or lime juice over the powder until it's completely covered, and let it sit for fifteen to twenty minutes. When you're ready, take the shot—but keep in mind that while this method masks the taste of the shrooms, its real purpose, according to seasoned psychonauts, is to make the trip shorter and more intense than eating the shrooms on their own. There's a lack of scientific evidence for this, but the hypothesis is that the juice breaks down the mushrooms before they enter your system, rendering the psilocybin and other compounds more bioavailable and allowing you to feel their effects more quickly.

MUSHROOM TEA

Psychonauts say that shroom tea is easier on the stomach than eating mushrooms straight, which can cause nausea as they're kicking in. However, steeping shrooms in tea can also make their psychedelic effects set in more quickly. To make shroom tea, grind your desired dose in a coffee or cannabis grinder. We recommend adding ginger as it helps with nausea. You may also try adding other herbs that you find supportive, such as chamomile for digestion and anxiety. Transfer the mushroom powder and any other herbs to a mug; we like to put them in a tea ball or tea bag first so they don't have to be strained out later (or eaten). Pour just-boiled water over the mushrooms and herbs, cover, and let steep for about fifteen minutes. Add honey if you want, and enjoy!

PB&J, PIZZA, AND MORE

To mask the taste of the shrooms, you can simply squish them into a peanut butter and jelly sandwich, scatter them atop a slice of pizza, or add them to another dish of your choosing. Just keep in mind not to eat too heavily. It's not recommended to shroom on a full stomach as it can contribute to nausea and also reduces the potency of your experience.

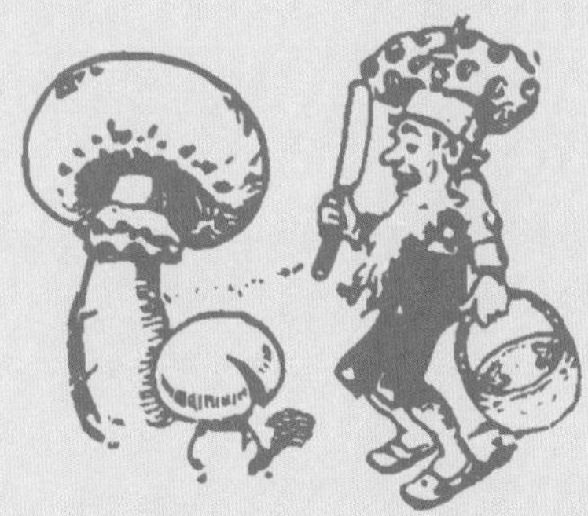

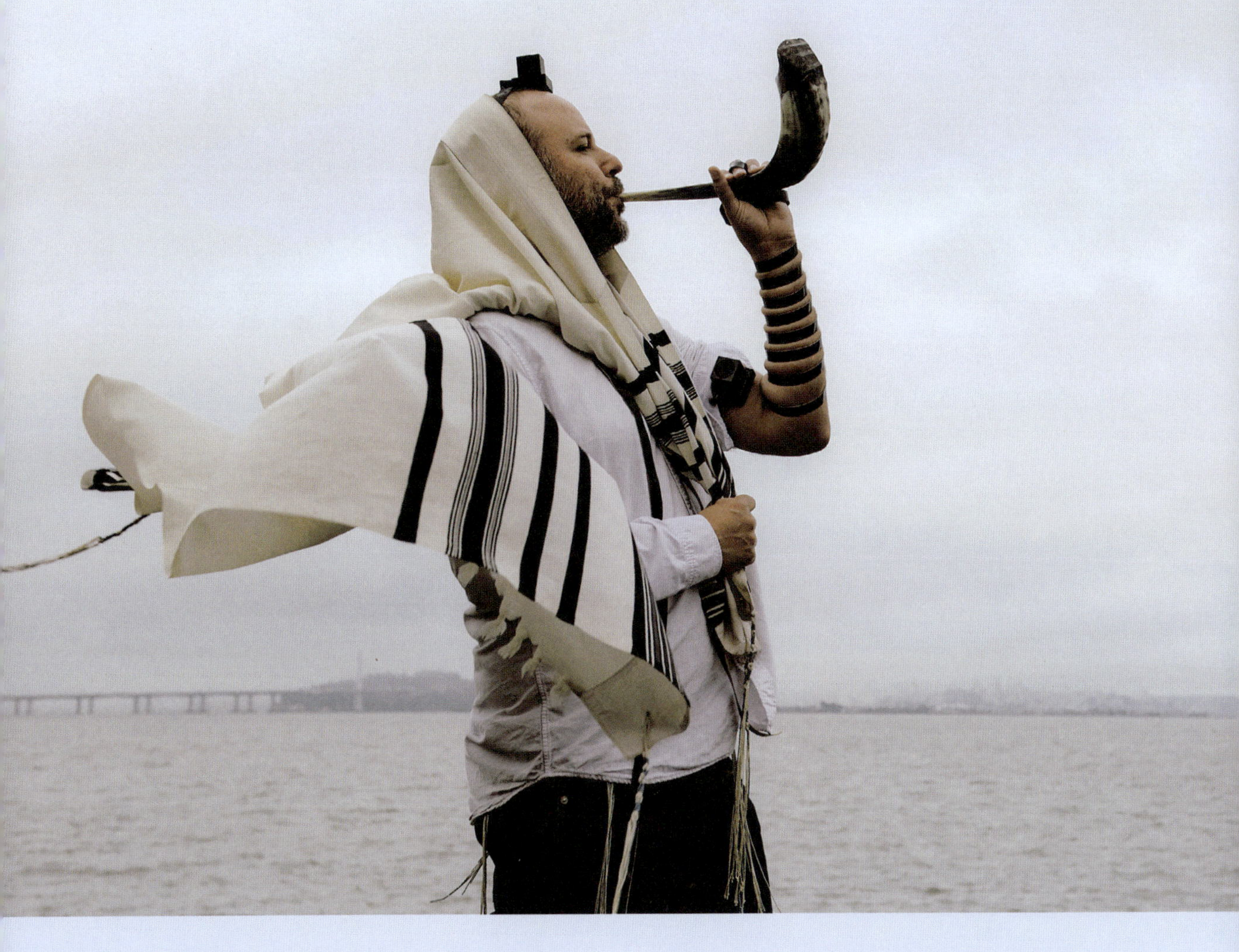

BEYOND THE JOURNEY

SHROOMS FOR RELIGIOUS LEADERS

A growing number of religious leaders are expressing burnout, a feeling of being disconnected from the reason they initially began to lead their congregations. Researchers at Johns Hopkins University investigated whether a mystical experience—occasioned by psilocybin—might help reignite their passion. They gave psilocybin to priests, rabbis, and imams who had never had a psychedelic experience before. A significant number of participants reported that, in their journeys, they reconnected with a higher power, experiencing the spiritual qualities of their trip through the language and symbolism of their unique faith traditions. One participant in this study, Rabbi Zac Kamenetz, has since been influential, alongside many underground facilitators and advocates (including author Yoseph Needelman-Ruiz, Natalie Ginsberg of MAPS, and DoubleBlind's own Madison Margolin), in reigniting a religious movement blending psychedelic practice into Jewish ritual.

INDIGENOUS WISDOM AND STEWARDSHIP

THE MAZATEC

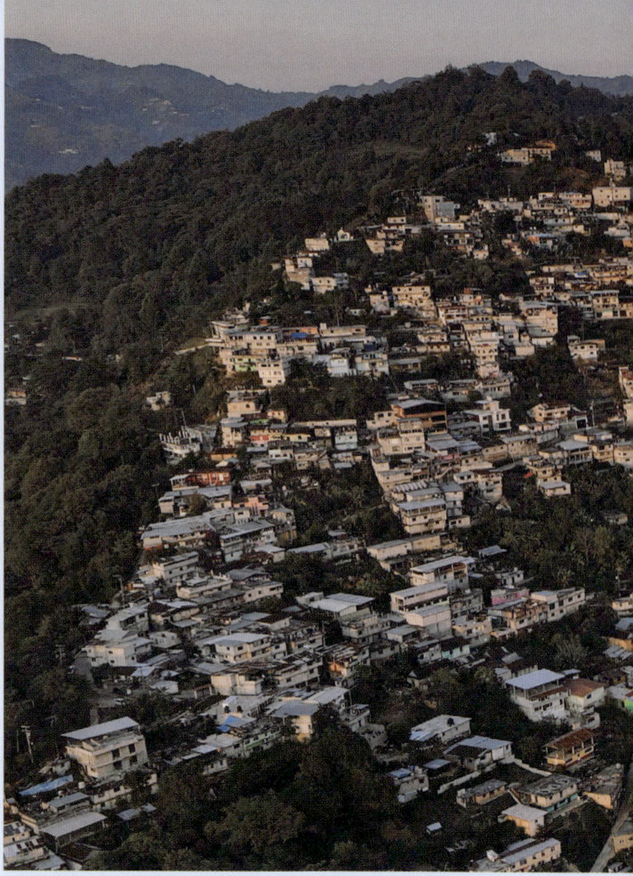

For centuries, and as an aspect of their culture, religion, and identity, the Mazatec have used mushrooms—which they refer to as *ndi xij'to* (little things that sprout from the ground)—and other psychoactive plants to cure physical, mental, and spiritual ailments.

There are specific periods and days where mushroom ceremonies are carried out, and healing is only one aspect of them; the ritual and community practice of these ancient traditions is also considered a form of resistance of the Mazatec people to capitalist modernity and outside influence.

Mazatec curanderos (healers) do not attribute the therapeutic effects of mushrooms to psilocybin. Instead, says Mexican anthropological researcher Dr. Sarai Piña Alcántara, they consider the mushrooms a deity, a conscious being believed to have a spirit, voice, and intention. Upon ingesting the mushrooms, they believe the deity possesses the person's body. "The mushroom is [also] a communication bridge with the spiritual world and other beings such as *chikones* [guardians of different natural places]," explains Piña.

This excerpt comes from a story reported for DoubleBlind's print magazine by Robyn Huang.

Above: An aerial view of Huautla de Jiménez, the economic, political, and religious center of the Mazatec region with more than 10,000 inhabitants.

Right: Curandera Margarita López combines various elements of traditional pre-Hispanic Mazatec culture with Catholicism. She chants in the Mazatec language to Catholic saints, all while guiding patients through their journey with the use of tobacco smoke, incense, eggs, and other divinatory tools.

Pages 96–97: Mazatec artist René Alvarado Martinez forages for mushrooms on a ranch in the Sierra Mazateca.

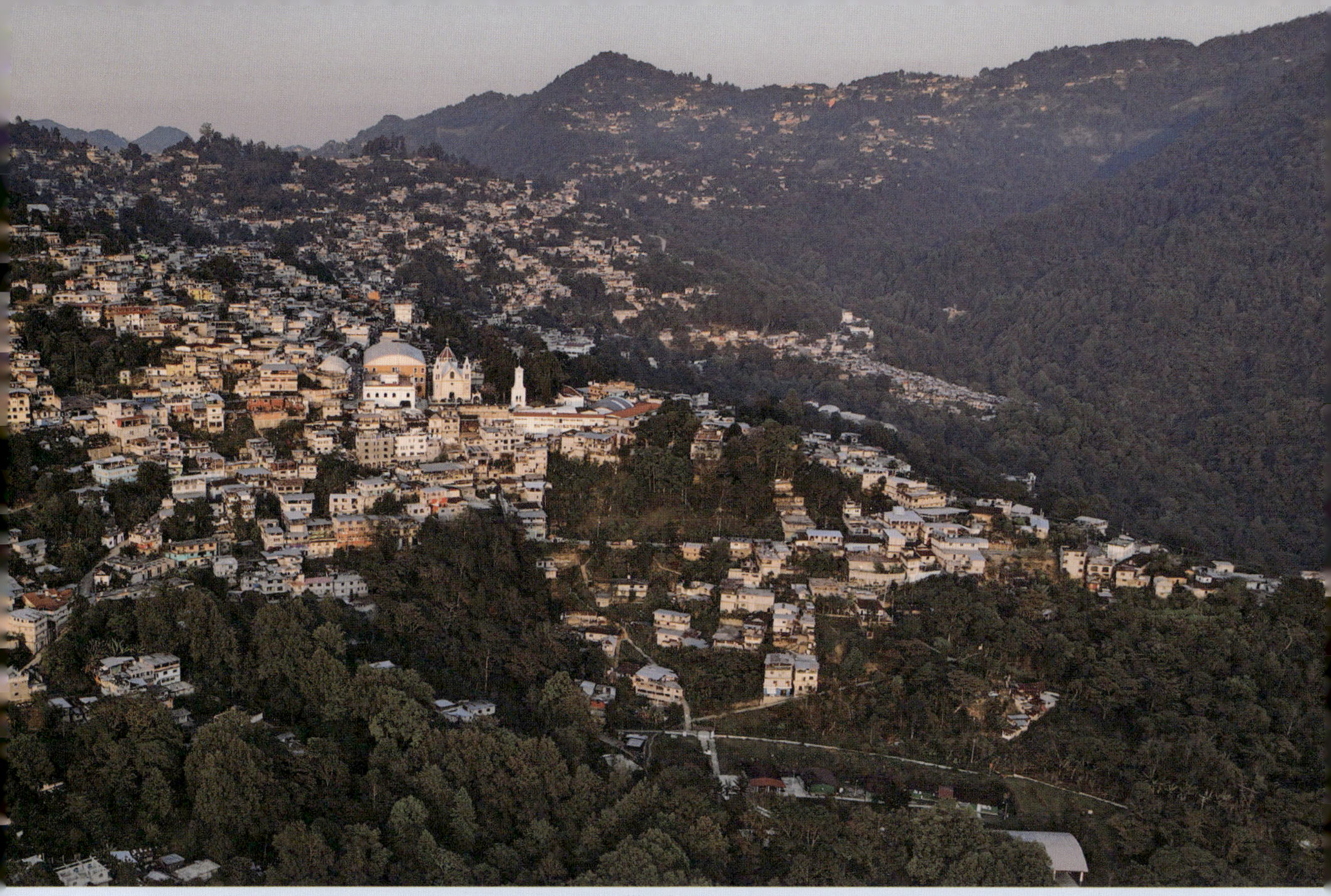

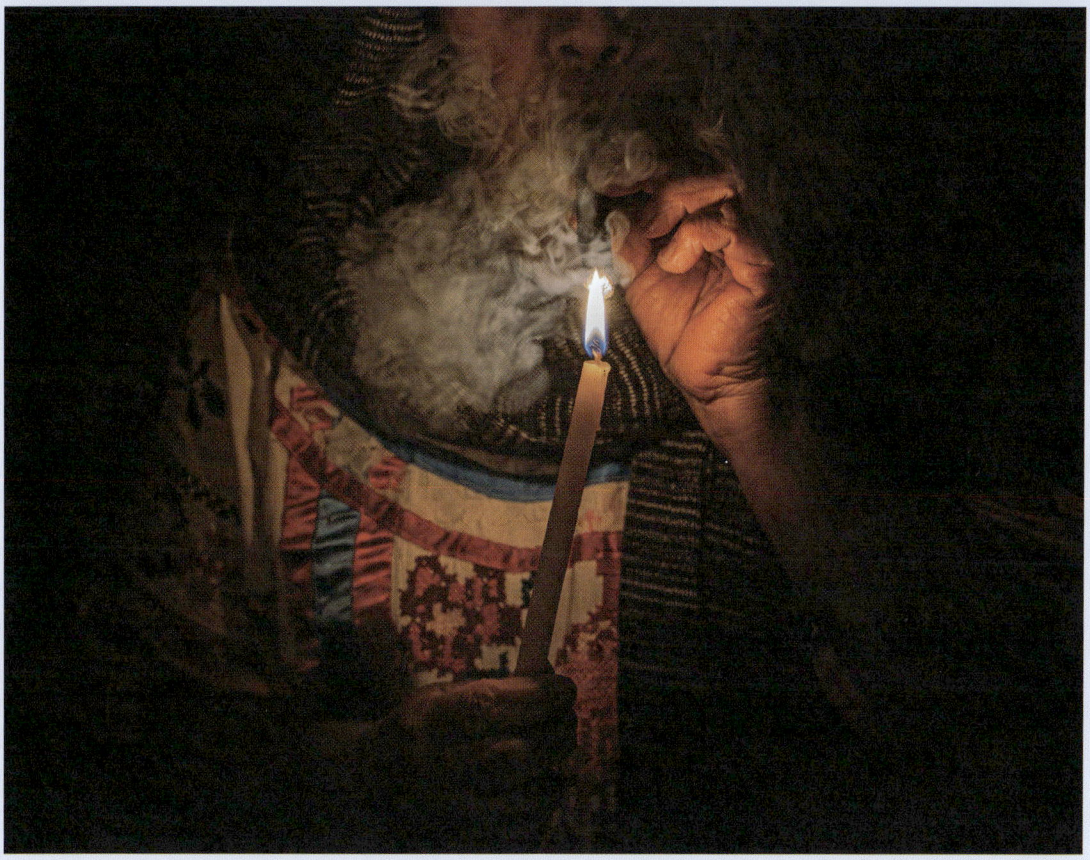

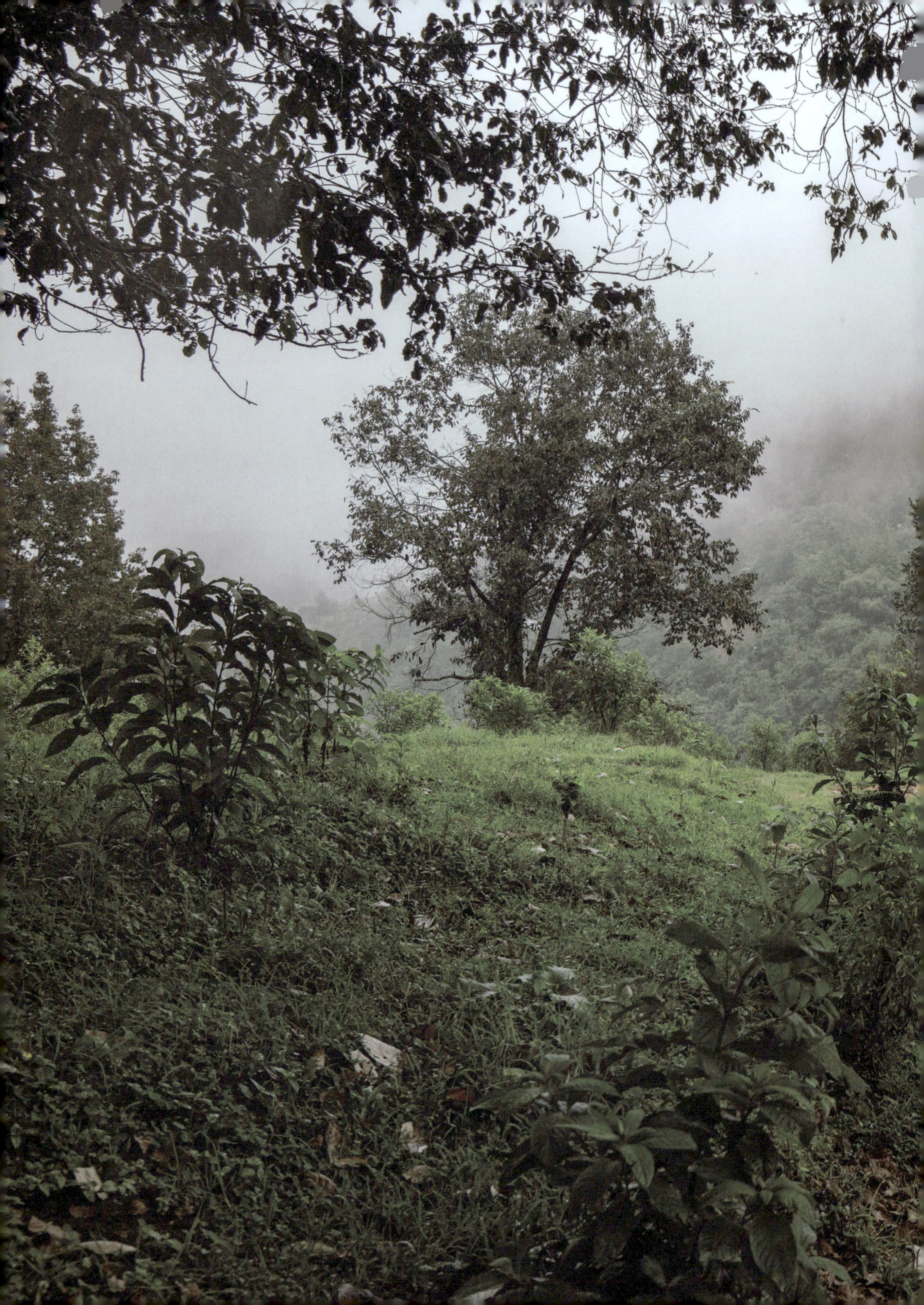

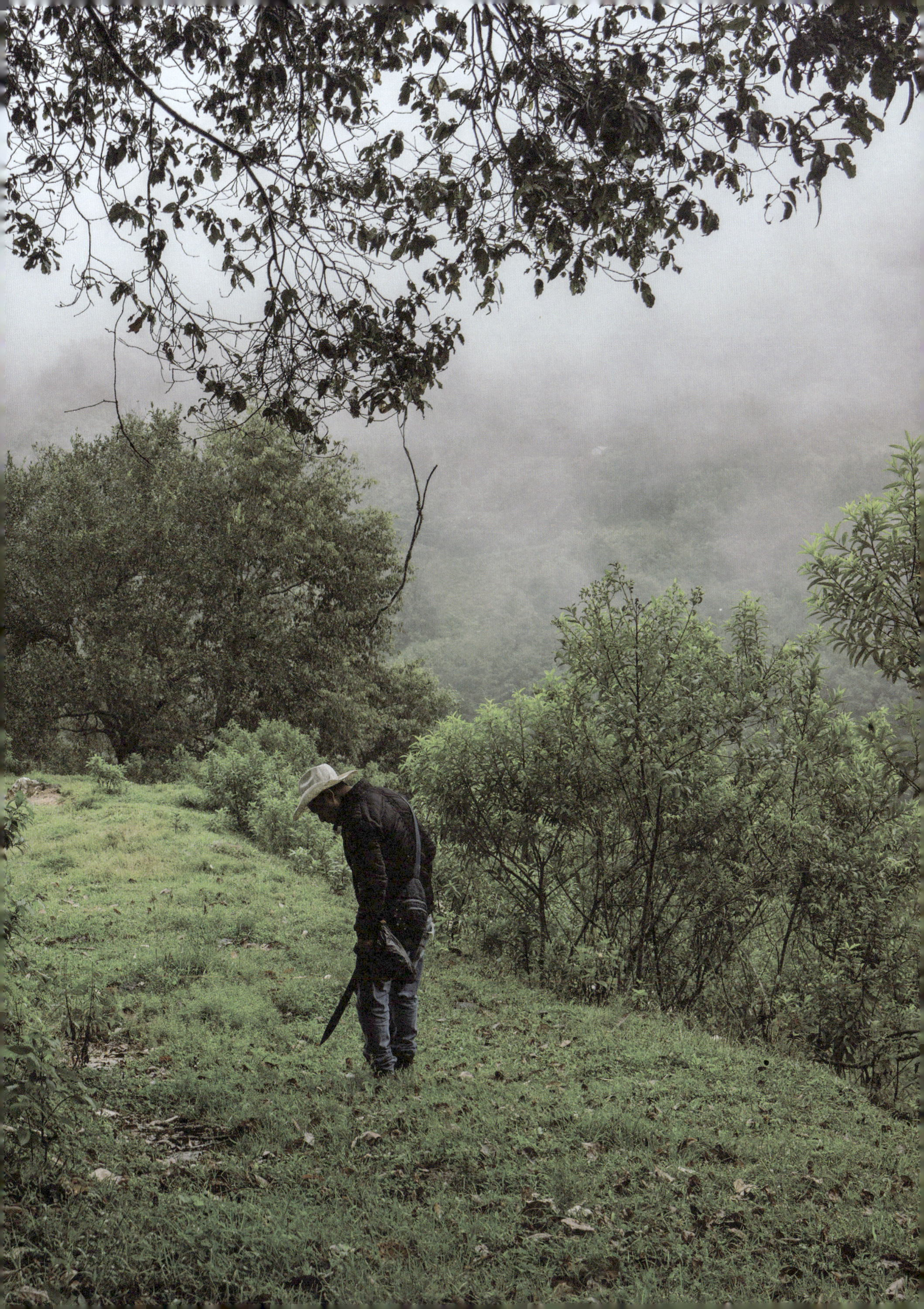

Risks and Contraindications

Physiologically speaking, mushrooms are relatively safe. This isn't to say that folks have not seriously injured themselves or died while on shrooms because their judgment was impaired and they did something careless (although many, many more people have done so under the influence of legal substances such as alcohol), but there are no serious contraindications for the average healthy adult. All classic psychedelics produce a transient increase in heart rate and blood pressure, so if you have a cardiovascular condition, it's recommended that you consult with a psychedelic-competent medical professional before taking mushrooms. It's also a good idea to get cleared to journey by a therapist or doctor if you're taking medications, especially for a specific disease or condition, but generally speaking, most common medications do not pose any risks or contraindications. The biggest risk with shrooms, really, is that they can be psychologically destabilizing if you're not prepared or properly supported before, during, and after the journey—more on this in chapters 2 and 4.

Magic mushrooms are considered to have a low abuse potential. In fact, a number of studies have shown them to be helpful in treating addictions to alcohol, nicotine, cocaine, and other substances. But as is the case for other classic psychedelics, such as LSD, it is easy to build a tolerance to them. If you were to shroom for a few days in a row (which is not recommended, as it's best to give yourself time to process each trip; see chapter 4), it would take a greater amount each time in order to feel the same effects. That said, taking shrooms will not create a physical dependence, and stopping any classic psychedelic (shrooms, LSD, DMT) will produce no withdrawal symptoms.

Still, there are psychological risks associated with shrooming. With any psychedelic, people who have a personal history of mental illness, especially schizophrenia, bipolar disorder, or psychosis, should approach tripping cautiously. The same caution is advised for anyone who has a family history of mental illness, especially if the person in question is a first-degree relative, meaning a parent or sibling.

If you're on SSRIs (selective serotonin reuptake inhibitors) or SNRIs (serotonin-norepinephrine reuptake inhibitors), a number of psychedelic professionals—whether therapists or staff at a retreat center—will encourage you to taper off these meds, with the help of your prescribing doctor, before journeying. This is because some hypothesize that an SSRI or SNRI might dull the potency of the experience; others warn of the risk of serotonin syndrome. That said, both these risks are far from definitive—and research has found that being on an SSRI does not always diminish the trip. Additionally, tapering off an SSRI or SNRI comes with its own considerations and risks, including side effects, that should be considered carefully with your doctor.

Generally, mushrooms magnify whatever is happening inside you. That can go in various directions. It can bring your shadow, as some call it, to the surface, forcing you to face that which needs to be healed. It's impossible to predict what you may realize while under the influence of shrooms—or any psychedelic. The revelations may be specific and circumstantial (such as "I need to leave my job" or "I need to go to therapy with my partner") or they may be more amorphous and internal (such as "I need to work on how I speak to myself" or "I need to cultivate deeper patience for others"). Moreover, because mushrooms can be highly unpredictable, they may cause panic or anxiety, especially in crowded, hectic, or overwhelming environments. All in all, tripping can be a vulnerable experience, so it's best to prepare in advance, set intentions, and cultivate a set and setting that can serve as an effective vessel for your journey.

Final Thoughts

When the journey is over, in addition to doing your own integration work, it's a good time to start thinking about how you can more meaningfully participate in giving back to the mushrooms, which, hopefully, gave you a lot.

Psilocybin mushrooms are not just a tool for individual healing—they are part of a much larger ecological and cultural web. One powerful way to contribute is by supporting organizations like the Fungi Foundation, which advocates for the integration of fungi into conservation policy worldwide. This pioneering nonprofit works to ensure that fungi are recognized and protected as essential to the health of ecosystems. By donating to or amplifying the work of such organizations, you help build a global movement that respects fungi's ecological importance.

Similarly, Esperanza Mazateca, a collective led by Mazatec people in Oaxaca, Mexico (see page 218), focuses on preserving Indigenous knowledge surrounding psilocybin mushrooms while supporting the community's socioeconomic well-being. Engaging with or supporting their work directly uplifts the stewards of these sacred traditions. Their efforts ensure that the benefits of the growing interest in mushrooms are not one-sided but shared with those who have long relied on and protected these medicines.

On a more personal level, reciprocity can start with how you interact with mushrooms in the wild. If you forage, do so responsibly by taking only what you need, avoiding overharvesting, and ensuring that the integrity of the habitat remains intact. Use local guides to help you properly identify mushrooms and avoid harming nonpsychedelic species or fragile ecosystems. Responsible foraging ensures that mushrooms can continue to thrive for future generations.

Growing your own mushrooms is another way to engage in reciprocity. It allows you to cultivate a direct relationship with mycelium, the sprawling underground network that mushrooms emerge from. This practice not only deepens your understanding of fungi's life cycles but also lessens the pressure on wild populations. Consider the act of growing as a collaboration—one that nurtures your healing while honoring the living intelligence of mycelium.

Finally, approach mushrooms with reverence and curiosity, acknowledging them as beings with their own spirit and role in the ecosystem. Building a relationship with mycelium isn't just about taking; it's about listening, learning, and finding ways to give back. Whether it's through supporting conservation efforts, protecting natural habitats, or cultivating fungi at home, reciprocity with mushrooms offers a way to honor the wisdom they provide while ensuring their enduring presence in the world.

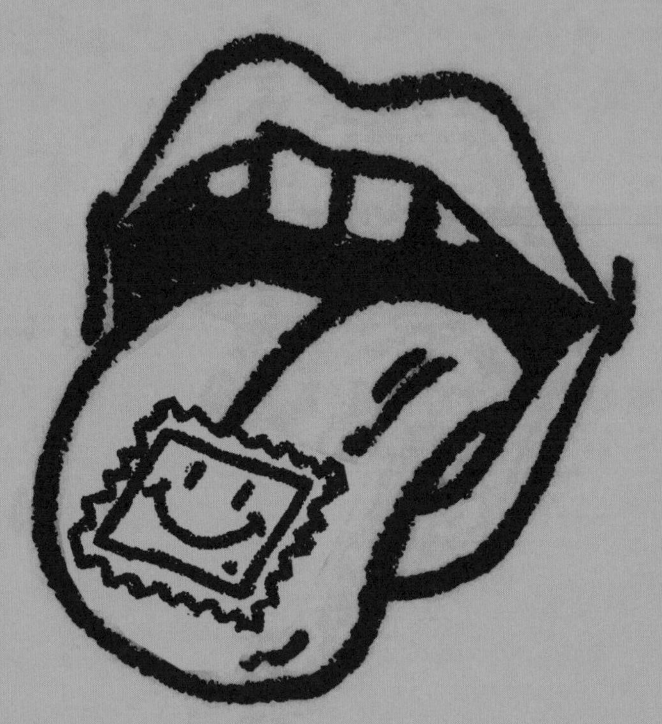

CHAPTER 6

LSD

LSD (lysergic acid diethylamide), or acid, is probably the quintessential psychedelic, in part because it fueled the psychedelic revolution of the 1960s. Countless icons and pioneers, from the Beatles to Steve Jobs, were shaped by acid and its influence on culture, innovation, therapy, and beyond.

Despite its popularity, how acid works—and why it inspires such profound spiritual experiences and creative revelations—remains a magical mystery. Even Albert Hofmann, the Swiss chemist who discovered LSD, described acid as "medicine for the soul," the type of language scientists—back then and today—try to stay far, far away from. Nevertheless, as most people who have done the stuff will tell you, its mystical qualities are undeniable.

LSD is commonly thought of as a drug made in a lab. It's true that it's a synthetic compound, but it's also derived from an alkaloid found in the ergot fungus. Interestingly, Reverend Danny Nemu, author of *Science Revealed* and *Neuro-Apocalypse*, hypothesizes that the manna, or "bread from heaven," that sustained the Israelite tribe during their forty-year exodus from Egypt contained ergot. Fast-forward thousands of years, and in 1938, LSD—for the first time in an isolated format—makes its debut in Basel, Switzerland, in the laboratory of Albert Hofmann, a chemist working for the pharmaceutical company Sandoz. Hofmann was looking to develop a stimulant to treat respiratory issues, but after testing LSD on sedated animals and finding that it did little more than make them twitch, he shelved the experimental compound. In 1943, he decided to revisit the compound, inspired by what he later characterized as a "peculiar presentiment" that it was worth looking into further. Little did he know it would go on to change the world, inspiring radicals and free thinkers, decades later, to challenge, well, just about everything from the nuclear family and the 9-to-5 job to the necessity of war.

From the lab, LSD eventually made its way into the hands of everyone from researchers to the CIA, which looked into its use as a "truth serum" during experiments, infamously known as MK-Ultra, in which they investigated whether the drug could be used for mind control. Throughout the 1950s and '60s, LSD became popular as a tool in therapy, from the offices of hip Hollywood practitioners who used it for stars like Cary Grant to the experiments of Harvard psychologists like Richard Alpert (later known as Ram Dass) and Timothy Leary.

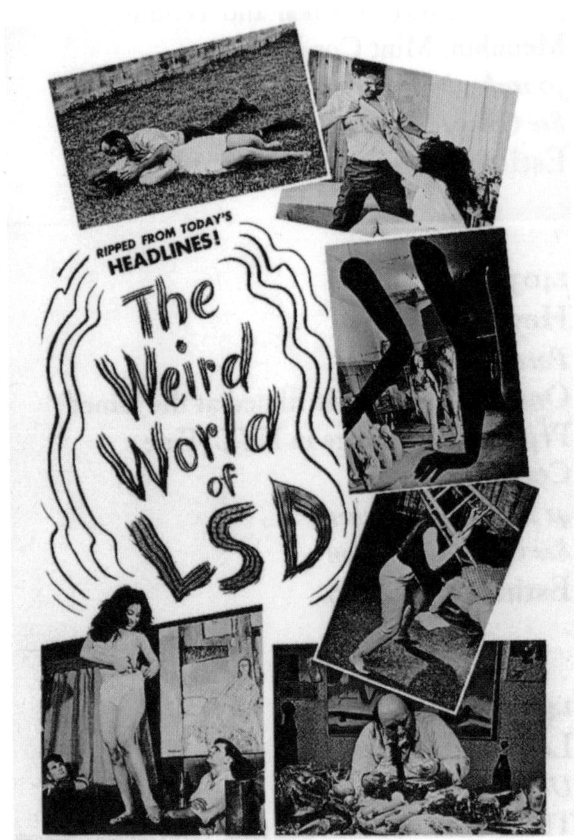

Leary went on to become an LSD evangelist, fueling the 1967 Summer of Love and propelling the tension between the powers-that-be and the youth generation. He, alongside other proponents such as chemist Owsley Stanley, a.k.a. Bear (who was also the sound engineer for the Grateful Dead), became targets of federal law enforcement in its effort to crack down on hippie renegades who stood in opposition to mainstream culture and politics. LSD became the secret ingredient inspiring the essence of music festivals like Woodstock, literature like Ken Kesey's *One Flew Over the Cuckoo's Nest* and later Tom Wolfe's *Electric Kool-Aid Acid Test* (about Kesey's Merry Pranksters), and even Alcoholics Anonymous, as one of its founders, Bill Wilson, had been influenced by the compound. Some credited LSD with helping social consciousness evolve, but others feared that it would corrupt society and undermine authority, especially in the context of Vietnam War protests. And so LSD was made illegal.

Above: LSD poster from 1967

Following pages: Timothy Leary at the League for Spiritual Discovery, an LSD-based meditation center in Greenwich Village, New York City, 1967

Because LSD was the Trojan horse of the counterculture, it carried a particularly strong stigma among politicians and the mainstream media. That's the reason why, when psychedelic science picked up again in the early 2000s—after a decades-long halt—researchers chose to focus on psilocybin instead of acid; they just thought they'd be up against less, from a publicity standpoint. (That, and the trip is about half as long, so the therapy would be cheaper.) But in the late 1950s, '60s, and '70s, both psilocybin and acid showed promise for many of the same conditions—depression, anxiety, alcoholism, and beyond. Today, LSD continues to be one of the most popular psychedelics of choice in the underground, though still significantly less so than psilocybin, but for a completely different reason than its absence from research: Pretty much anyone with a half-decent green thumb can grow shrooms, whereas acid requires the skills of a chemist.

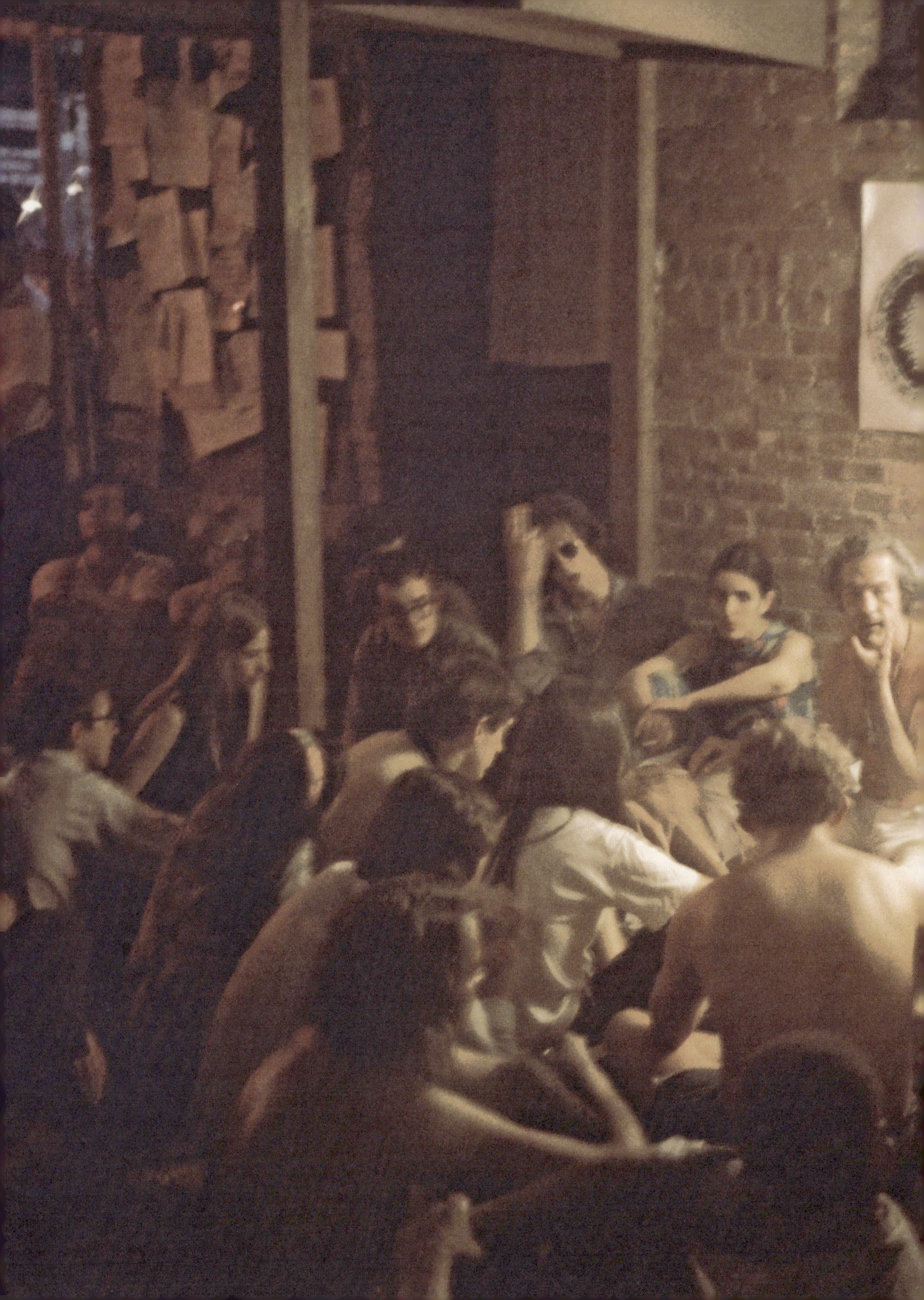

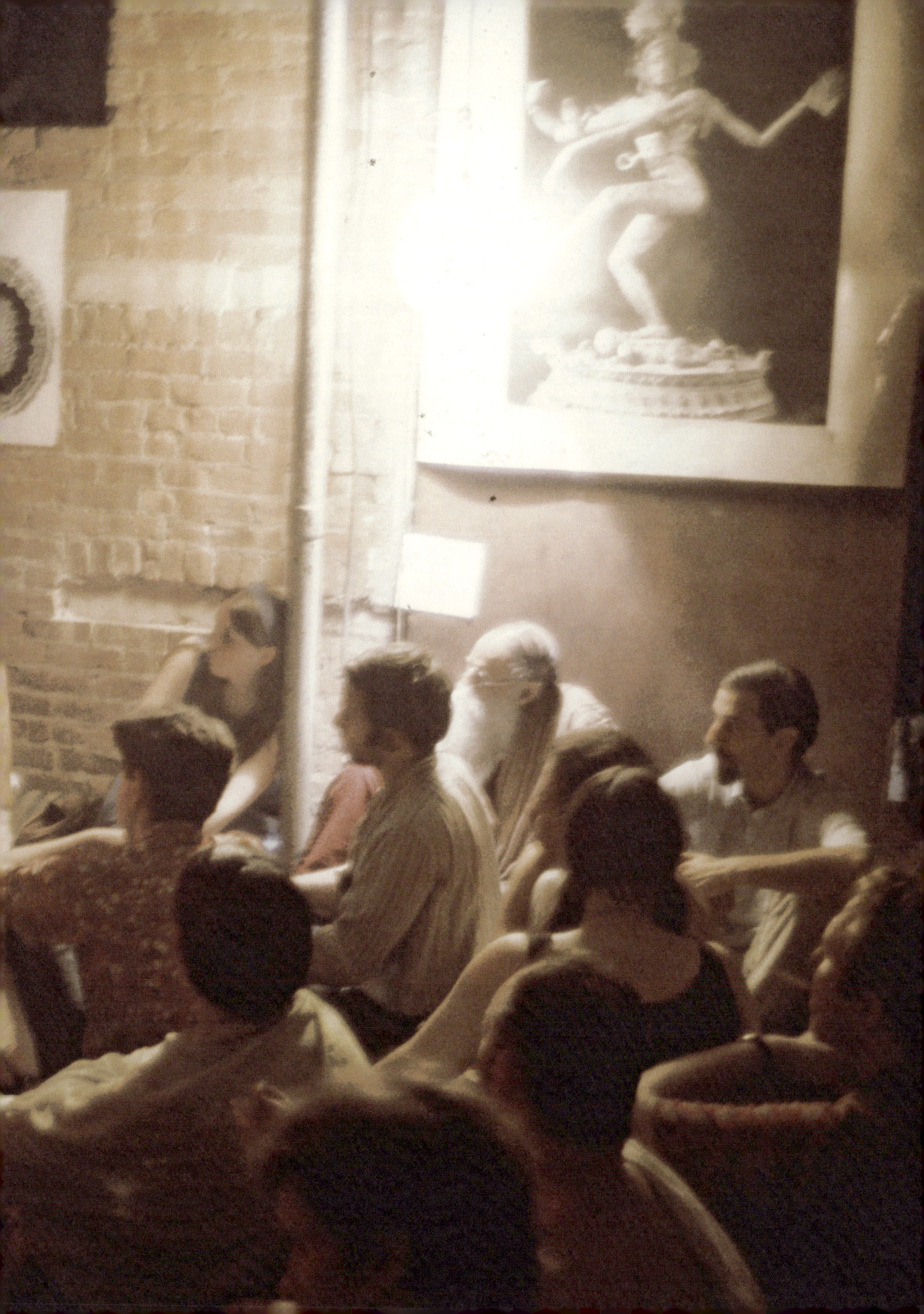

Testing Your LSD

Because of the unregulated nature of the underground market for synthetics like LSD (yes, we're still talking about Schedule I prohibited substances), it's hard to know that what you're getting is what you think it is. That is, unless you have a drug testing kit. But be warned: There are a lot of testing kits out there, and not all of them are reliable or legitimate. That's why you should be sure to get your drugs *and* your drug testing kit from a trustworthy source. While we can't recommend an acid dealer, we can recommend where to find an LSD testing kit: DanceSafe, a harm reduction nonprofit that offers kits via its website.

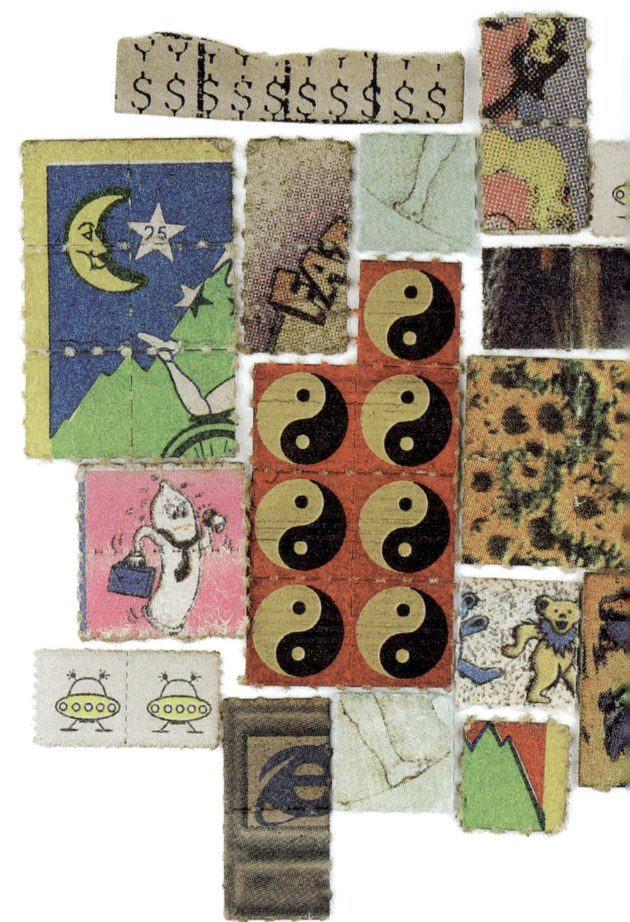

Drug testing kits work via reagents—chemicals that turn certain colors when they come into contact with certain chemicals. While reagents can't detect every chemical or tell you the absolute purity of the drug you have, they nonetheless can confirm the presence, or lack thereof, of LSD (or MDMA, or whatever it is that you're testing) as well as potential adulterants, such as fentanyl.

LSD Dosage

So you want to trip on acid but don't know how much to take? Well, a "standard" dose of LSD may vary depending on who you ask, but it generally ranges between 75 and 200 micrograms, with 100 mics being about the average. A microdose of a psychedelic is usually considered one-tenth of a full dose, so in the case of LSD that's about 10 micrograms. We'll get into microdosing in more detail in chapter 12, but if anything noticeably trippy is happening (i.e., the walls are melting, or it seems like your cat is smiling at you in a strangely poetic way), then, sorry, but you've taken more than a microdose—it happens to the best of us. Anything above 15 mics is when you should start feeling the effects; 25 to 75 mics is considered a light dose, and please, folks, don't do anything above 300 mics unless you're prepared for a wild ride. Truly, it's just not necessary and generally not recommended if you don't have a lot of experience and have worked your way up in dosage.

Dosing LSD can be tricky because it comes in various forms that can be hard to measure, so, as with all psychedelics, take less and gradually increase—especially if it's your first time buying from that guy who knows that guy. In general, LSD is prepared as a liquid, which can be taken straight or dropped onto tabs of a blotter paper (about 100 micrograms per tab). It can also come in the form of a gel or gel tab.

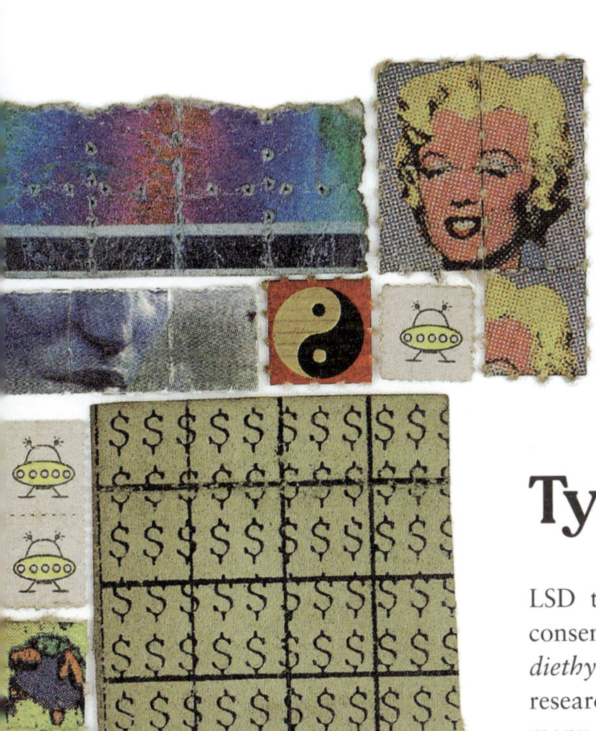

Types of LSD

LSD terminology can be confusing because there isn't much consensus around it. Technically, *LSD* stands for *lysergic acid diethylamide-25*—and *acid* is slang that, according to our best research, first appeared in the US lexicon by 1965. But acid has many, many names. Sometimes the term used to refer to acid will tell you what form it's in, such as *blotter* or *dots*. Sometimes a name refers to legend and lore about the particular chemist or place where a form of acid was first synthesized. Other names—like *lucy*, *battery acid*, and *electric Kool-Aid*—arise from popular culture. Much like it is with cannabis, the term a person uses to refer to LSD often says more about their generation than what's in the drug itself.

BLOTTER

Acid is a unique drug for many reasons. Not only is it partially synthetic, but you don't typically swallow a pill or make tea out of this potent psychedelic. Instead, micrograms of liquid LSD are dispensed onto an absorbent paper, called blotter paper, hence the nickname *blotter*. Some of these blotter sheets are works of art, with elaborate designs printed on them.

ORANGE SUNSHINE

Orange Sunshine (or California Sunshine) is the creation of Nicholas Sand and Tim Scully, who just might be the most well-known LSD chemists in history—other than Albert Hofmann, of course. It made its debut in San Francisco in 1967 and eventually made its way around the world. It typically came in small, round orange tablets known for their bright color and consistent potency.

WINDOWPANE

Blotter tabs are the most common way to take acid. Yet they're certainly not the only way—especially if you were tripping in the '80s. Windowpane acid is an alternative to blotter tabs that uses gelatin as a base. It earned the name *windowpane* because the clear, square gel tabs resembled tiny windowpanes. Some underground chemists reportedly poured LSD-laced gelatin into plastic fluorescent light diffusers—the kind with a grid pattern used in office ceilings—using them as molds to form evenly sized squares.

DOTS

Don't let the name fool you—an acid microdot has nothing to do with microdosing. A microdot is a tiny, pressed pill made with either crystal or liquid LSD and filler.

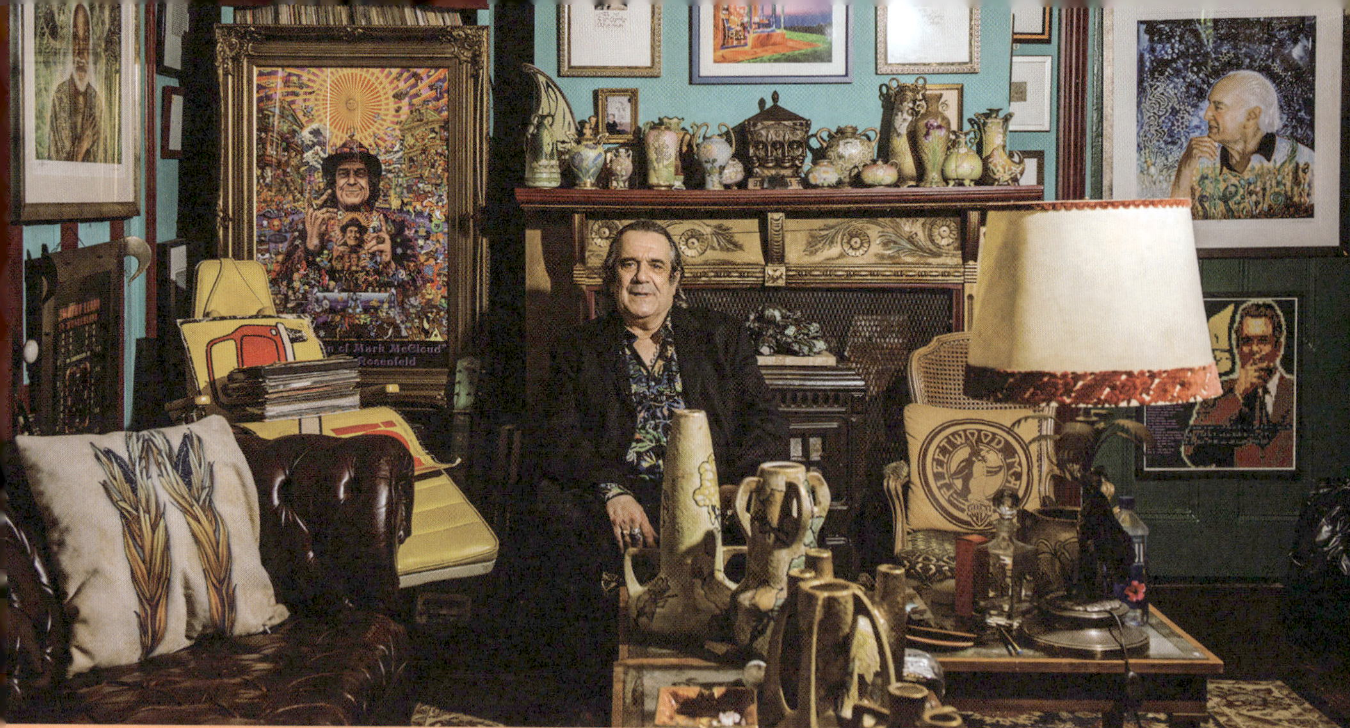

BEYOND THE JOURNEY

INSIDE THE ACID MUSEUM

When you step through the front door to Mark McCloud's Victorian mansion in the Mission District of San Francisco, untouched by the cycles of the seasons and decades past, time seems to stand still. The couch is worn in from visitors who've come to survey McCloud's 30,000 tabs of acid, framed behind glass and hidden from the outside world by black velvet drapes—meant to block out natural light, but lending an eerie air to the decrepit place. Imagery of skulls and the devil, portraits of Timothy Leary, Ram Dass, and Albert Hofmann, and prints of sayings like "LSD: Let's Stop Destruction" or "LSD: See Your Travel Agent" clutter McCloud's living room, home to what he claims is the largest collection of LSD blotter sheets in the world.

In the 1960s, prior to the criminalization of LSD in the United States, sensationalistic stories about people jumping out of windows while tripping fueled the hysteria that caused Richard Nixon to sign the Controlled Substances Act. McCloud is among the few people who actually *did* fall out of a window while on LSD—and survived to tell the tale. "I was pre-med at Santa Clara, and I took a bunch of Orange Sunshine, and accidentally go out a seventh-story window at this place called the Swing Building," he recounts, detailing the sound of his bones crushing as he plunged to his face. "I got into the magical enterprise of dying on LSD," McCloud says. "And I know that the only reason I came back is that I was on acid—I could navigate the extremely infinite pathway of what was then called the Rainbow Bridge, the voyage between life and death, corporal and discorporal, dying and coming back to life. That's the miracle of the mulligan."

In golf (which McCloud says the Scottish invented as "an excuse to hunt for mushrooms"), a mulligan is a second chance, a magical event that is "the mercy of a do-over." Declared dead on the spot, while tripping through the whole ordeal, McCloud experienced the journey of his soul leaving his body, making a first stop in Hell before ascending to Heaven, where he was offered another shot at life in his body. And so McCloud made his home a shrine to LSD "to thank it for saving my life," he says. "The smallest way I could pay my debt was by showing off the glory of the manufacturers' vision expressed by the blotter itself."

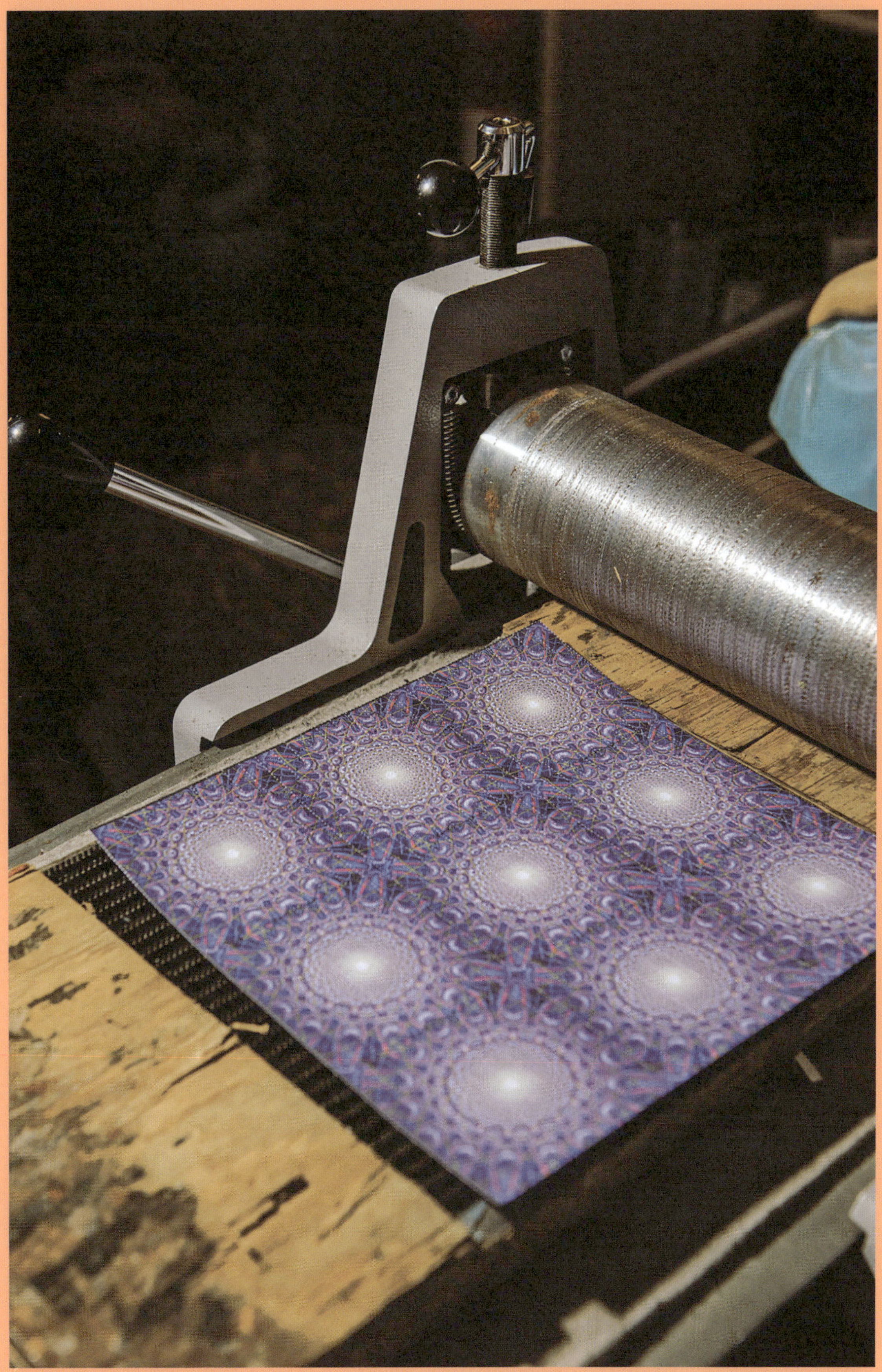

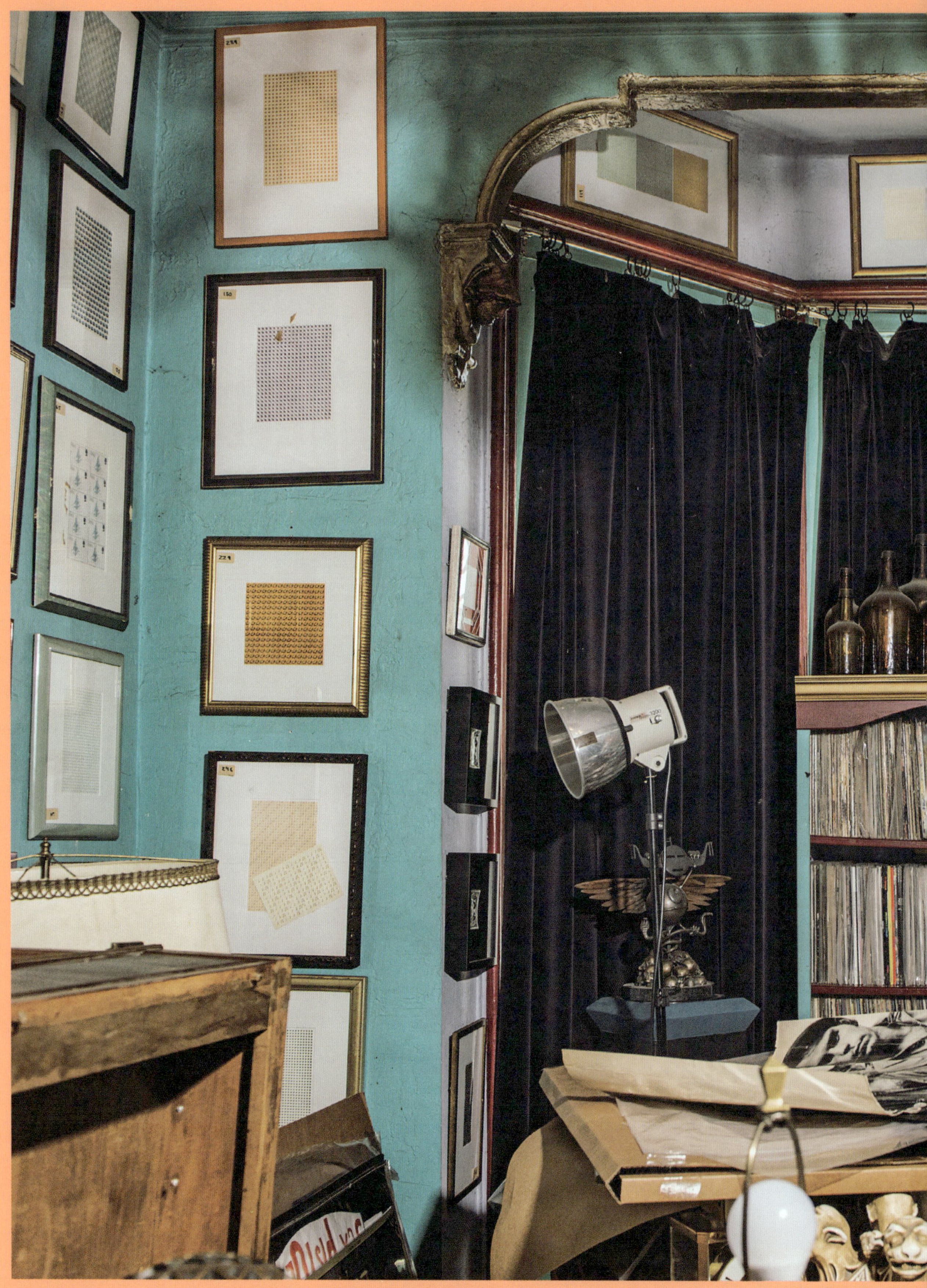

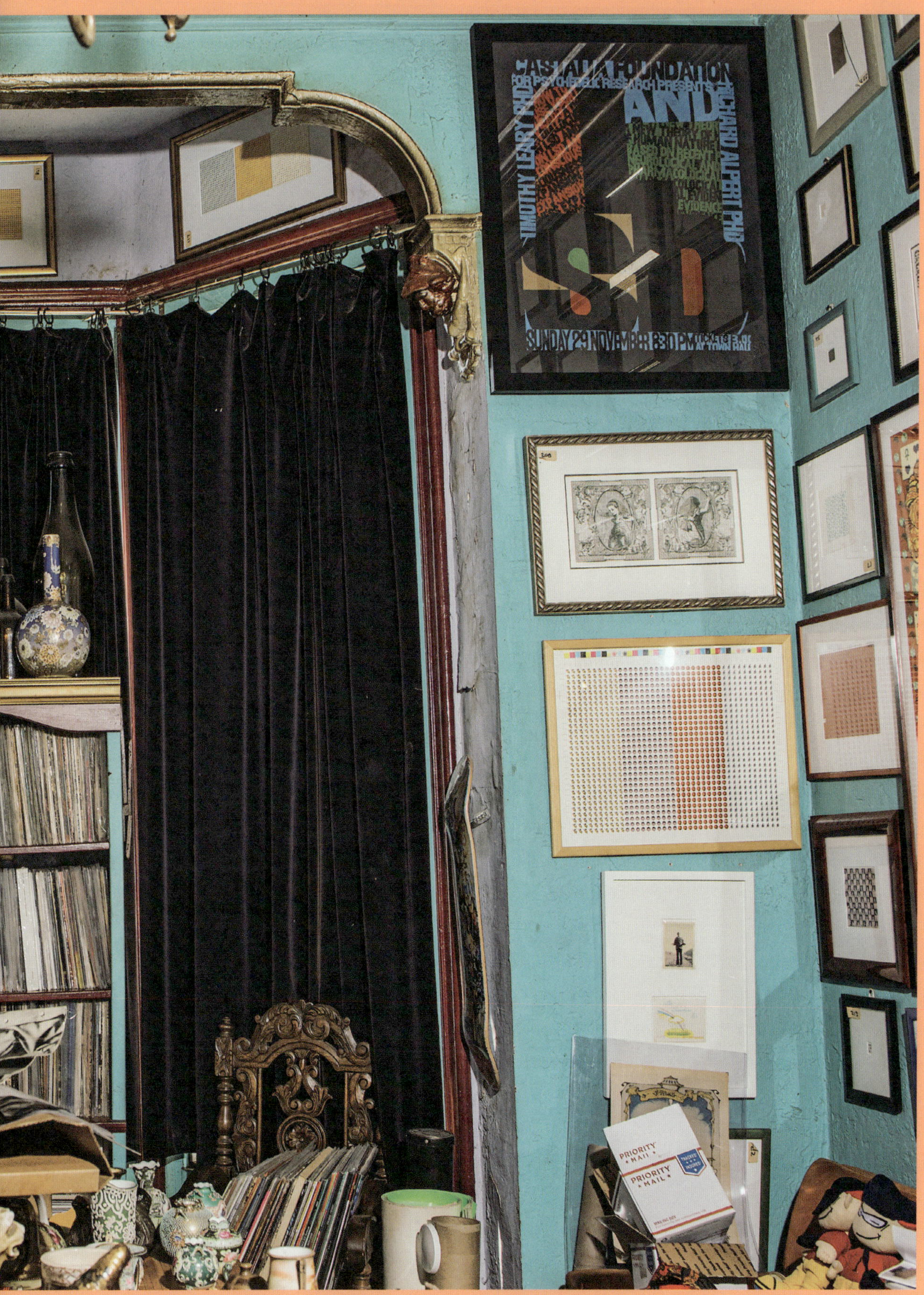
FOR PSYCHEDELIC RESEARCH PRESENTS
TIMOTHY LEARY PHD
AND
RICHARD ALPERT PHD
SUNDAY 29 NOVEMBER 8:30 PM
PRIORITY MAIL
PRIORITY MAIL

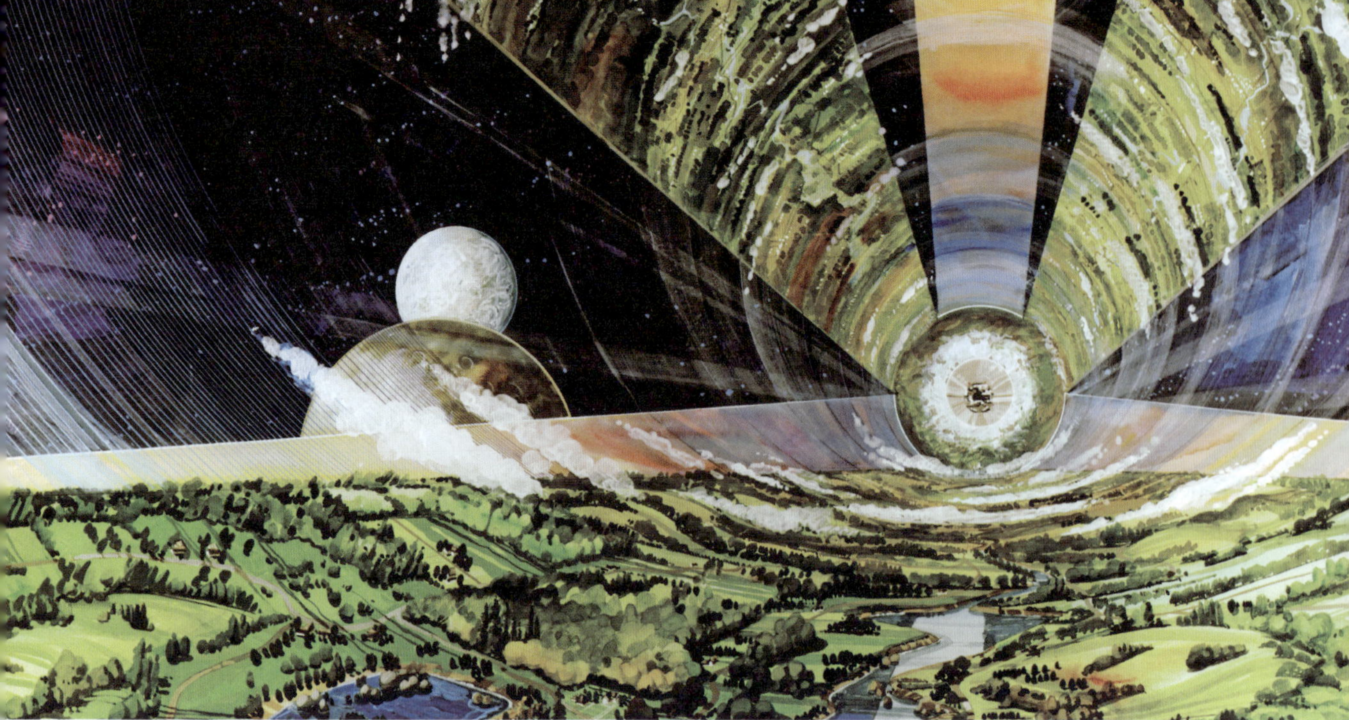

What's an LSD Trip Like?

Dreamy and dreadful, playful and pensive, blissful and bizarre, everything at once, and totally beyond description—it's hard to articulate what an acid trip is really like.

The standard effects of LSD are both sensory and visual and can include intensified perception of colors, visions of stationary objects "breathing" or vibrating, and a distorted perception of shapes, sounds, and sense of time and space. Acid can be a lot of fun in stimulating, social environments, or it may cause paranoia or social anxiety and be better suited for quiet time at home or in nature. It depends on the person, the day, and the specifics of the environment (see chapter 2). While tripping on LSD, someone might be more sensitive to specific environments or people, or their belief systems may be altered altogether, which could affect how they engage with their surroundings. Some people love to party on acid—to go to concerts or cruise around festivals—and they find that's true for them pretty much every time they do it. Other people discover that the effects depend on where they're at in their life, and some people can't imagine why anyone would want to trip anywhere other than somewhere quiet, private, and serene.

If you've never dropped acid before, we'd recommend starting somewhere where you can let loose—where you're surrounded by people you trust—and seeing how it makes you feel. Otherwise, you might end up being that person who steps into a port-o-potty for quiet at a festival and then locks themselves in accidentally. (Not joking, that's a thing and you won't die, but we wouldn't recommend it either.)

LSD can often be unpredictable, and in addition to inducing a wide range of emotions and strong sensations (joy, anxiety, panic, euphoria, paranoia, fascination, and more), it can also cause physiological sensations like increased heart rate, elevated blood pressure, dilated pupils, loss of appetite, and changes in body temperature regulation. Like shrooms, LSD is generally considered safe for healthy adults; any physiological symptoms are temporary and should pass. That said, just like with any psychedelic, if you're concerned, then it's better to be safe and to consult with a psychedelic integration therapist ahead of time. Find more information on potential risks and contraindications on page 118.

How Long Does Acid Last?

A typical LSD trip lasts around eight to twelve hours—depending on the dose, how you're feeling (physiologically and psychologically) that day, and the quality of the acid. The effects of the LSD usually come on within twenty to ninety minutes after you take it. Note that even after you've "come down" from acid, the next day or few days may be considered part of the "afterglow" (for more on this, see page 135).

This is a Tripping 101 tip for all psychedelics, but especially acid because it lasts so long: Look at a clock when you take the drug and write down the time. When you're tripping, sometimes ten minutes can feel like an eternity and at other times it can fly by—but if you know, generally, that it takes a couple hours to peak and that you'll start coming down after six to eight hours, it can really help in those moments when you feel like you've fallen into a timeless, spaceless void.

If you find yourself wishing the trip would just be over already, sorry, there's not much that can be done other than to remember that *you got this*. Breathe, change the music, go outside if you're inside or vice versa, take a bath or shower (if you feel you can do so safely). It's all about relaxing and coming back to your intention or "why" for having the experience in the first place. And remember: You're on a drug, and you will be back to normal eventually (even if it doesn't feel that way). In fact, in just a few hours, you'll probably be laughing at that time you thought the moment you were in was never going to end.

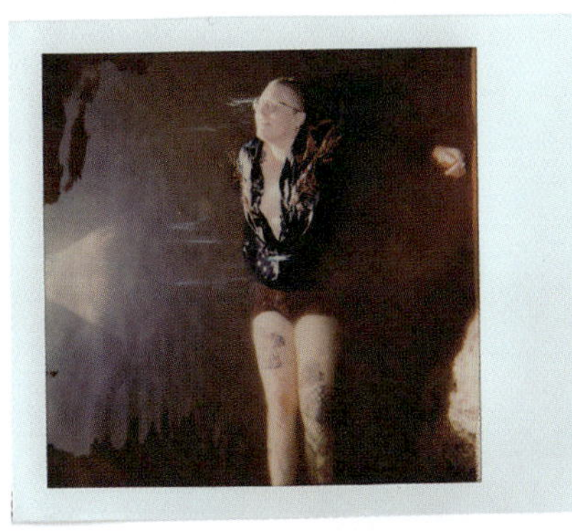

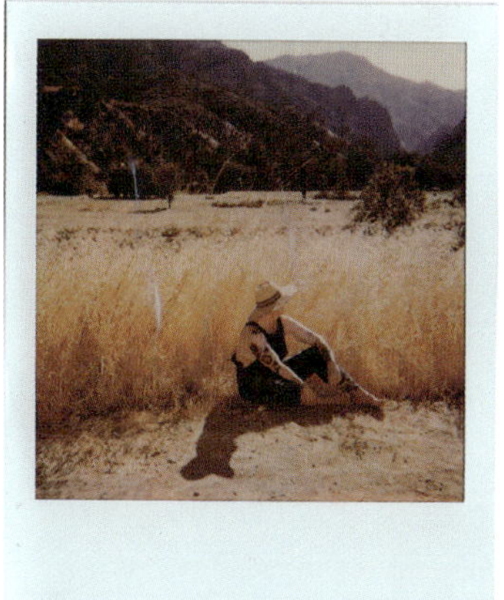

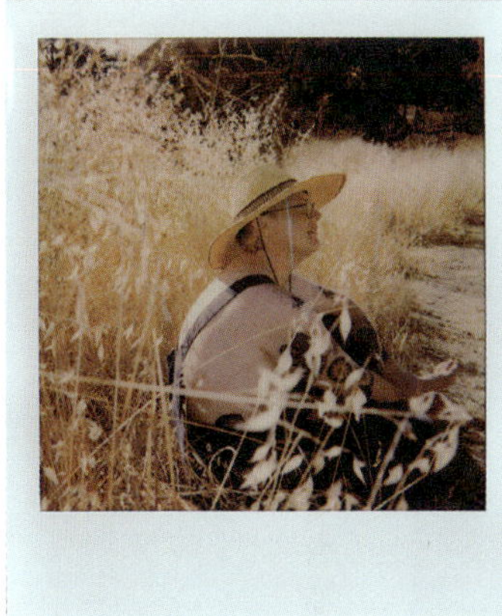

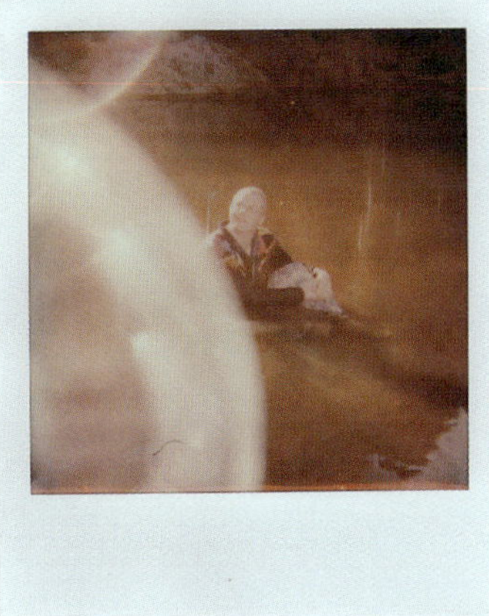

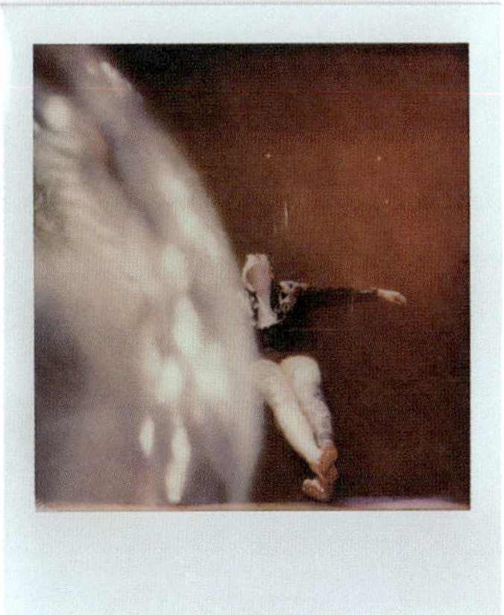

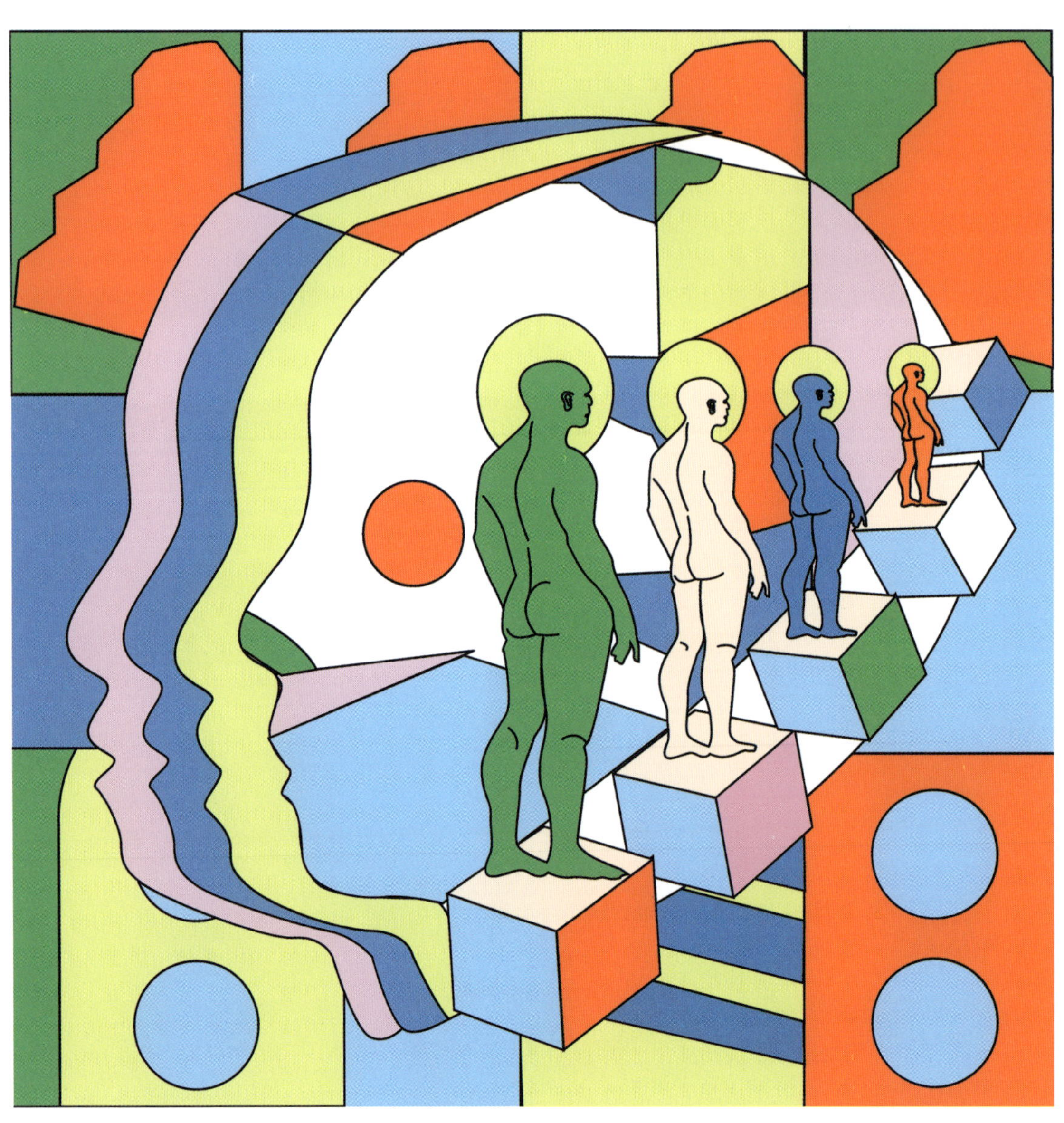

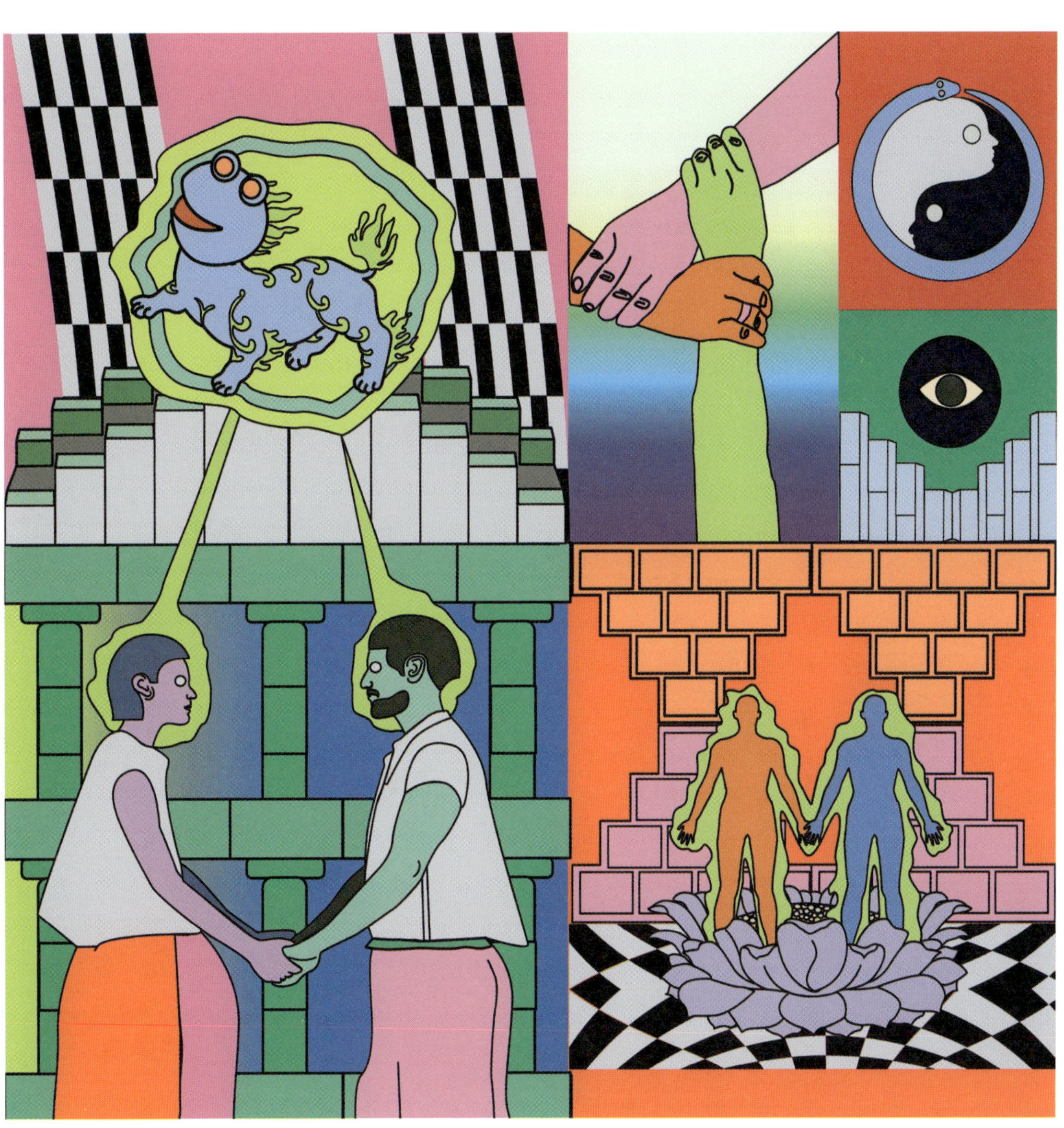

1P-LSD

When drugs become prohibited or controlled, underground chemists often get to working on making analogs. The compound 1P-LSD (1-propionyl-lysergic acid diethylamide) is an example of that—and it sits, much like other psychedelic analogs, in a gray area in the United States. It can be purchased online and marketed as a "research chemical" or "novel psychoactive substance," but, technically, it's not legal to take it because of a federal law that prohibits the consumption of drugs that are similar to drugs that are federally illegal. LSD and 1P-LSD are remarkably similar in chemical structure, differing only in a small group of atoms. Experienced users report extremely similar—even identical—effects from both substances. While it's not common, there is the chance that some compounds sold as 1P-LSD will be fake and/or adulterated, and unfortunately, LSD drug-checking kits don't work for this closely related alternative.

BEYOND THE JOURNEY

BICYCLE DAY

Every year on April 19, devoted psychonauts celebrate Bicycle Day—the LSD holiday, akin to 4/20 for cannabis, in honor of the first intentional acid trip ever, taken by chemist Albert Hofmann. After first stumbling upon it, Hofmann didn't try to synthesize LSD again for five years. Then, on April 16, 1943, he reproduced the compound in his lab for further pharmacological investigation. He must have absorbed a small amount through his fingertips because he began to feel strange and left work early that day. When he got home, he "sank into a not unpleasant intoxicated-like condition, characterized by an extremely stimulated imagination," he describes in his 1979 memoir *LSD: My Problem Child*. "I perceived an uninterrupted stream of fantastic pictures, extraordinary shapes with intense, kaleidoscopic play of colors."

Intrigued and suspecting that his experience might have had something to do with the LSD, three days later Hofmann intentionally dosed himself with 250 micrograms of acid (about 2.5 times what has since become the "standard" dose) at around 4:20 in the afternoon (go figure). The LSD shook him up; he began to hallucinate and struggled to speak "intelligibly." The laboratory turned out not to be the ideal setting for his experience, so he asked his assistant Susi Ramstein (who became the first woman to take LSD) to help him get home. At that time in Basel, Switzerland, where Hofmann lived and worked, no cars were allowed on the road due to World War II restrictions, so he and Ramstein rode their bikes back to his house as his trip kicked in. While Hofmann's first acid trip was nothing short of terrifying—spiraling, demonic insanity and sensations of death—the next day he felt refreshed and better than ever. "The world was as if newly created," he wrote. "All my senses vibrated in a condition of highest sensitivity, which persisted for the entire day."

As the cultural influence of psychedelics, including LSD, grows again within the United States and beyond, Bicycle Day is typically celebrated with panels of psychedelic experts, dance parties, comedy shows, and beyond.

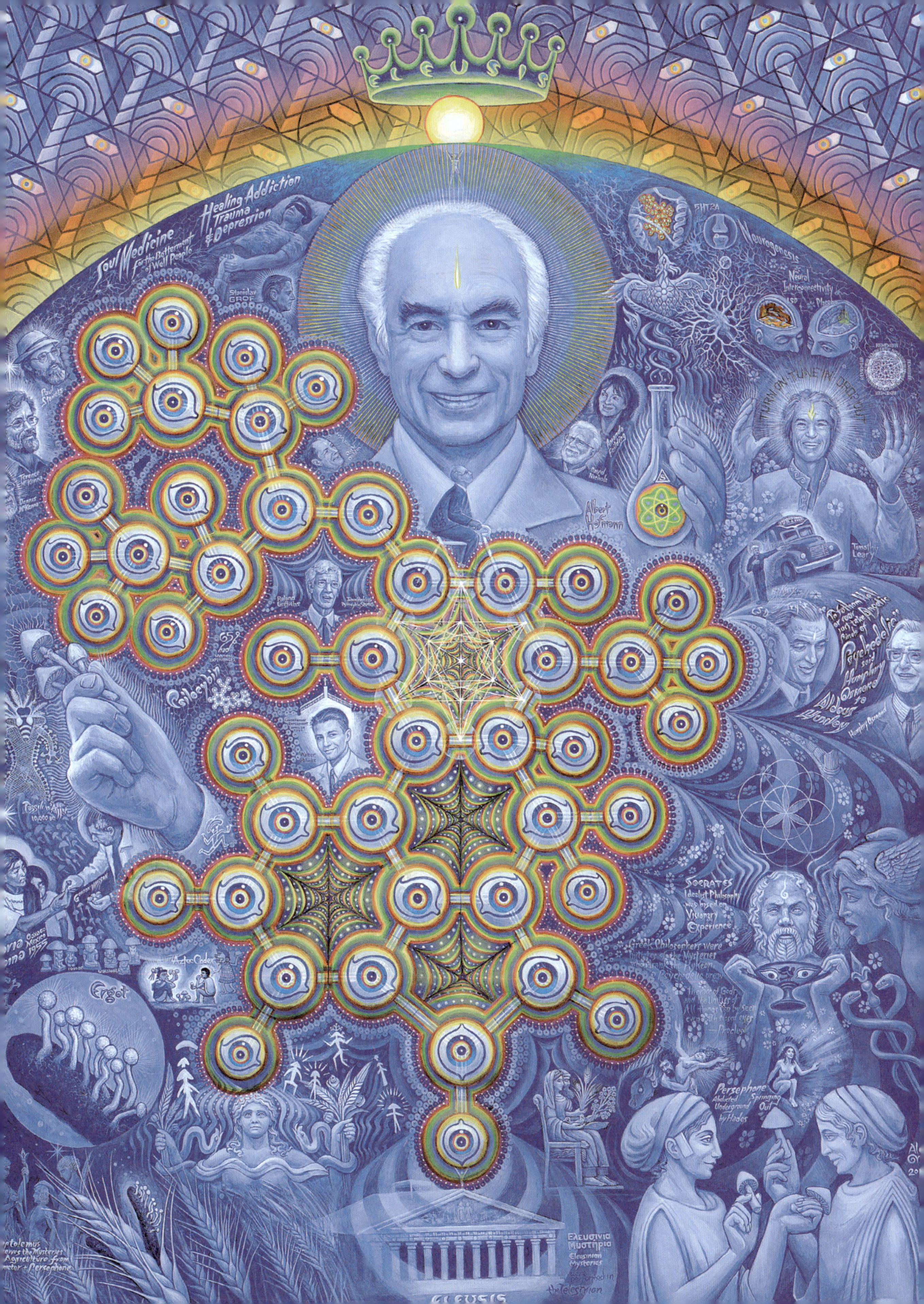
ELEUSIS
Soul Medicine
for the Betterment of Well People
Healing Addiction Trauma & Depression
Stanislav GROF
Neurogenesis
Albert Hofmann
Timothy Leary
"To fathom Hell or soar Angelic just take a pinch of Psychedelic" said Humphry Osmond to Aldous Huxley
Humphry Osmond
Psilocybin
Ergot
Aztec Codex
SOCRATES
Idealist Philosophy was based on Visionary Experience
Persephone
Abducted Underground by Hades
Springing Out
ELEUSIS

Risks and Contraindications

Acid can be transformative, but it's not for everyone. The risks are the same as they are with the other classic psychedelics, shrooms and DMT. For starters, if you have an underlying mental health condition or family history of schizophrenia, bipolar disorder, or psychosis, you may want to avoid it altogether. Indeed, psychedelics in general could magnify whatever's going on in your psyche, including stuff that's beneath the surface of everyday consciousness—this applies even to people who don't have any specific mental health conditions. (For instance, it's possible when you're tripping to suddenly encounter feelings and memories from a past breakup or death of a loved one that you may not have realized was still affecting you in the present day.)

While no one has ever lethally overdosed from LSD (and there's a record of folks taking thousands of hits all at once, albeit accidentally), it is extremely potent. LSD is so strong that an average dose is measured in mere micrograms! Definitely do not drive or operate heavy machinery while you're tripping, since your balance, motor skills, and coordination could be impacted. Don't do it, kids. If you have a cardiovascular condition, seek screening and medical supervision during the experience from someone trusted.

LSD (like other psychedelics) could trigger psychosis or manic episodes. This, however, is often the result of underlying or undiagnosed mental health conditions, in combination with an unsupportive set and setting (see chapter 2). In other scenarios, LSD could cause flashbacks, which are both rare and spontaneous. It could happen in the days, weeks, or even years after the experience. In other circumstances, LSD (as well as other hallucinogens like psilocybin) has been associated with HPPD (hallucinogen persisting perception disorder)—basically persisting patterns or trails after the other effects of the substance have worn off.

As far as contraindications go, for a person on a drug like an SSRI or SNRI, there's a chance that the acid will not affect them as strongly, although there's limited research proving this definitively. Generally, though, LSD is physiologically safe in combination with other substances, and if you've properly prepared for the experience, you should feel comfortable relaxing and knowing that you are safe, even if you start to feel physically unwell.

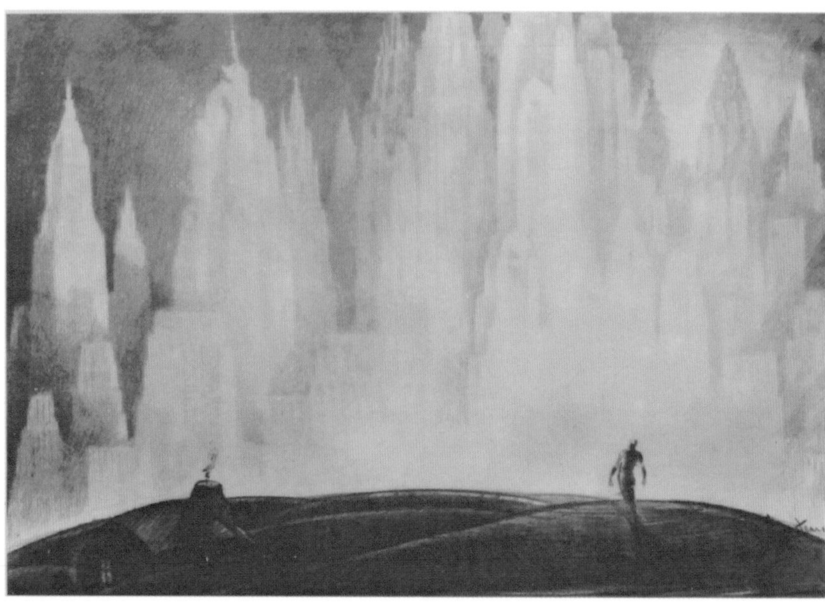

Final Thoughts

As mentioned in chapter 1, it can be trickier, but not impossible, to partake in reciprocity efforts with synthetic compounds. One way to do this is to spend time thinking about and integrating the significance of any experiences you might have had regarding what's sometimes referred to as "unitive consciousness" on LSD. While all psychedelics can be deeply spiritual, LSD in particular is known for inspiring mystical experiences that make a person feel like the boundaries between them, other people, the universe, and basically everything have dissolved. It can feel incredibly meaningful when you're experiencing it, but once you come back down to earth, it can be easy to revel in the shifts in your mood without reflecting on how you might leverage that sensation of interconnectedness to show up more meaningfully for others. One way you can do this, if you feel inspired, is to bring these profound moments of unity to your integration community or therapist and think about actionable steps to take in your life accordingly, whether that's volunteering, beginning to compost, or just making more of an effort to say hi your neighbors. Perhaps these seem like simple suggestions, but they can help you stay connected to your journey and also sustain the positive shifts in mood that you experience directly after your trip.

Reciprocity with LSD also can mean giving back to the community, culture, and environment that make its use possible. Support harm reduction initiatives like DanceSafe, which offers education and drug testing to ensure safer use, and advocate for policy reform to reduce stigma and expand access to research. Because of LSD's cultural baggage, it's been left out of decriminalization initiatives that focus on natural psychedelics such as shrooms and ayahuasca. If you've been transformed by acid, you can get involved in reform efforts to change that. By helping our culture foster a deeper respect for this substance, you can help build a future where LSD's transformative potential is recognized and responsibly integrated into society, alongside other psychedelics.

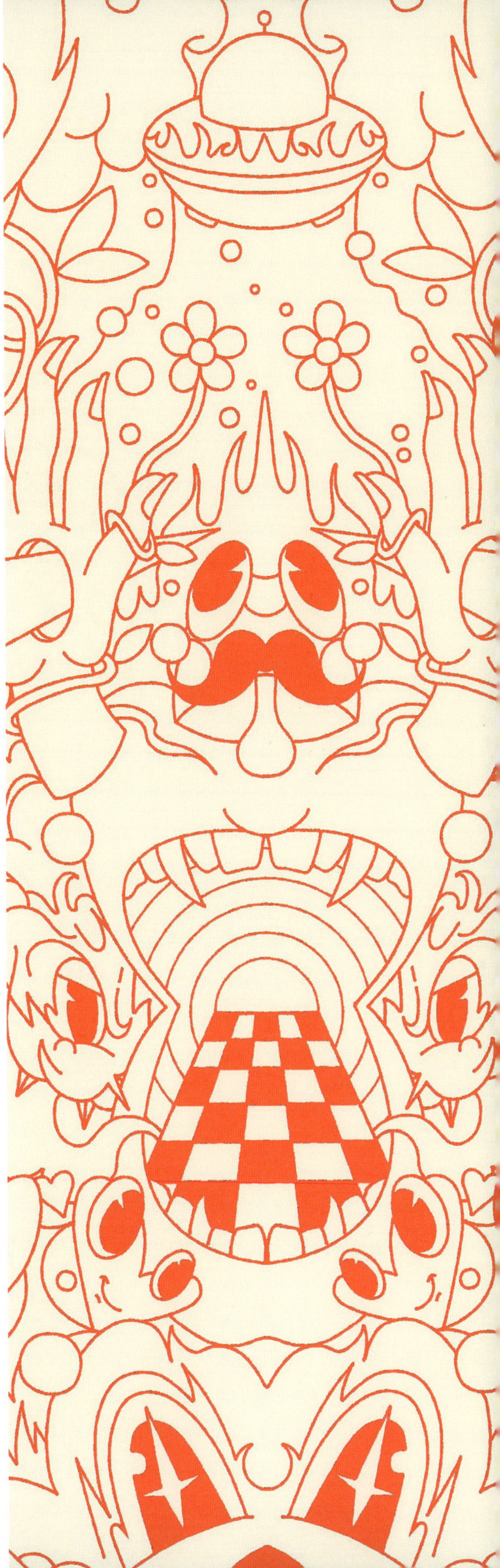

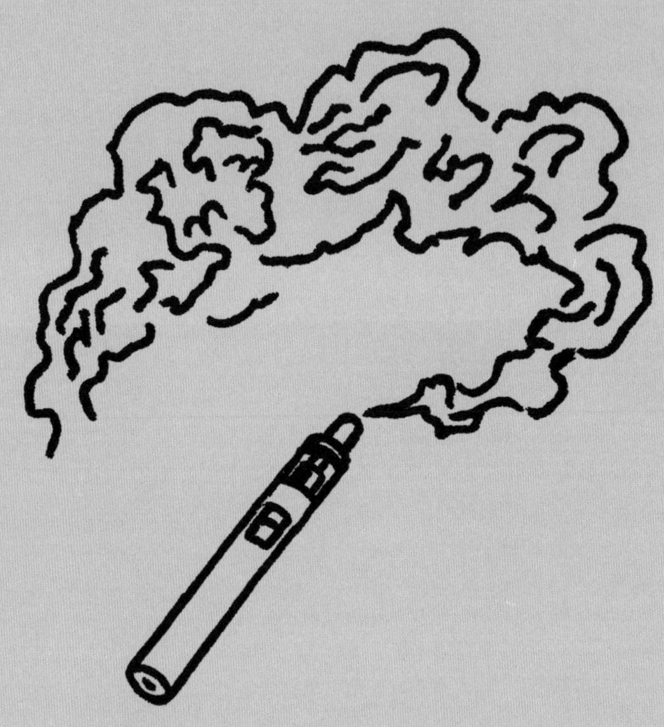

CHAPTER 7

DMT

Meet dimethyltryptamine, or DMT—a rocket ship offering a tour of the universe, aliens and all. This potent substance comes in many forms, from synthetic to organic, and occurs naturally within certain plants and even the mammalian brain. Yes, you read that right: DMT lives endogenously inside your very own brain. Now put that in your pipe and smoke it. You might've heard that DMT also plays a role in the most extraordinary of human experiences, including death and dreaming. We're sorry to tell you that even though this myth has been passionately proliferated by psychonauts for generations, there's no evidence it's true. But what we *do* know is that smoking DMT is so profound that it's led a lot of people to believe—whether there's science to back it or not—that this theory is plausible.

There are many ways to imbibe DMT. Most commonly, it's taken as a crystal or powder extract that can be smoked or vaped for a quick yet intense experience. If you're offered the opportunity to do DMT like this or you hear people just talking about "DMT," this is most likely what they're referring to. It's also what we'll be referring to in this chapter when we talk about the experience of vaping or smoking DMT (i.e., the duration, uses, how to prepare, and so on). In its plant form, DMT has been in use for millennia (perhaps since the beginning of humankind) in ceremonial or ritualistic contexts. Most famously, DMT is the main psychoactive compound found in ayahuasca. To make DMT orally active, it must be combined with a monoamine oxidase inhibitor (MAOI)—a substance that blocks the body's natural enzymes (called monoamine oxidases) from breaking down DMT in the gut before it reaches the brain. In ayahuasca, the MAOI comes from the ayahuasca vine, a.k.a. the caapi vine, which is harvested from the *Banisteriopsis caapi* tree. This vine is brewed together with a DMT-containing plant. In Peru and Brazil, the DMT-containing plant is usually *Psychotria viridis*, known as chacruna. In Ecuador or Colombia, the DMT-containing plant will more likely be *Diplopterys cabrerana*, also known as chaliponga, and this brew is technically called yagé (although some people still refer to it as ayahuasca, and we'll do so for ease in this book). In the regions in and around Iquitos, Peru, there's overlap, and you may get either combination. (See chapter 8 for more on ayahuasca.)

Similarly, in the Middle East, plants such as acacia, which contains DMT, and Syrian rue, which contains MAO inhibitors that allow the DMT to become orally active, have historically been used in combination; acacia in particular makes various appearances in biblical texts as an element of religious rituals and as entheogenic incense. Some posit that the burning bush encountered by Moses was an acacia shrub.

Two other forms of DMT are changa or yopo. Changa, an invention of the early 2000s, consists of smokable herbs spiked with DMT and an MAO (monoamine oxidase) inhibitor. When smoked, changa offers a gentler experience than crystalline DMT or ayahuasca; visuals are possible, as is an emotional release, but it's generally not as intense. Yopo, by contrast, is a powerful psychedelic snuff made from the seeds of the *Anadenanthera peregrina* tree and used for millennia, with archaeological evidence tying its ancient use to communities in Peru, Colombia, Venezuela, the Caribbean, and beyond. It contains bufotenine as its primary psychoactive ingredient, along with trace amounts of DMT and sometimes 5-MeO-DMT (a similar compound). When yopo is insufflated, its effects come on quickly and typically last for five to fifteen minutes.

You may also encounter 5-MeO-DMT and 4-AcO-DMT. As noted, 5-MeO-DMT is similar to but not the same as DMT (see page 184). Of all the substances mentioned here, 4-AcO-DMT is, despite its name, the only one that isn't a form of DMT. Rather, 4-AcO-DMT is more closely related to psilocybin; in fact, it is sometimes referred to as "synthetic shrooms" because it's thought that, like psilocybin, it's converted to psilocin in the body.

Because of the short duration of DMT when smoked and vaped, it's sometimes referred to as the "businessman's trip." Although we can't imagine anyone ever actually did this, the idea is that it's short enough that someone could, in theory, have an entire journey during their lunch break. Despite the brevity, the experience can be just as profound as that of longer-lasting psychedelics such as LSD and shrooms. In fact, DMT has a cult following of psychonauts because it offers a peek into what feels like a distinct realm, with visuals and beings that seem to appear only for people on this particular substance. So don't be fooled and think to yourself, "It's only fifteen minutes." It may be the craziest fifteen minutes of your life.

What's a DMT Trip Like?

The sensation of smoking DMT is often spoken of as a "blastoff" because the effects kick in so quickly and intensely. It may start with a beating heart and a sudden loss of your sense of time and space. Within a matter of moments, you may feel as if you're being transported into another realm, replete with its own entities and other visual components.

DMT trips are known for their swirling, colorful, kaleidoscopic visuals that may manifest as patterns or superimpose themselves atop other real-world imagery within your visual purview. For this reason, it may be less disorienting as well as more profound to keep your eyes closed.

DMT is often referred to as the "spirit molecule" thanks to its highly entheogenic nature, and indeed, a DMT experience may lead to a loss of your regular sense of self, a sense of oneness with the surrounding world, and, in some cases, ego dissolution. Some people find that after a profound experience with DMT, they feel newly connected to their identities, bodies, and relationships. It's also not uncommon for self-identified atheists to reevaluate their spiritual philosophies after a DMT trip.

Although there remains little scientific explanation for the phenomenon, many people who take DMT report seeing elves, spirits, aliens, angels, or other nonhuman entities. The DMT spirit world is indeed a mystery to behold, and many say that such entities communicate information to their observer. What they communicate and how is idiosyncratic, but often these moments are among the most profound of the DMT experience.

Ethnobotanist Terence McKenna described these entities as "machine elves" or "clockwork elves," although they look different to different people. As psychedelic researcher Rick Strassman observed, "The function of the beings is to communicate, and what they communicate is information. Their shape or form may contain information, but more importantly, there is an exchange, a relationship between the observer and the beings, sometimes verbal, sometimes nonverbal. Then it's up to our mind, our intellect, to describe the communication, to extract meaning from it."

According to a survey of more than 2,500 participants, led by psychedelic researcher Alan Davis and published in the *Journal of Psychopharmacology* in 2020, most DMT consumers interact with DMT entities via intuitive, emotional, or telepathic means and report that these entities seem real, like messengers of a deep and hidden truth. For many, it can be a hallmark or life-changing experience, with positive impacts on mood, well-being, and life perspective.

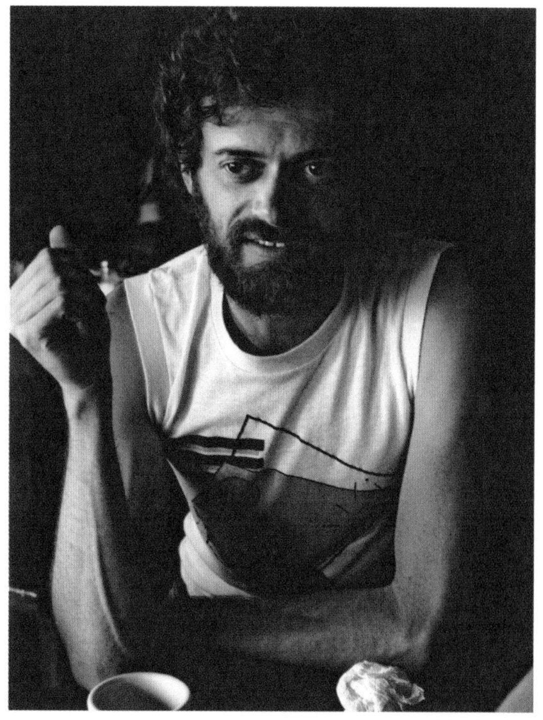

Terence McKenna at the Esalen Institute in June 1984

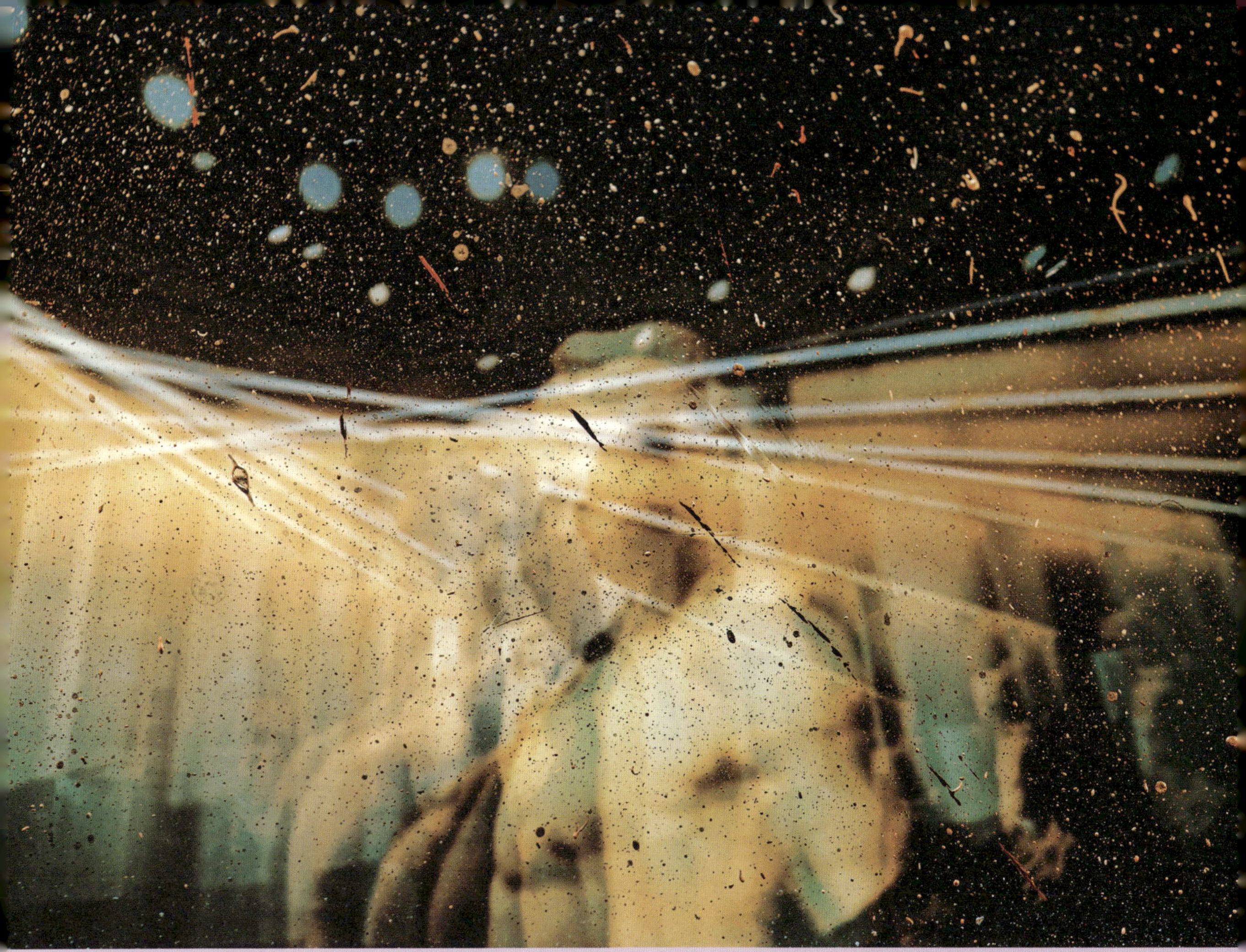

BEYOND THE JOURNEY

DMT ELVES

A group of researchers who believe the entities encountered on DMT have wisdom to share have created a way to extend the DMT experience so people can spend more time in those realms and bring back their insights. Their program, called DMTx, extends the duration of the DMT experience through continuous intravenous (IV) infusion, making it last for up to a few hours. Allegedly, during one of these experiences, the entities themselves told one of the participants how to optimize the infusion methodology—and it worked.

So who are these mysterious entities—these "machine elves" or "clockwork elves"? What do they look like? They aren't identical for everyone, but they're often described as part cosmic jesters, part alien architects, and all-around mischief-makers. These cheeky, kaleidoscopic beings seem to inhabit a realm of impossible geometry, where everything shimmers, pulses, and dances with purpose. They can be hyperintelligent, endlessly curious, and slightly bonkers, flitting around like interdimensional mechanics fixing the fabric of reality—or maybe just playing with it for fun. Travelers report that the elves might "speak" to you, not in words, but in some dazzling telepathic code of pure meaning that leaves your human brain hilariously inadequate. Are they trying to teach you universal truths, or are they just pranking you with cosmic puzzles? No one really knows. But one thing's for sure: Encountering the machine elves is like being dropped into the middle of a psychedelic Cirque du Soleil, with you as the baffled yet awestruck guest of honor.

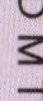

How Long Does DMT Last?

When DMT is smoked or vaporized, the onset is almost instantaneous; you begin to feel the effects almost immediately. This rapid onset is followed by an intense peak that occurs around ten minutes after intake. During this peak, it's common to experience vivid visuals, profound shifts in perception, and a complete sense of immersion in the experience. The overall duration of a smoked or vaporized DMT trip is relatively brief, typically around thirty to forty minutes.

By contrast, DMT taken as part of an ayahuasca brew has a much slower onset, usually taking thirty to sixty minutes to begin. The peak effects are more gradual and sustained, lasting for two to four hours, and the overall experience can continue for four to eight hours.

The short-lived effects of vaporized DMT make it distinct among psychedelics, offering a rapid and powerful experience without requiring the extended commitment of substances like LSD or psilocybin. While the general consensus among the psychedelic field is to never take a trip lightly, the shorter duration can be nice if you're incredibly busy and don't have many hours to devote to the experience, or if you're hoping to lean on a friend or family member to hold space for you.

DMT Dosage

The amount of DMT used significantly influences the intensity of the experience. Smoked or vaporized doses generally range between 10 and 40 milligrams. For beginners or people seeking mild effects, a lower dose of 10 to 20 milligrams can induce subtle changes in perception and light visual distortions. More experienced users aiming for a "breakthrough" experience—a complete departure from reality—commonly do doses closer to 25 to 40 milligrams.

When smoking DMT, the dosage is typically measured by the weight of the crystals or powder being used. People often weigh the substance using a milligram scale to ensure accuracy. When using a vape pen, determining the dose can be more challenging, as it depends on the concentration of DMT in the vape liquid and the volume of each inhalation. While some underground vape cartridges include information on the concentration (e.g., milligrams of DMT per milliliter of liquid), they don't usually provide guidance on how many drags are needed to reach a certain dose. In most cases, you just have to take slow draws, waiting for five to ten minutes between each one to ensure you don't accidentally do way too much.

Be wary that some vapes are much more potent than others. Some are very mild and need to be hit upwards of ten times in order for you to feel anything resembling a classic DMT experience, with visuals and a shift in consciousness. A few hits on a mild DMT vape pen can be relaxing, almost like having a glass of wine or smoking some cannabis. Other DMT vape pens are much stronger and can get you to a place of disassociation after just a few inhalations.

For those using ayahuasca, in which the DMT is made orally active by being combined with MAO inhibitors, the dosage is harder to measure precisely. Ayahuasca dosages are typically determined by the concentration of DMT and MAO inhibitors in the brew, which can vary widely depending on the preparation. See chapter 8 for more details.

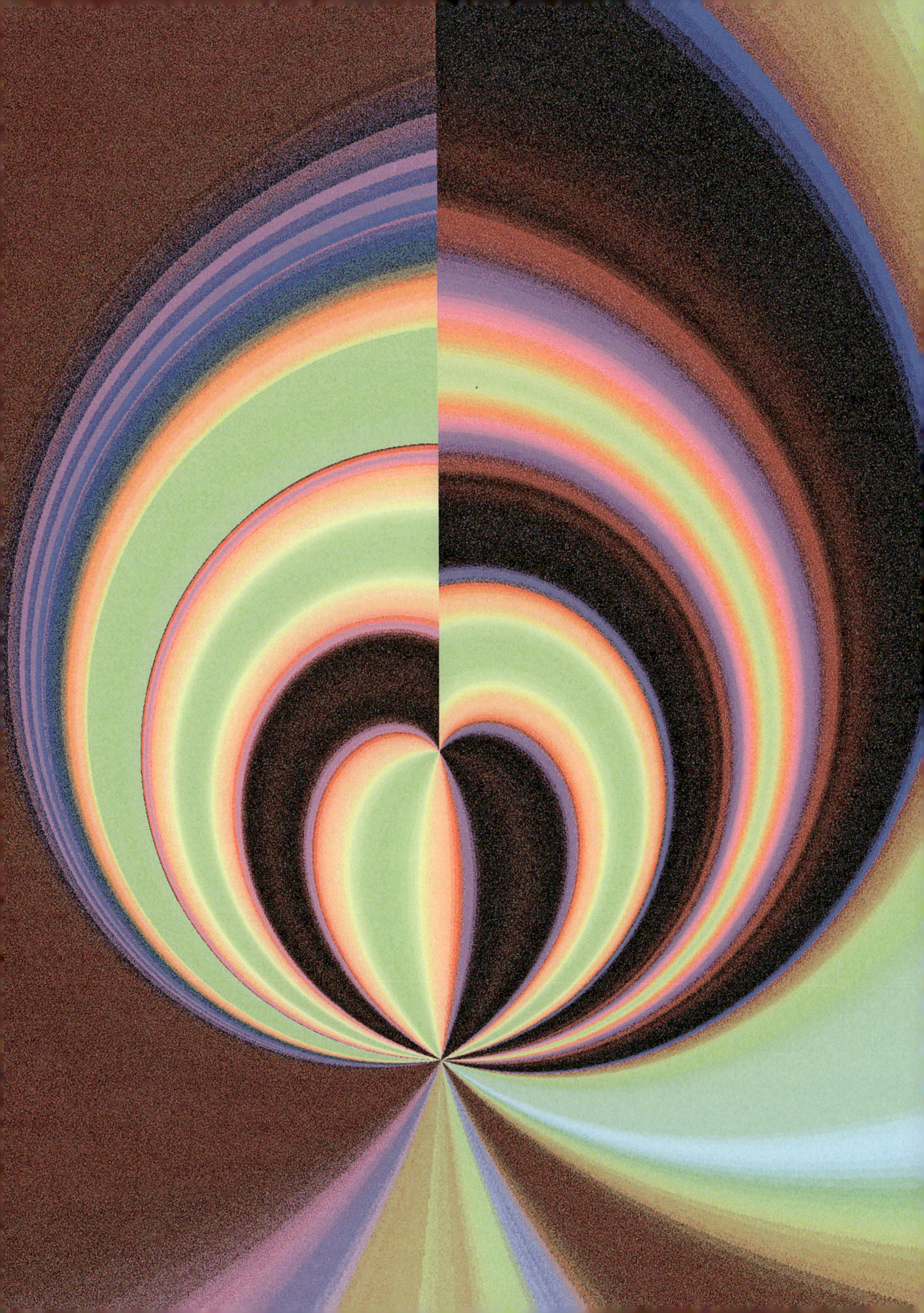

Risks and Contraindications

Although DMT is one of the shortest-acting psychedelics, it is also one of the most potent, which comes with both physical and psychological risks. On a physical level, smoking or vaporizing DMT can cause an increase in heart rate and blood pressure. This makes it unsuitable for people with heart conditions, high blood pressure, or other cardiovascular issues. Anyone with such conditions should avoid using DMT unless cleared by a medical professional.

Psychologically, DMT's rapid onset and intensity can be overwhelming, particularly for people with little experience in altered states of consciousness. If you have a personal or family history of psychotic disorders, such as schizophrenia or bipolar disorder, exercise caution, as DMT can exacerbate symptoms or trigger psychotic episodes. Some people report experiencing temporary anxiety, paranoia, or delusions during the trip. In rare cases, repeated or excessive use of DMT has been associated with the development of a messiah complex—a person's delusional belief that they have been divinely chosen or possesses unique insights meant to change the world. While this phenomenon is not exclusive to DMT and can occur with other psychedelics, it underscores the importance of responsible use and self-awareness.

Careful consideration of set and setting (see chapter 2) is crucial to mitigating risks. A chaotic or negative environment can amplify fear or anxiety during the trip. As is the case with other classic psychedelics, if you're on an SSRI or SNRI, consult with a trusted professional about the best way forward. By approaching DMT with respect, preparation, and caution, users can help ensure a safer and more meaningful experience.

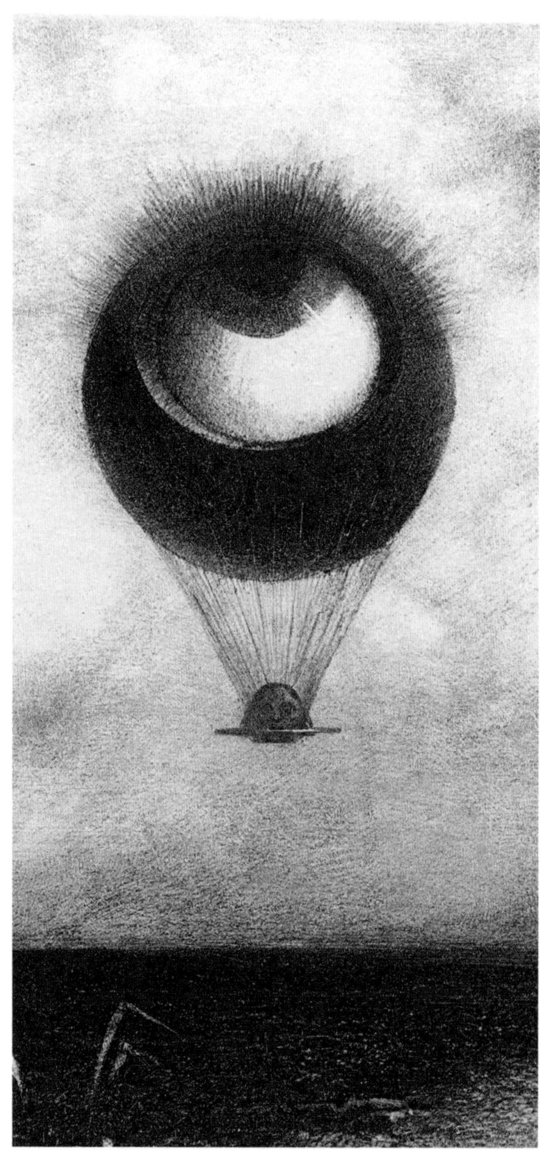

Final Thoughts

DMT can be a profound teacher, offering journeys that challenge our understanding of the very nature of reality and self. While vaped or smoked DMT is generally synthetic, you can engage in reciprocity by learning about and supporting the stewards of DMT-containing medicines like ayahuasca and yopo. Their wisdom reminds us that these experiences are not just personal but part of a broader ecological and cultural tapestry. More to come on this in the next chapter.

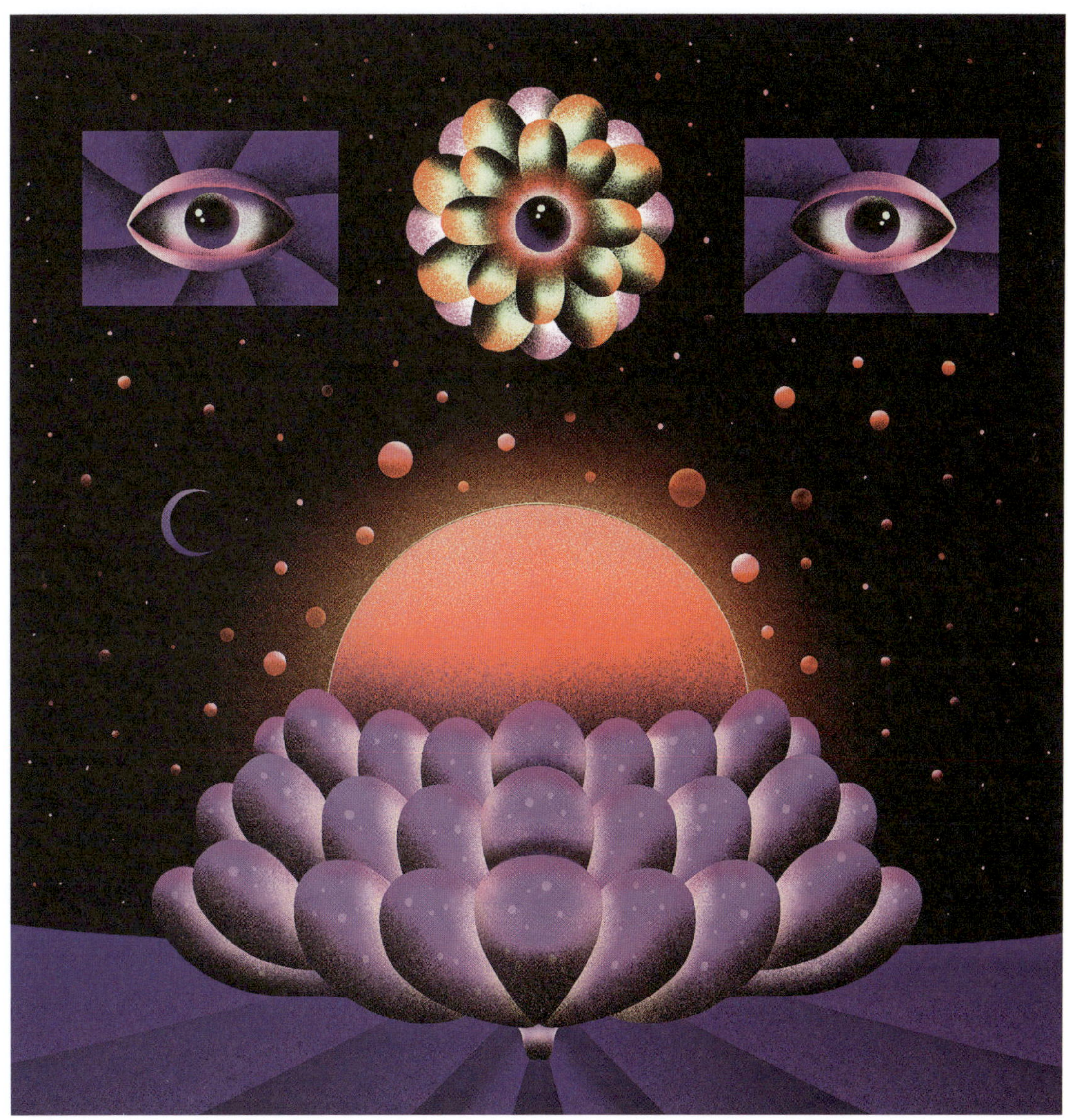

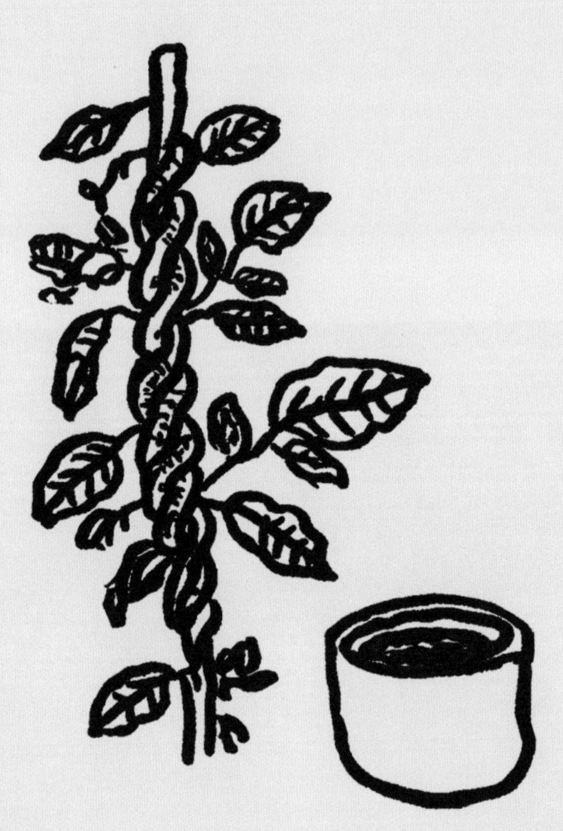

CHAPTER 8

AYAHUASCA

If you pay attention to pop culture and mainstream media, you may have noticed that people these days are talking about ayahuasca, a DMT-containing brew from the Amazon that is usually available to foreigners (i.e., anyone without an ancestral tie to it) only in a ceremony with a trained facilitator or shaman. The term *ayahuasca* derives from the Quechua language and means "vine of the soul" or "vine of the dead," and it refers to the ayahuasca or caapi vine from the *Banisteriopsis caapi* tree. In order for a brew to be considered ayahuasca, it must be prepared with the *B. caapi* vine. To make the ayahuasca brew, the caapi vine is combined with a DMT-containing plant, typically *Psychotria viridis* (otherwise known as chacruna) or *Diplopterys cabrerana* (otherwise known as chaliponga), depending on the region of the Amazon where it's being made. If the caapi vine is combined with *D. cabrerana*, the brew is technically yagé, although retreat centers and facilitators still often call it ayahuasca, if only because that name is better known. We'll do that here, too, for the sake of simplicity, as best practices for preparation, vetting your facilitator, and beyond are widely applicable.

The synergy between these indigenous Amazonian plants is what gives ayahuasca its profound effects. DMT on its own is not orally active because, when ingested, it is broken down by monoamine oxidase (MAO) enzymes in the liver and stomach, preventing it from entering the bloodstream. However, the bark of the *B. caapi* vine contains natural MAO inhibitors, which prevent the enzymes from breaking down the DMT, allowing it to bypass this metabolic barrier and deliver its psychedelic and spiritual effects over the course of several hours. Without this precise combination, the transformative experience ayahuasca offers wouldn't be possible.

While the brew has blossomed in popularity over the past decade, people have been visiting the Amazon in search of it for generations. It started becoming mainstream, so to speak, in the late 1990s and early 2000s, when celebrities such as Sting and Tori Amos spoke about their experiences, and when ayahuasca retreat centers and chapters of the Brazilian Santo Daime church began to proliferate around the world, which made the experience more accessible. By the 2010s, ayahuasca was growing significantly in Hollywood as an alternative therapy, touted by celebrities such as Chelsea Handler, Megan Fox, and Lindsay Lohan.

As a result of this attention, there's now a booming ayahuasca tourism industry in Peru, Colombia, Costa Rica, and beyond—and a booming underground in cities from Los Angeles to Berlin. But while the mainstream has only just seemed to catch on, ayahuasca has been used by Indigenous tribes in South America for thousands of years for healing, divination, and connection with the spirit world.

By some estimates, this ancient brew is incorporated into at least a hundred different traditions, and each group has its own unique rituals centered around it, intertwined with their culture and spiritual beliefs. Some of the earliest writings about ayahuasca in modern history were published beginning in the 1850s by Ecuadorian geographer Manuel Villavicencio, and he was followed by English botanist Robert Spruce, who encountered its use among Tucano, Guahibo, and Zápara tribes. In the 1950s, renowned ethnobotanist Richard Evans Schultes engaged in field studies of ayahuasca, reigniting Western interest in it. Many ethnobotanists and anthropologists followed in Schultes's footsteps, documenting the traditional use of ayahuasca, including Wade Davis, Luis Eduardo Luna, Kathleen Harrison, and Terence and Dennis McKenna. A small group of them brought clippings of the ayahuasca vine to Hawaii for cultivation, and today, much of the brew being served in the United States and beyond originates there.

While the use of ayahuasca today varies, the Indigenous groups who are most likely to be found facilitating ayahuasca ceremonies for foreigners in the Amazon or in their own country are the Shipibo-Conibo, the Huni Kuin, the Yawanawá, the Cofán, the Siona, and the Secoya. If you sit in a ceremony with a facilitator who is not Indigenous Amazonian but trained in the Amazon (which, in our opinion, is a requisite), they're likely to have been trained by one or more of these groups.

It's important to note that there is no one right way for ceremonies to happen—and we would be doing a disservice to you and these varied traditions if we laid out too many specifics here and primed people for a ceremony setup that may, ultimately, be very different what they experience. The most important thing is to find a facilitator you trust and then to follow their instructions. Ceremonies can be in the evening or during the day. They can involve music throughout or occur in complete silence. Sometimes participants are asked to sit up straight in their floor seats, while in other cases lying down is permitted or dancing is welcome. We'll offer some generalities, but take them with a grain of salt and know that it's best to not come into ceremony, or any psychedelic journey, for that matter, with too many preconceived notions and expectations.

What's an Ayahuasca Trip Like?

Ayahuasca's effects can vary from hour to hour, journey to journey, and person to person. The brew can make you feel nauseated or elated, heavy or light, in your body or out of body. It can make you shake or want to sit still; it can cause you to see visuals or hear echoes. Nearly anything is possible. One of the most well-known effects of ayahuasca is that it can make a person "purge"—which people in the global ayahuasca community sometimes refer to as "getting well." This oftentimes looks like vomiting, which can happen at any point during the journey and, often, multiple times throughout the experience. "Purging" can also involve sweating, a sudden urge to go to the bathroom, shaking, crying, or a number of other physical and emotional releases. Again, we don't want to set too many expectations here—or instill unnecessary fear—so we'll just say that, generally, purging is considered not an unfortunate side effect of the experience but a critical component of the healing process, bringing forth negative or challenging energies and helping a person release them. We'll also say that it doesn't happen to everyone.

The ayahuasca itself is a thick, brown liquid that looks much like molasses. It is often poured from a carafe, like a pitcher or mason jar, into a small cup, such as a shot glass. In most ceremonies, you'll have the opportunity to drink multiple cups throughout the night, and how much you drink will be entirely dependent on you and that particular ceremony.

The journey may dig up past traumas; it can bring people face-to-face with their wounds and the parts of themselves that they typically avoid looking at. For others, the experience may feel highly spiritual, enabling them to connect with what feels like a divine entity. People often report experiencing this entity or the spirit of the plant as a wise feminine energy, which is why ayahuasca is sometimes referred to as Grandmother or Mother Ayahuasca in the global ayahuasca community. Whether or not you believe there's truly a spirit living in the plant, people report again and again that it feels like they can communicate with the plant—that they can ask it questions or make requests of it that shape their experience.

In general, the community of foreigners who drink and serve ayahuasca have their own ways of engaging with this ancient brew, from an entire genre of "medicine music" (which you can find on Spotify) to lingo. But it's important to remember that these frameworks don't pertain to all traditions or Indigenous ways of understanding. Instead, they're products of the commodification, globalization, and evolution of ayahuasca in a modern context.

---

ayni
(Quechua; also spelled ayniy or aini)
noun

the principle, originating among Andean communities in Peru, Ecuador, and Brazil, that everything in the world is interconnected

According to the principle of ayni, we don't simply give or receive but are always partaking in exchanges of energy that affect ourselves, others, our communities, and our planet. To engage in the practice of ayni is to prioritize reciprocity—that is, to actively seek ways to give back and to move through the world with an understanding that all of our actions—big and small—have implications. In the context of plant medicines, this often means being mindful of where our medicine comes from, who is administering it, and how we can support the communities that have preserved the knowledge around them for generations.

How Long Does Ayahuasca Last?

The length of an ayahuasca journey can vary widely, depending on the ceremony. It typically lasts anywhere from four to six hours. It may take thirty minutes to an hour for any detectable effects to settle in.

While the acute, consciousness-imploding experience of ayahuasca may last for only several hours, individuals can walk away from the experience feeling a deep psychological shift that is long-lasting. Some experience an "afterglow" in the months following; the afterglow phenomenon is unique to each individual, but psychiatrist Walter Pahnke described it in a paper published in *Current Psychiatry Therapies* in 1970 as an "elevated and energetic mood with a relative freedom from concerns of the past and from guilt and anxiety" and an increased willingness "to enter into close interpersonal relationships." It's important to note, however, that, as is the case for all psychedelics, ayahuasca is not a panacea. Following an experience, a person may feel destabilized and like their life is more challenging. Someone else may feel like the ayahuasca didn't do anything for them at all. There have been reports of people drinking multiple cups of ayahuasca during a ceremony and not feeling it. Really, anything is possible.

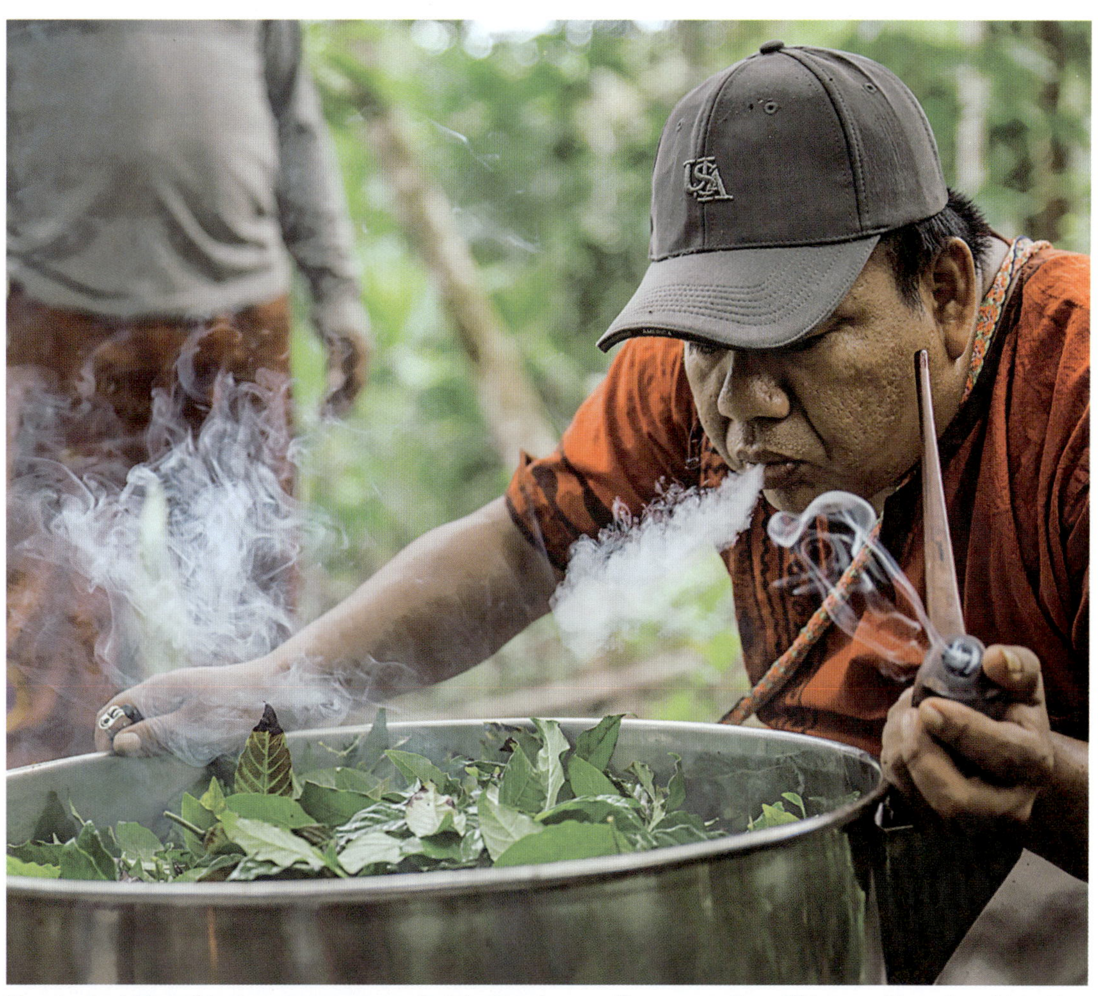

Maestro José López Sánchez prepares a new batch of ayahuasca. The preparation of this sacred brew is restricted to trained healers who have completed extensive initiation and study.

INDIGENOUS WISDOM AND STEWARDSHIP

THE ASHÁNINKA

The Asháninka are considered one of the largest Indigenous groups in the Amazon, with the majority living in Peru and some residing in Brazil. They utilize various plant medicines in their spiritual practices, and ayahuasca is central to their traditions. Historically, the Asháninka have been known for their fierce independence and resistance to domination. They fought against early Incan conquest and then entered into diplomatic relations and alliances with the Inca. Throughout the generations since, they've faced repeated external threats. Notably, the Shining Path (Sendero Luminoso), a Maoist guerrilla group, invaded Asháninka territories in the 1980s, leading to widespread violence, displacement, and the loss of thousands of lives. The Asháninka organized self-defense strategies, contributing to the expulsion of Shining Path militants from their lands. Their strong sense of freedom and readiness to defend their territory reflects a deep commitment to their land and way of life.

Unlike the case with the Shipibo-Conibo (discussed on the following page), you are unlikely to encounter a retreat center where Asháninka are serving ayahuasca to foreigners. "We want respect, because our culture is strong," writes Ash Ashaninka, an Asháninka activist and leader, in a poem on deforestation. "It is ancestral, we are older than the Bible."

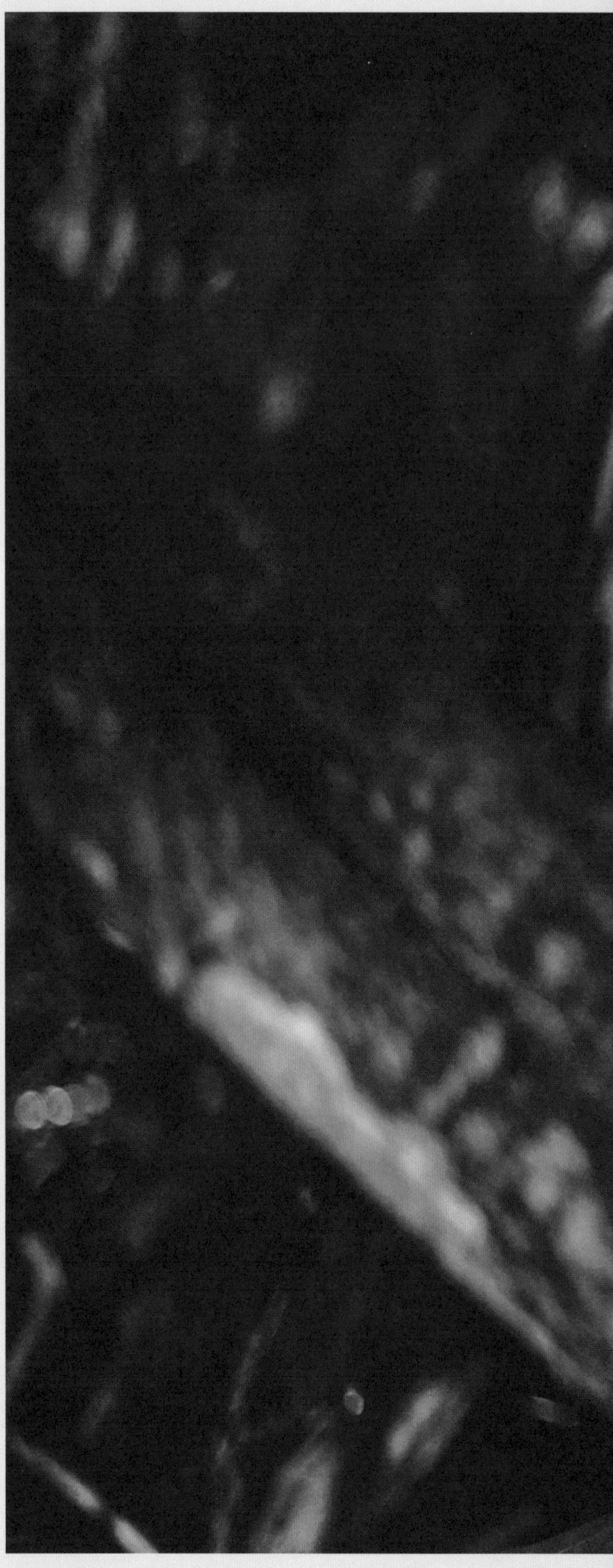

Chayeki Tinkavo, president of the Asháninka and Mashiguenga Indigenous Self-Defense Committee of the Apurímac River Valley, in Otari, Peru, on September 19, 2021

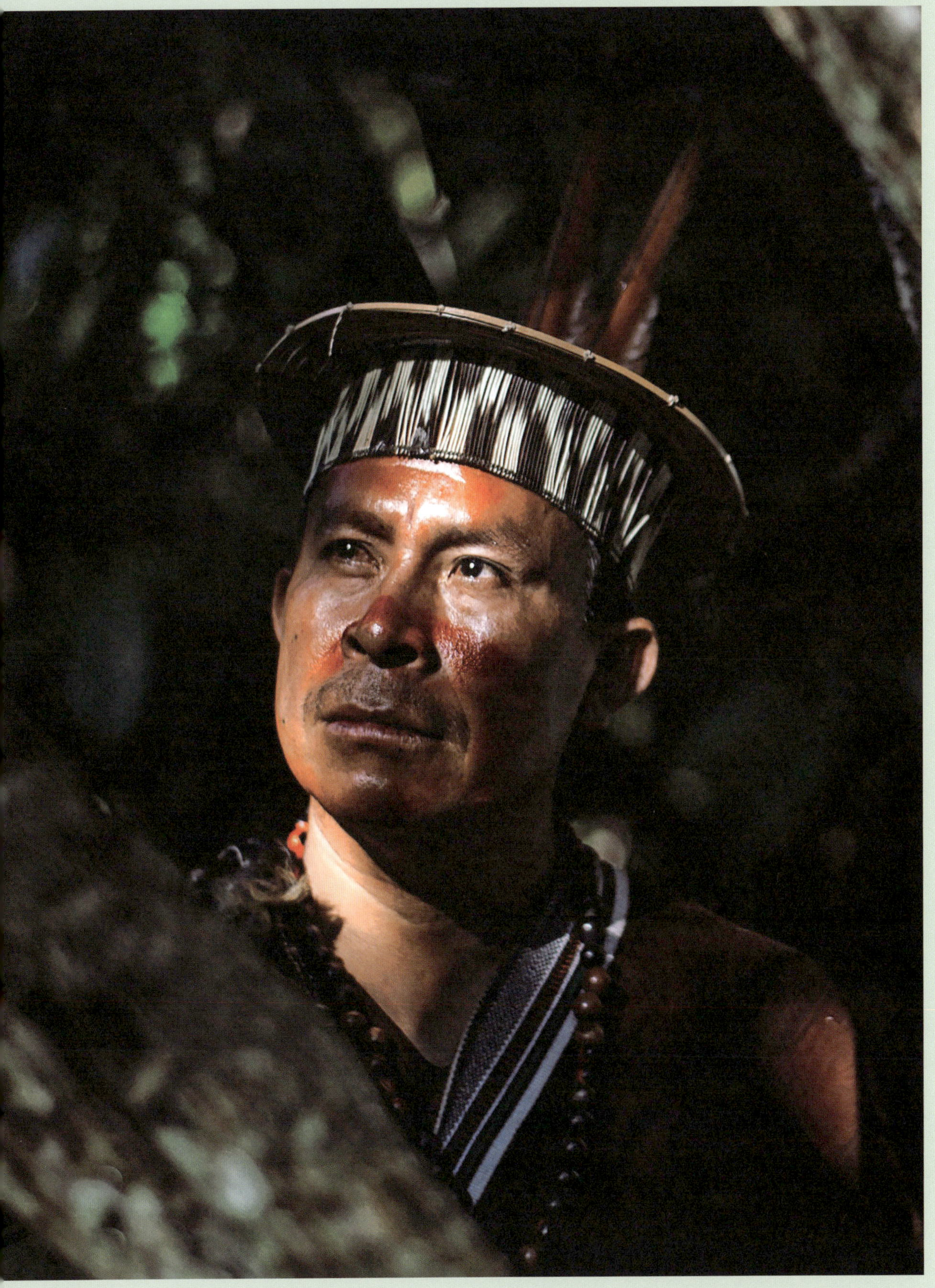

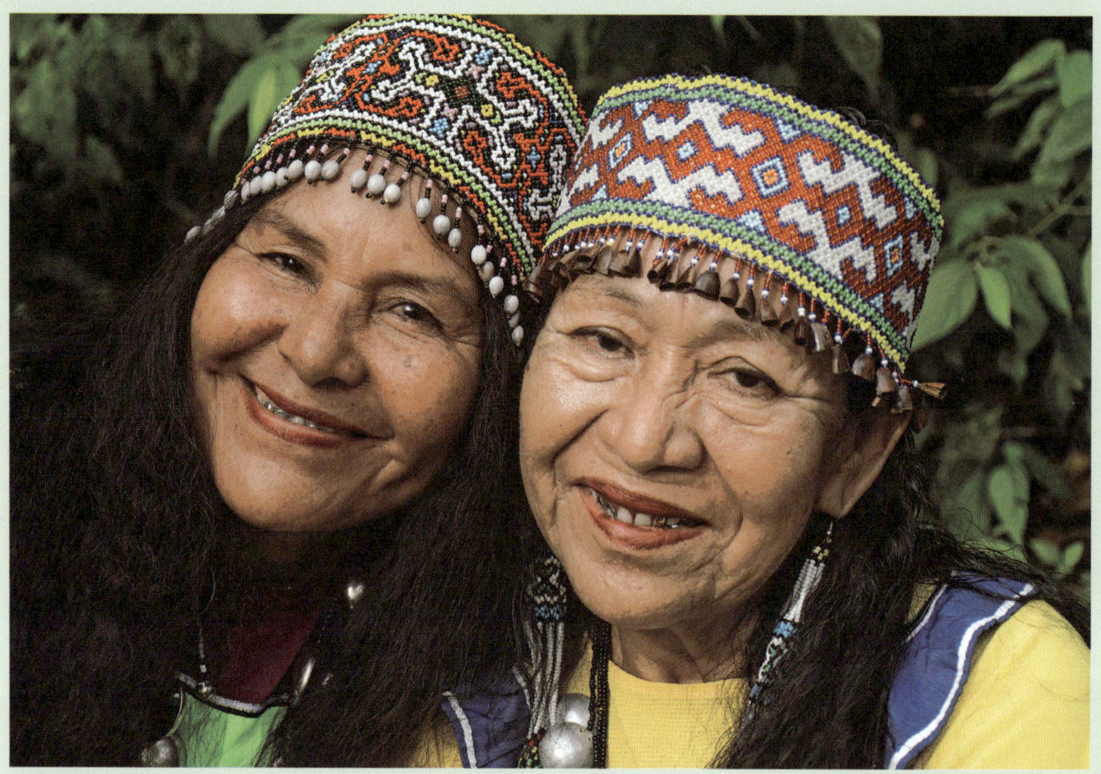

Maestras Teresa and Laura, female Onanyabo (wisdom keepers/healers) at the Temple of the Way of Light in Peru

Pages 140–141: Maestras Laura, Lila, Kati, and Teresa preparing themselves and the ceremonial maloka (space) before an ayahuasca ceremony at the Temple of the Way of Light. In this photo, the maestras are cleaning and aligning themselves, and protecting the ceremony space. These traditional shamanic preparations are carried out before every ceremony and are crucial to safely and responsibly work with ayahuasca.

INDIGENOUS WISDOM AND STEWARDSHIP

THE SHIPIBO-CONIBO

In the Shipibo-Conibo tradition, the shamans (known as curanderos or curanderas) believe that traditional sacred songs do as much healing as the ayahuasca. This group, scattered over a large area of Amazon jungle in Brazil, Ecuador, and Colombia, as well as Peru, says that these sacred songs, called ikaros, are gifted to them by the plants while the shamans are in long periods of isolation and training in how to hold ceremony. The songs can be enchanting and eerie—and sometimes a shaman will sing a particular song to a particular person because they are sensing that it is what they need to hear to heal. It's hard to describe, but many say it feels like the ikaros are doing spiritual surgery on them, activating and potentiating the ayahuasca as it moves through their body and healing specific areas that require attention.

"The plants tell me which ikaro to sing to which person," says Rojelia Velera Gonzales, a sixty-three-year-old healer who has been serving ayahuasca for thirty years. "Then, the ikaro comes to the body of the person. It penetrates their body and it heals them."

The Shipibo-Conibo (often referred to as the Shipibo for short) are also known for their intricate woven tapestries, which are said to be visual representations of these songs. Whether sitting in ceremony with a Shipibo shaman or in another tradition, the music can be one of the most profound parts of the experience.

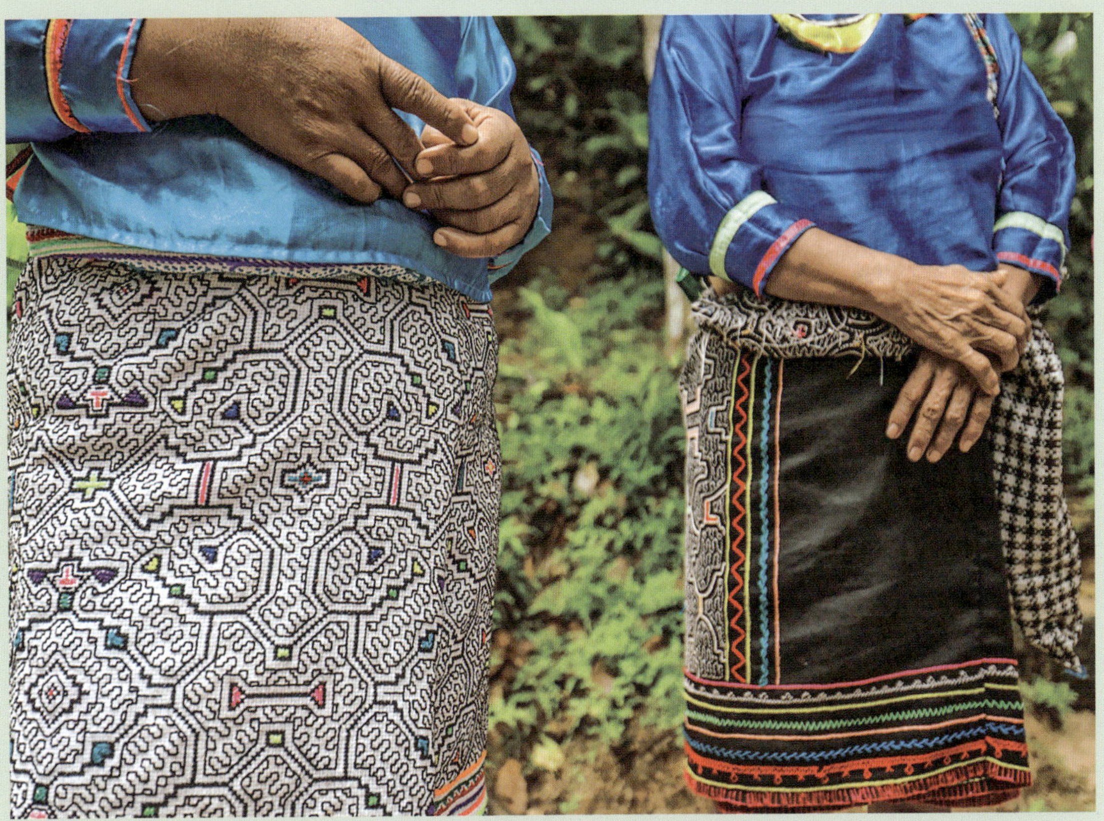

Handwoven skirts featuring designs known as kené, which hold deep spiritual and healing significance within the Shipibo culture

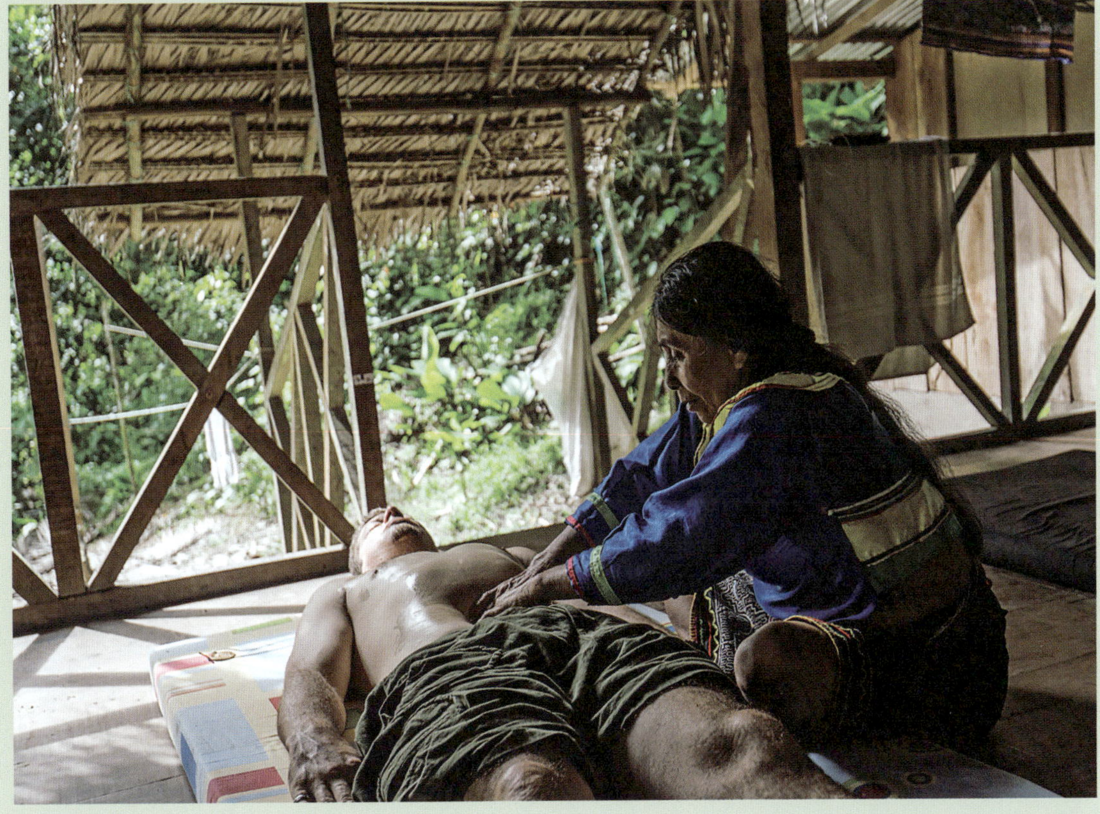

Maestra Rojelia giving a massage to extract negative energies from the body of a patient, an integral part of the Shipibo medical tradition

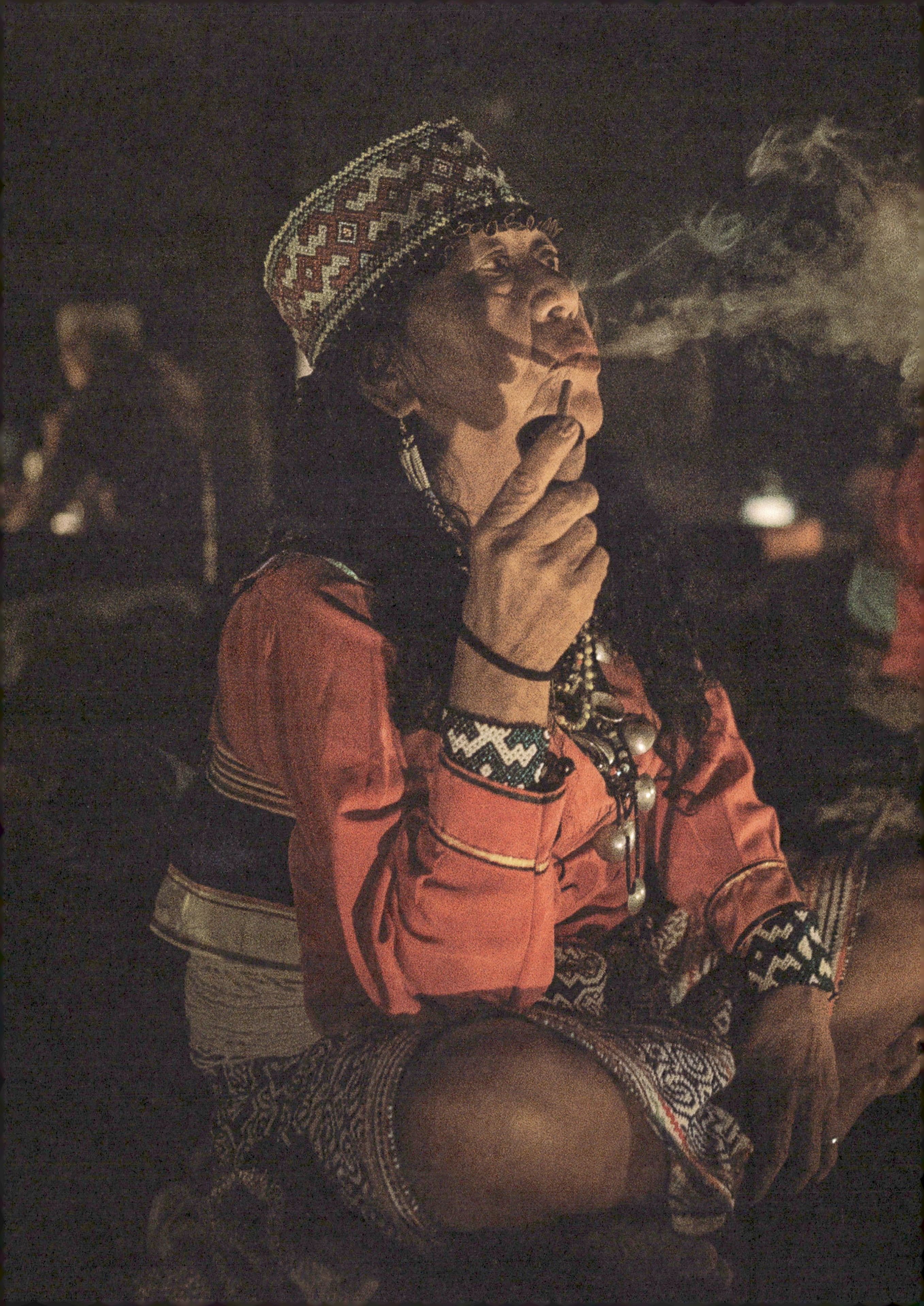

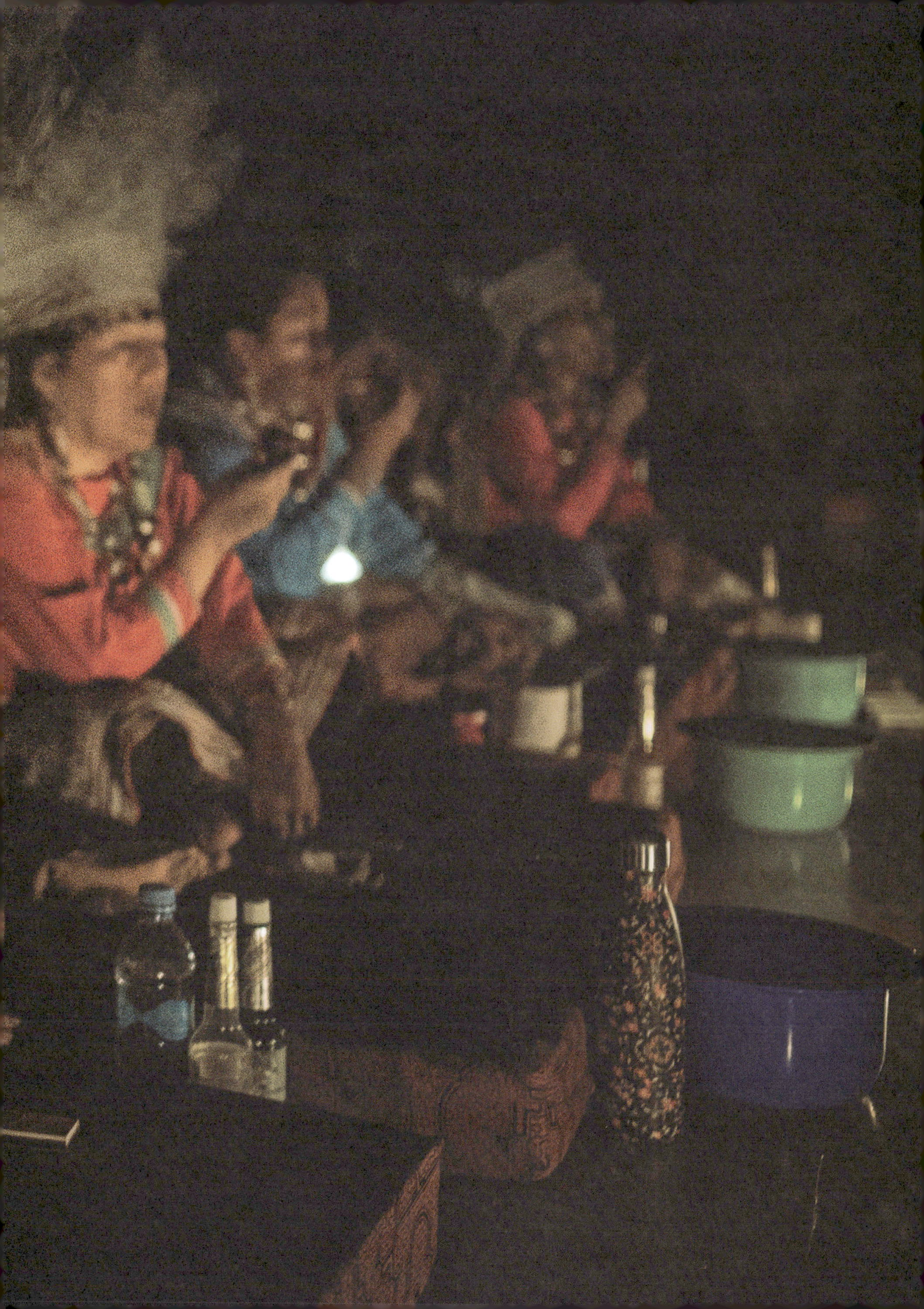

How to Know If You're Ready

Ayahuasca has a reputation for being more intense than other psychedelics, such as shrooms and LSD. In fact, a lot of folks who have tripped many times on other substances are afraid to sit in an ayahuasca ceremony. This is, in part, because people don't like to vomit (though, as addressed on page 134, purging is actually considered an important part of the healing process in many traditions). It's also because ayahuasca is considered to be more challenging, with the potential for uncomfortable emotions and thoughts. Describing the ayahuasca experience, one 2016 study published by *Frontiers in Pharmacology* on the therapeutic potential of ayahuasca noted, "Participants frequently confront their innermost fears: fear of insanity, fear of death, paranoid thoughts or the despair of cosmic loneliness and outcast. Distressful somatic symptoms such as dizziness, diarrhea, nausea, and vomiting may also arise and become an essential part of the process." It's true: Ayahuasca isn't for the faint of heart. But we also want to challenge this narrative that it's always harder than other psychedelics, because it's not that simple. Ayahuasca can offer a gentle and loving experience, and other psychedelics, such as shrooms, can be challenging. That said, embarking on an ayahuasca journey is a significant commitment requiring introspection, intention, and preparation. So, how do you know if you're ready?

INTENTIONS: This isn't so different from what you would do with any other psychedelic. Ask yourself *why* you want this experience and what you hope to explore or get out of it. (For more on setting an intention for your trip, see page 49.)

MENTAL AND PHYSICAL HEALTH: We talk more about risks on page 150, but generally, be sure on an emotional level that you are willing or prepared to confront deep-seated traumas, fears, and other potentially uncomfortable feelings.

DIETA: In the days to weeks before your ayahuasca ceremony, the server will likely recommend that you abstain from certain foods and activities.

RESEARCH: Learn about the different ayahuasca traditions, practices, and space holders available to you. Ask yourself whether you want to sit with a community you know and see on a regular basis, or whether you'd prefer a new social environment. With ayahuasca in particular, make sure that you have friends, family, or a therapist who will be available to you following the experience. It can be challenging to sit in a ceremony, have an intense journey, and then suddenly find yourself back in your old environment with no one to talk to.

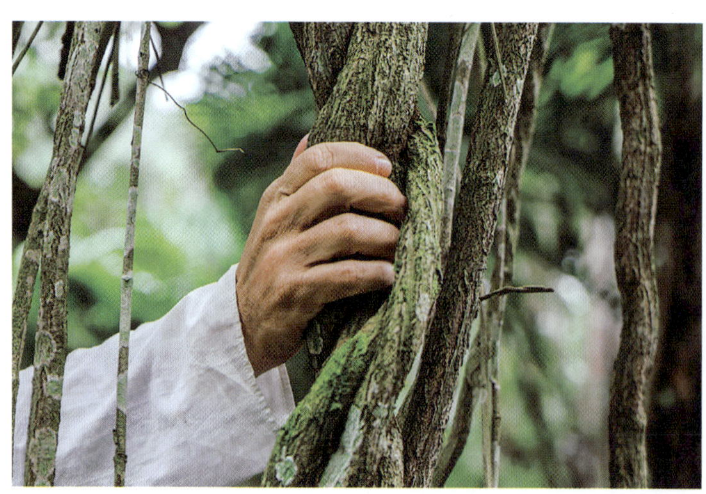

A guest at the Temple of the Way of Light holds an ayahuasca vine. Since 2012, the Temple has focused on the sustainable production and preservation of this sacred plant, planting over 3,000 vines on its grounds.

THE AYAHUASCA DIETA

The term *dieta* refers to a period of restriction—typically three to seven days, but sometimes as long as fourteen—with regard to diet, intimacy, and substances in order to cleanse the body and spirit in preparation for an ayahuasca journey. It's often advised, too, that the dieta continue for a period of time following the journey. Below is a general outline of what you might find in a dieta, but, as with other parts of the ceremony, recommendations will vary depending on the facilitator.

MOST FACILITATORS WILL ASK YOU TO AVOID:

- Alcohol
- Drugs, including cannabis
- Red meat
- Sexual activity, including with yourself

SOME FACILITATORS WILL ASK YOU TO ALSO AVOID:

- Caffeine
- Processed foods
- Sugar
- Dairy products
- Spicy foods
- Salt

MOST FACILITATORS WILL RECOMMEND THAT YOU CONSUME:

- Fresh fruits
- Cooked vegetables (steamed or boiled)
- Whole grains
- Herbal teas (noncaffeinated)

SOME FACILITATORS WILL RECOMMEND THE FOLLOWING:

- Engage in gentle exercise, like yoga or walking
- Practice meditation or mindfulness
- Avoid or limit screen time

Now, again, we want to provide the disclaimer here that different facilitators approach the dieta in many different ways, so the best thing you can do is to find someone you trust and listen to them. Don't bother trying to find definitive information about the dieta online because it doesn't exist and what's there can be confusing. A Western facilitator will often send a lot of recommendations that can feel overwhelming, especially for a first-timer who doesn't want to do anything wrong and suffer the consequences, but others may be much more relaxed about it.

We're not going to lie, a dieta that requires no salt means it's pretty hard to get anything savory to have flavor. You're better off going in a sweet direction with honey and fruit—or adding tons of herbs to your dishes. If you're in the midst of a dieta and find yourself thinking, "I can't eat anything and everything tastes like mush," try our favorite recommendations: smoothies and cold-pressed juices; yogurt with honey, dates, fresh fruit, and sunflower seeds; and a piece of fish with lemon and herbs.

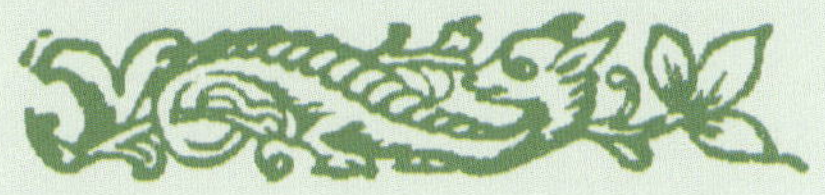

THE WORK OF WOMEN

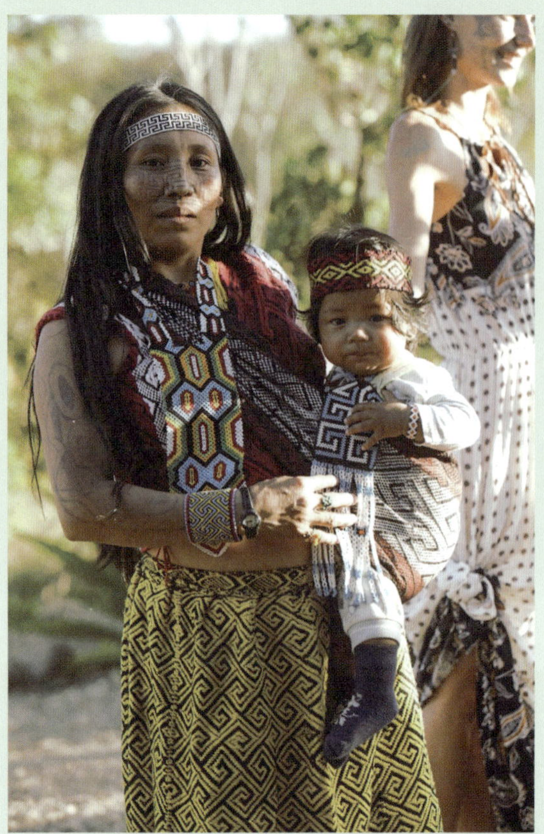

Rita Huni Kuin, age twenty-nine, doesn't know how long her village—and the other Huni Kuin villages surrounding it—has been patriarchal. No one, including her elders, seems to know either. It is a common belief, however, among the Huni Kuin, an Indigenous group in the Brazilian and Peruvian Amazon, that work was done more collectively among men and women prior to European colonization during the rubber boom at the turn of the nineteenth century.

For as long as Rita and her elders remember, though, the women in her village, Aldeia Chico Curumim, have not had a voice politically nor been recognized internationally for their contributions to the preservation of Huni Kuin culture. Huni Kuin men have traveled around the world, serving ayahuasca, speaking on behalf of their communities, and selling glass bead necklaces and weavings made by the women for decades, but often the female makers of these crafts were not credited or compensated equitably—until now.

In early 2022, women across thirty-six Huni Kuin villages along the Jordão and Tarauacá rivers in Brazil formed the first association intended to give them a voice, locally and globally. The association, named Ainbu Dayá, or "work of women" in Hatxã Kuin, the language of the Huni Kuin, was established with the support of Living Gaia, a nonprofit that was founded in 2013 by Alexandra Schwarz-Schilling, a German entrepreneur and coach who was inspired by the Huni Kuin and her transformative plant medicine experiences. "Until recently, [the women] were doing a great job of bringing our culture forward, but we didn't have the visibility, it was only the men," says Rita, from her home in Jordão, a small city and the capital of the municipality of Jordão. "We want to show the world that the Huni Kuin women are here, that we have a voice, and that we are working to preserve our culture and support our communities."

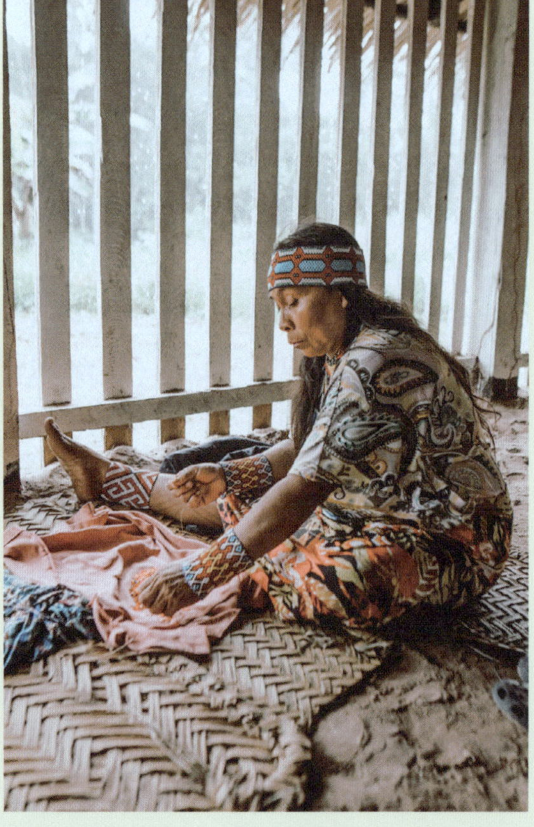

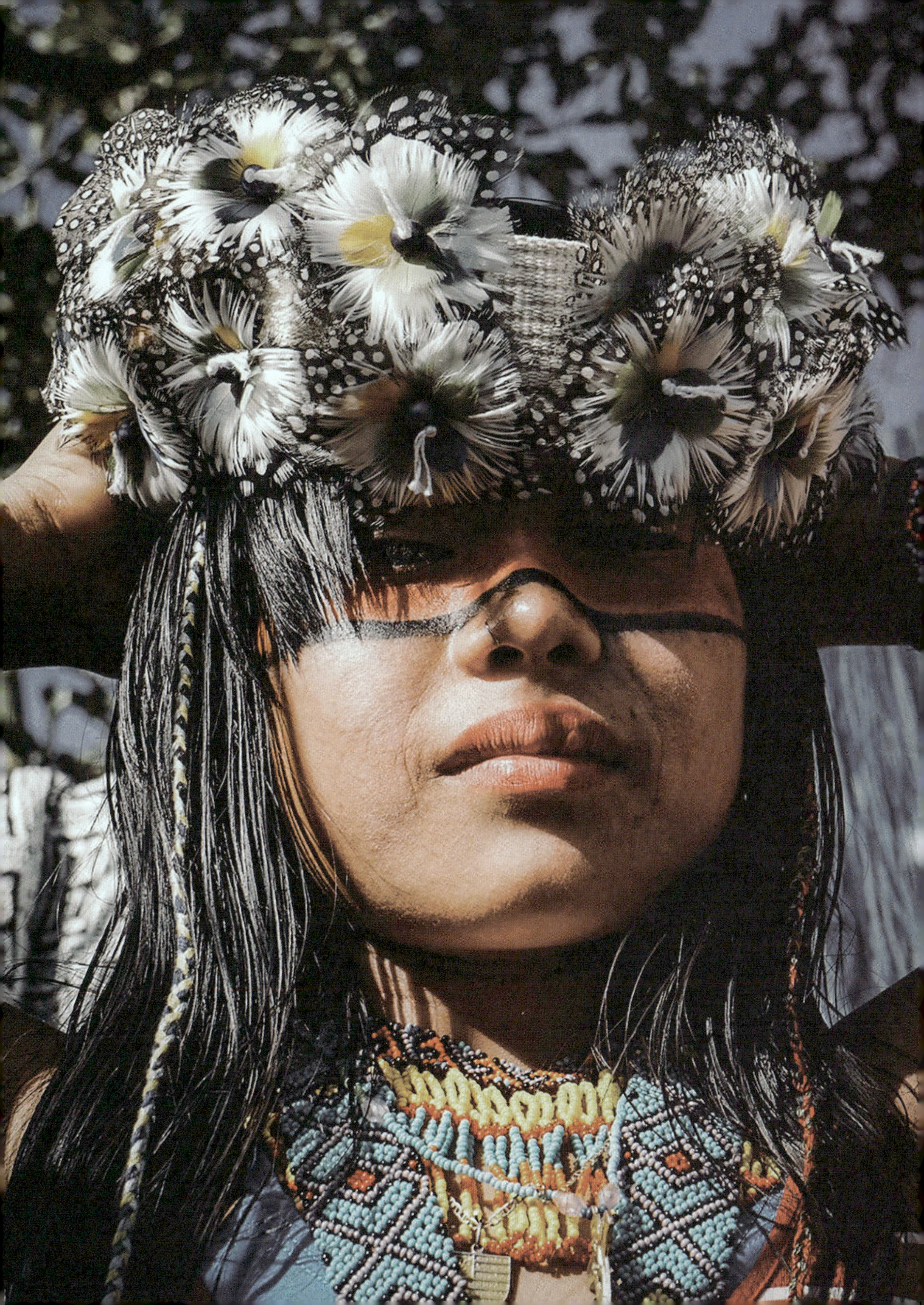

HOW TO FIND A VETTED RETREAT CENTER

Though some people may opt for a one- or two-night ceremony closer to home, typically ayahuasca is a multiday experience during which a group of participants receives the psychedelic brew under the guidance of a shaman, facilitator, or guide. These retreats can vary in length of time and cost, ranging from a few hundred dollars to thousands of dollars.

While ayahuasca retreats have grown in popularity in the United States, "ayahuasca tourism" has led many people to travel to Peru, Colombia, and other areas where local Indigenous groups have built an established tradition of ayahuasca use. In addition to the areas around Pucallpa, Peru, many retreat centers are located in and around Iquitos, Peru, and across Costa Rica. An ayahuasca experience at one of these Indigenous retreat centers will be very different from one undertaken with an underground practitioner in your home country or at a legal ayahuasca church such as the Santo Daime or the União do Vegetal (see page 148).

There's much to consider when choosing your ayahuasca retreat, though. Unfortunately, just because a retreat center has a well-designed website that makes it look credible doesn't mean that it is. In recent years, several well-funded retreats and clinics located abroad in beautiful, resort-like environments have been at the center of scandals, ranging from neglect of participants to wrongful deaths. If you're considering traveling abroad to a retreat center, ensure that you've found an ethical and safe one by asking these questions.

- **Is the ayahuasca retreat engaged in sacred reciprocity?**

  Indigenous communities have been drinking ayahuasca for thousands of years, so the booming interest in the substance has brought up tricky ethical questions. Sacred reciprocity calls for either supporting or giving back to the Indigenous communities with ancestral ties to ayahuasca, and a number of retreat centers are doing it right, such as the Temple of the Way of Light in Peru, which is the biggest employer of Shipibo people in their region and has a nonprofit, the Chaikuni Institute, that is working on environmental and social justice projects in the Amazon.

- **Are the facilitators transparent, clear communicators who welcome questions?**

  Responsible ayahuasca retreat centers understand that proper client intake is essential and will be readily accessible for consultation and queries. Someone from the retreat center should be willing to discuss your questions with you before you commit to a program. Indeed, some retreats require interested parties to fill out an application, so that they can vet the participants' safety and suitability for an ayahuasca ceremony. Good retreat organizers understand this need for vetting on both sides and should have questions for you as well. Also note that each ayahuasca journey is different, and ethical retreat facilitators should not guarantee specific results. They also should be able to lay out the sequence of events that compose the ceremony, guidelines and expectations for new participants, and how they will help participants integrate the journey afterward.

- **Who will lead the ayahuasca retreat, and what is their background?**

  The leaders of ayahuasca ceremonies have a wide range of titles: shaman, healer, facilitator, practitioner, ayahuasquero, curandero, and maestro, among others. Reliable retreats will provide detailed information about the ceremony leader's spiritual lineage tradition, their training, how many years they've been working with ayahuasca, and how long they've been leading ceremonies themselves. Find out whether there is a chance to connect one-on-one with the facilitator before or after the ceremony, and whether a translator will be provided to aid with communication if there is a language barrier. Unfortunately, the boom in ayahuasca tourism has increased the incidence of false, untrained, or unethical facilitators and retreat centers. Ethical retreats are aware of these scams and will be glad to provide you with their bona fides and assure you of the ceremony leader's credentials as well as your safety.

- **What is in the preparation we'll be drinking?**

  The liquid brew consumed during an ayahuasca ceremony is typically made with two ingredients: the ayahuasca vine (*Banisteriopsis caapi*) and a DMT-containing plant (either *Psychotria viridis*, otherwise known as chacruna, or *Diplopterys cabrerana*, otherwise known as chaliponga). The facilitators and/or retreat center should be willing to tell you what's in the brew you're drinking; if they don't, that's a red flag. There was a time when facilitators incorporated other ingredients into the brew, but that's not as common anymore. Also, do not drink a brew that has datura or toé in it. There have been some reports of unethical facilitators serving the brew with these compounds, which can cause terrifying hallucinations and, in some cases, hospitalization or even death. If a facilitator is adding these substances to the brew, it suggests a serious disregard for participant safety and traditional protocols.

- **What health conditions and medications are contraindicated for an ayahuasca retreat?**

  Good retreat centers require participants to fill out a mental health and medical history. Legitimate and responsible groups will always do a medical screening of participants; not being asked to do so is a major red flag. See more info on risks and contraindications on page 150.

- **What is the ratio of assistants/staff to participants during the ayahuasca retreat?**

  Ayahuasca ceremonies often last for hours, and participants frequently purge during them, whether through sweating, vomiting, or diarrhea. While there is usually only one ceremonial leader, there should be sufficient assistants to track everyone in the circle and to offer support to individuals if needed. Larger groups should provide more staff. At no point in the ceremony should you feel like you need support and not be able to easily find it.

- **How do the ayahuasca retreat facilitators support someone who is struggling during the ceremony?**

  Whether the challenges are physical or emotional, an ayahuasca journey can be a daunting experience. While distressing moments are often considered key to the releasing and healing aspects of the ceremony, it's good to find out in advance how facilitators support participants who are struggling.

- **What is the integration process after the ayahuasca retreat?**

  While integration therapy is recommended for all psychedelics, ayahuasca, in particular, is known for bringing challenging emotions and thoughts to the surface that you'll likely want help processing. Post-ceremony support is essential for participants to safely and securely process the visions, challenges, and insights of the ceremony. The healing journey that ayahuasca opens a person up to often only truly begins after the ceremony ends. The inner work that happens after the ceremony is key to fully digesting and incorporating the experience. Credible ayahuasca retreats will offer modalities and support for integrating your experience after the ceremony. It's important to note that many retreats and facilitators do not offer ongoing one-on-one support as they don't have the resources. That is something you should set up for yourself beforehand by finding a psychedelic integration therapist whom you connect with, even if it's just for a few sessions. But the retreat center and facilitator should be available for questions and to point you in the right direction.

BEYOND THE JOURNEY

LEGAL AYAHUASCA CHURCHES

Most Westerners who are interested in drinking ayahuasca for the first time don't know this, but there are actually two Brazilian ayahuasca churches with chapters in the United States, Europe, and beyond. The churches—Santo Daime and União do Vegetal (UDV)—originated in the twentieth century and combine Christian, African, and Indigenous elements. Their legality differs depending on the country and the church.

Santo Daime has faced legal challenges regarding the use of ayahuasca in the United States. However, certain branches have been granted legal protections, allowing them to conduct ceremonies in some states. Santo Daime chapters also exist in Canada and parts of Europe.

União do Vegetal achieved a major legal victory in 2006 when the US Supreme Court ruled in *Gonzales v. O Centro Espirita Beneficente União do Vegetal* that the church could legally import and use ayahuasca for religious ceremonies under the federal Religious Freedom Restoration Act. UDV now operates legally in several US states. Like Santo Daime, UDV also has a presence in Canada and in some European countries.

Some people may not feel comfortable with the elements of Christianity within the ceremonies of these churches. But, because they have legal protections in some states and countries, they are able to practice with less risk than Indigenous Amazonian facilitators, who have to practice completely underground when traveling outside their home countries.

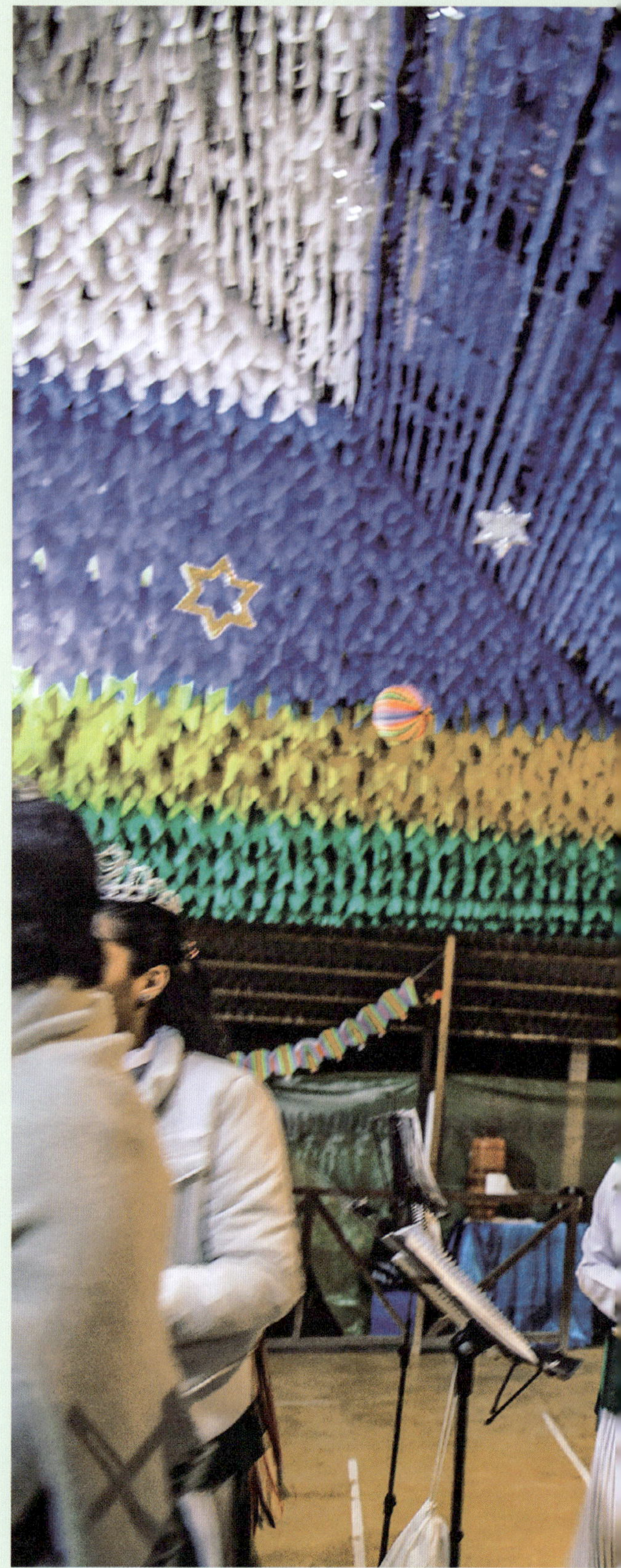

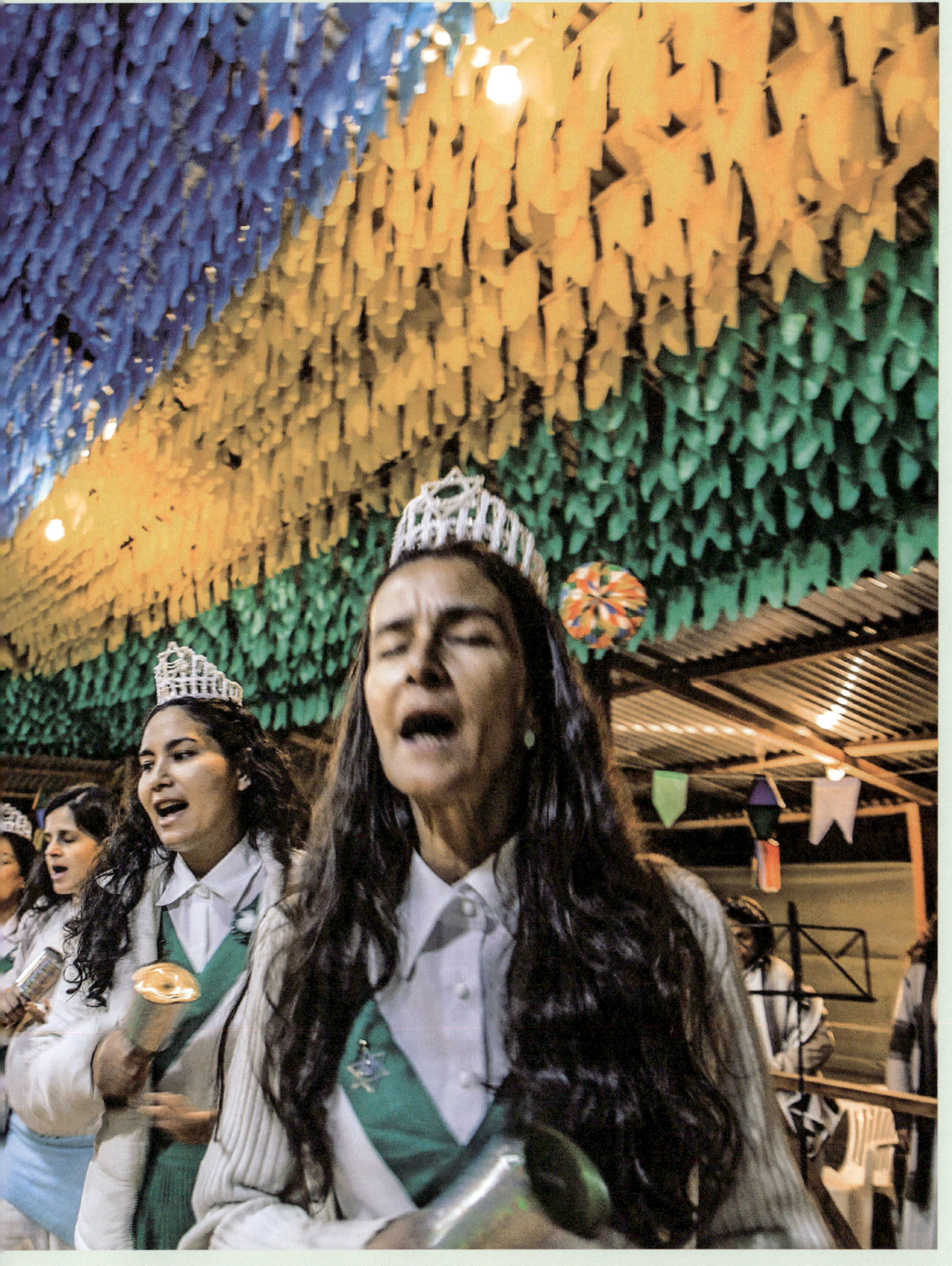

A Santo Daime ceremony in Brazil in 2014. The ceremony involves the singing of over 150 hymns and dancing for about twelve consecutive hours.

Risks and Contraindications

We want to start by saying that, if you're sitting with a responsible facilitator, they should ask you for your medical and psychological histories and flag any potential issues.

That said, anyone with cardiovascular disease, epilepsy, or liver and kidney issues will likely be advised to avoid ayahuasca due to the potential for complications. Personal or family history of mental health conditions like psychosis, schizophrenia, or bipolar disorder will also likely disqualify you.

Many common drugs are considered safe with ayahuasca. However, ayahuasca may cause issues and even medical emergencies when combined with certain prescription medications. We can't provide an exhaustive list and your trusted facilitator should be helping with this, but the active alkaloids in the ayahuasca vine—harmine and harmaline—are types of MAO inhibitors and are contraindicated with all the same medications that are contraindicated with MAO inhibitors. These include all antidepressants (which are MAO inhibitors or SSRIs), most anxiety medications, vasodilators, muscle relaxers, narcotic painkillers, and antihistamines. Some herbs, such as passionflower, St. John's wort, and kava, have the potential to increase the potency of the experience and are often considered contraindicated by facilitators.

These risks underscore the importance of treating ayahuasca with respect and caution. It's not just about ensuring a safe experience but also about honoring the centuries-old Indigenous knowledge that gave rise to this powerful medicine. Proper preparation, full transparency about your health, and choosing a reputable setting are nonnegotiable for anyone considering this journey. Perhaps the most important reason for all of this work is that you'll want to be fully at ease once you actually drink the medicine—and knowing you've done your due diligence ahead of time will help with that.

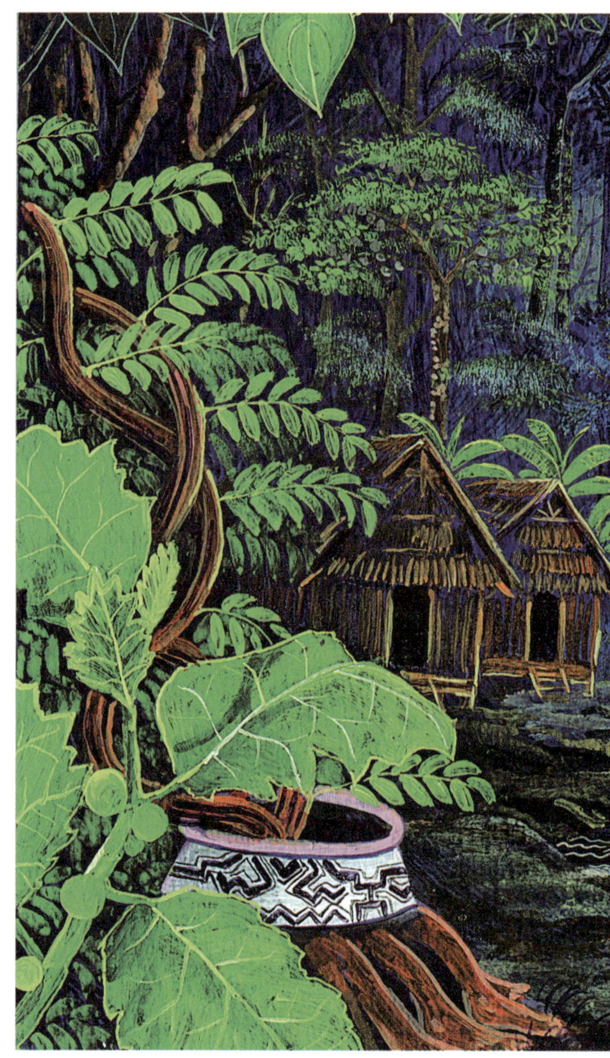

Final Thoughts

Of all the psychedelics we cover, ayahuasca is among the most complicated, given its rich, millennia-old cultural history. After you've had your first ayahuasca experience, in addition to doing your own integration work, there are many ways in which you can begin to support movements to preserve this sacred brew. The Chaikuni Institute at the Temple of the Way of Light in Peru works on reforestation and sustainable development projects related to ayahuasca, while the Indigenous Medicine Conservation Fund provides financial resources directly to Indigenous communities to ensure their sovereignty and stewardship. Similarly, UMIYAC (Union of Indigenous Yagé Doctors of the Colombian Amazon) represents a coalition of Indigenous healers working to preserve traditional medicine practices around yagé while advocating for the protection of their territories and cultures. Chacruna, a nonprofit organization, furthers this work by amplifying Indigenous voices, fostering cultural understanding, and advocating for equitable and ethical access to psychedelic plant medicines. You can find more information on all these groups in the additional resources section at the end of this book.

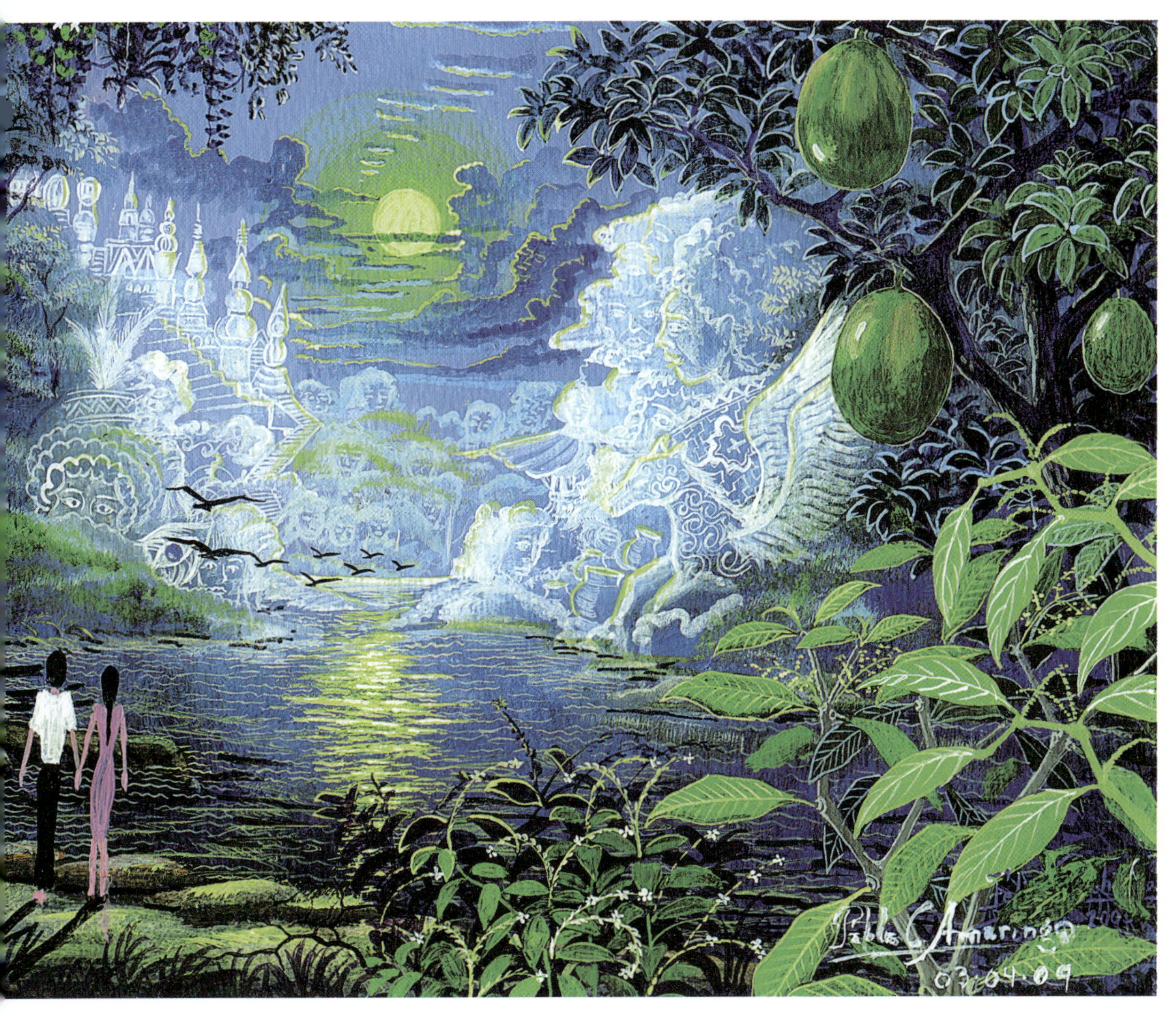

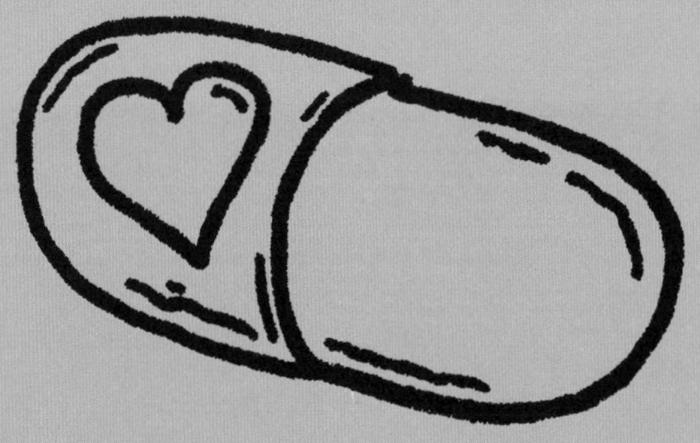

CHAPTER 9

MDMA

Most people who have done MDMA think of it as a party drug, and—we're not going to lie—it can be a lot of fun. But because it has this reputation, many people don't realize how therapeutic it can be if it's taken in a more intentional setting. MDMA (or, more formally, 3,4-methylenedioxymethamphetamine) is a drug that truly morphs to suit its environment.

MDMA was first discovered in 1912 when chemists working for the German pharmaceutical company Merck synthesized the compound in a larger effort to develop a medication to control bleeding. Much like LSD, once MDMA had been synthesized, it was left by the wayside until 1965, when chemist Alexander "Sasha" Shulgin rediscovered it. Shulgin had had a lifelong interest in chemistry and consciousness, fueled by a transformative experience on mescaline in the late '50s. This inspired him to try synthesizing and taking other similar psychoactives, including MDMA, which he had read about in existing chemical literature.

Headquartered in California's Bay Area, Sasha and his wife Ann Shulgin started a movement by introducing MDMA to psychotherapist Leo Zeff, who went on to treat more than 4,000 patients with MDMA and train 150 therapists to use it in their work. These therapists found it useful in facilitating communication, enhancing empathy, and helping patients work through relationship conflicts. In fact, its use as a tool in couples therapy earned MDMA its nickname the "love drug," thanks to its empathogenic or entactogenic qualities—meaning that it carries the power to conjure feelings of empathy, oneness, and/or emotional openness, especially in relation to another person or people.

By the early 1980s, MDMA had spread beyond the clinics and into the clubs, coming to be the starchild of the rave scene, thanks to its euphoric and empathogenic effects, in conjunction with its upper-like qualities, which made it easier for partygoers to stay up all night dancing and connecting with each other.

As its recreational use increased, however, so did the attention MDMA gained from government officials, and in 1985 the US Drug Enforcement Administration (DEA) criminalized it, pointing to concerns about its potential health risks and abuse—never mind its proven efficacy among therapists and scientists. MDMA became classified as a Schedule I controlled substance, alongside other compounds like LSD, cannabis, and heroin.

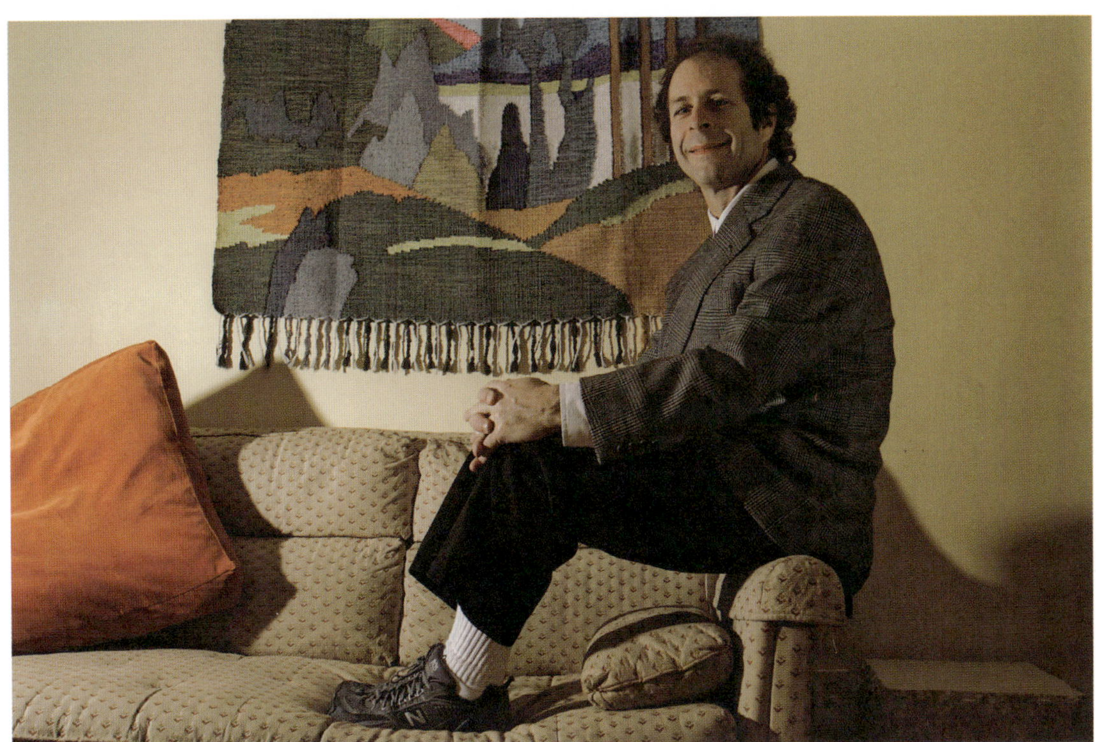

Rick Doblin, PhD, founder of the Multidisciplinary Association for Psychedelic Studies, photographed at his home office in 2004

Nonetheless, science and research around MDMA persevered, and in the year after it was outlawed, a young activist, scientist, and Harvard grad named Rick Doblin founded a then-little nonprofit called the Multidisciplinary Association for Psychedelic Studies, or MAPS, which worked to overcome regulatory barriers to explore MDMA's therapeutic potential. (MAPS has since established a for-profit arm for the development of MDMA called Lykos.)

In 2017, MDMA was given "breakthrough therapy" status by the FDA, accelerating the possibility of approval for its use in the treatment of PTSD. In a historic and unexpected move, the FDA rejected approval of MDMA in 2024, but advocates are still hopeful it will receive approval in the coming years both in the United States and in other countries, such as the Netherlands and Israel. In addition to official clinical trials in the United States and other countries, MAPS also launched a limited program, approved by the FDA, that allows a small number of sites across the United States to offer MDMA-assisted psychotherapy for PTSD prior to full FDA approval. It's important to note, however, that if/when MDMA becomes approved as a medication for PTSD, what will become legal—and more specifically, rescheduled—is an entire protocol that involves therapy in addition to taking the substance, as well as the requirement for a doctor's prescription. In other words, no, you won't be able to just walk into a pharmacy and buy MDMA, and most therapeutic work (especially outside the bounds of clinical supervision) will remain underground until widespread decriminalization takes hold.

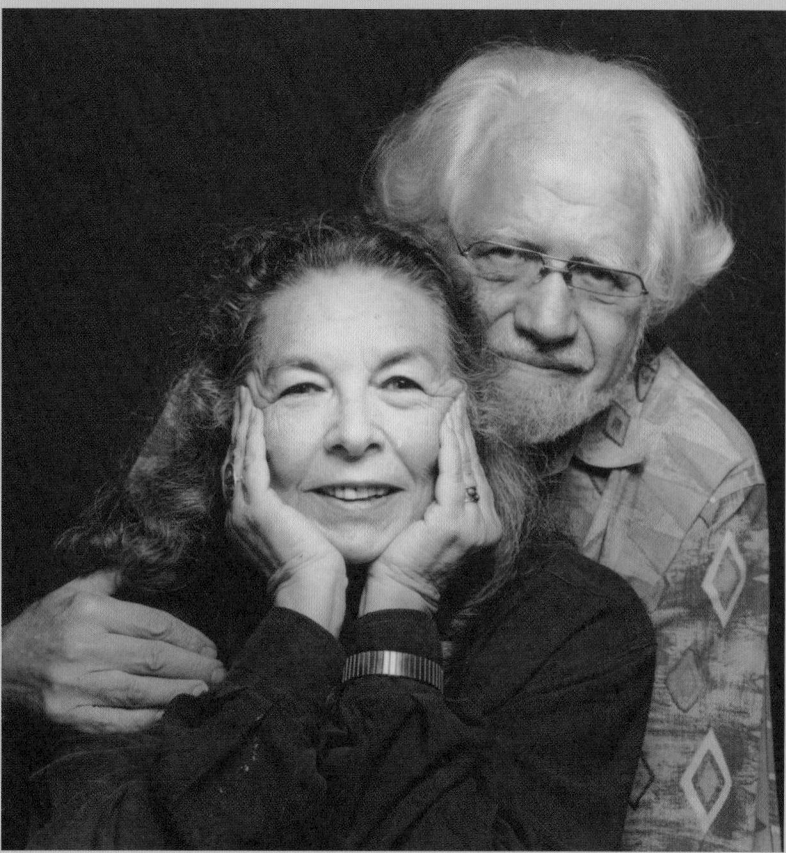

Ann and Sasha Shulgin were married for more than thirty years, partners in both life and work. Sasha, a chemist, synthesized and explored hundreds of psychoactive compounds, while Ann focused on their therapeutic potential. Together, they coauthored *PiHKAL: A Chemical Love Story* and *TiHKAL: The Continuation*, works that intertwined their scientific discoveries with their love story.

BEYOND THE JOURNEY

THE GODFATHER OF ECSTASY AND HIS FARM

Perched upon a hilltop in Lafayette, California, overlooking Berkeley and San Francisco Bay, is a charming, rustic shack that happens to be the modest birthplace of more than two hundred novel psychoactive substances. The ramshackle laboratory is where biochemist Alexander Shulgin, known by his nickname Sasha, spent much of his time synthesizing some of today's most popular and obscure psychedelics, from MDMA to the whole 2C series (2C-B, 2C-I, 2C-T-2, 2C-T-7, and so on). Needless to say, the lab looks like a midcentury mad scientist's lair because, well, that's basically what it was.

Sasha and his wife Ann's land was a hub for Bay Area bohemians, artists, and academics alike, from LSD chemist William Leonard Pickard to astronaut Buzz Aldrin to psychologist Richard Miller. On Easter and the Fourth of July, Sasha and Ann would often host picnics and get-togethers at the "Shulgin Farm," home not only to Sasha's lab but also the cottage where he was born, hand-built by his father, a refugee of the Russian Revolution. During moonlit gatherings, Sasha experimented with psychedelics on himself and a small group of self-selecting friends. Not quite an actual farm, the property features flowers of all kinds, cacti, and verdant foliage offering shade to a dusty stone pathway leading from the main house to the lab—which was licensed by the DEA and the State of California, although it was still raided in 1994.

Today, Sasha and Ann's daughter Wendy and others are committed to keeping the Shulgin legacy alive. Shulgin's lab, later formalized as the Alexander Shulgin Research Institute, continues researching new psychedelics and rediscovering compounds from his vault. The farm also hosts events. Count us in.

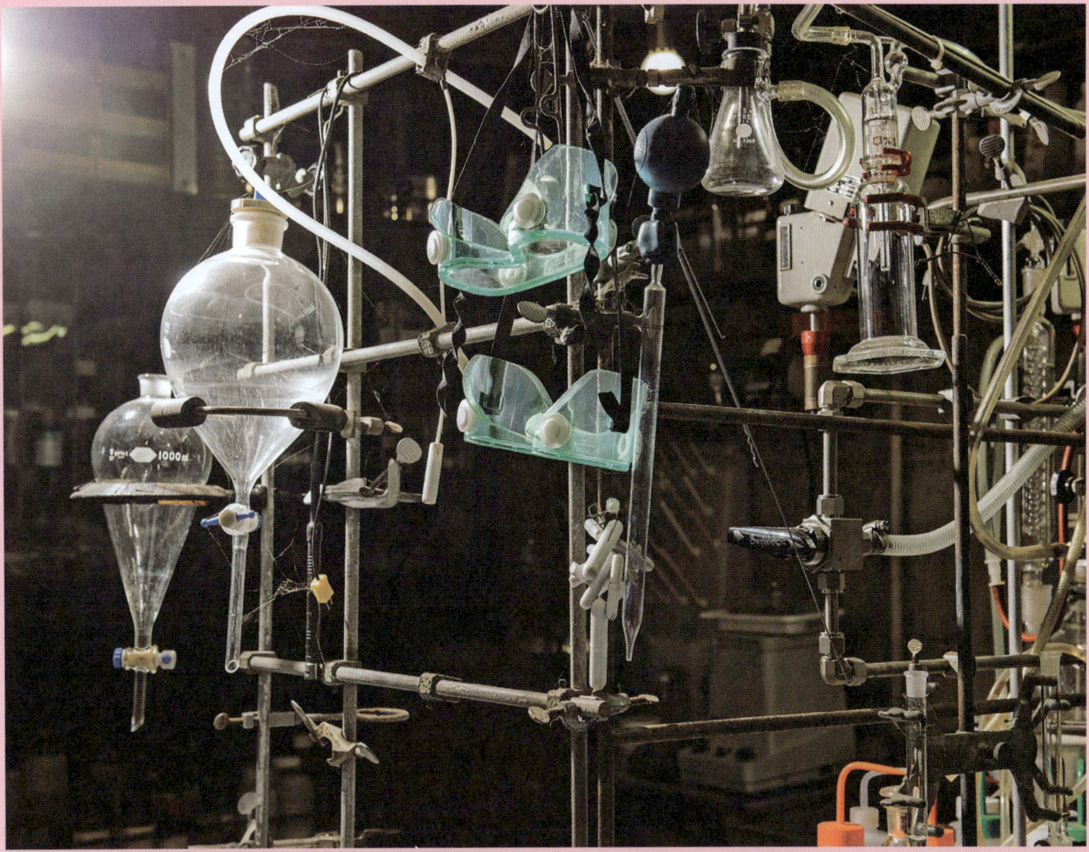

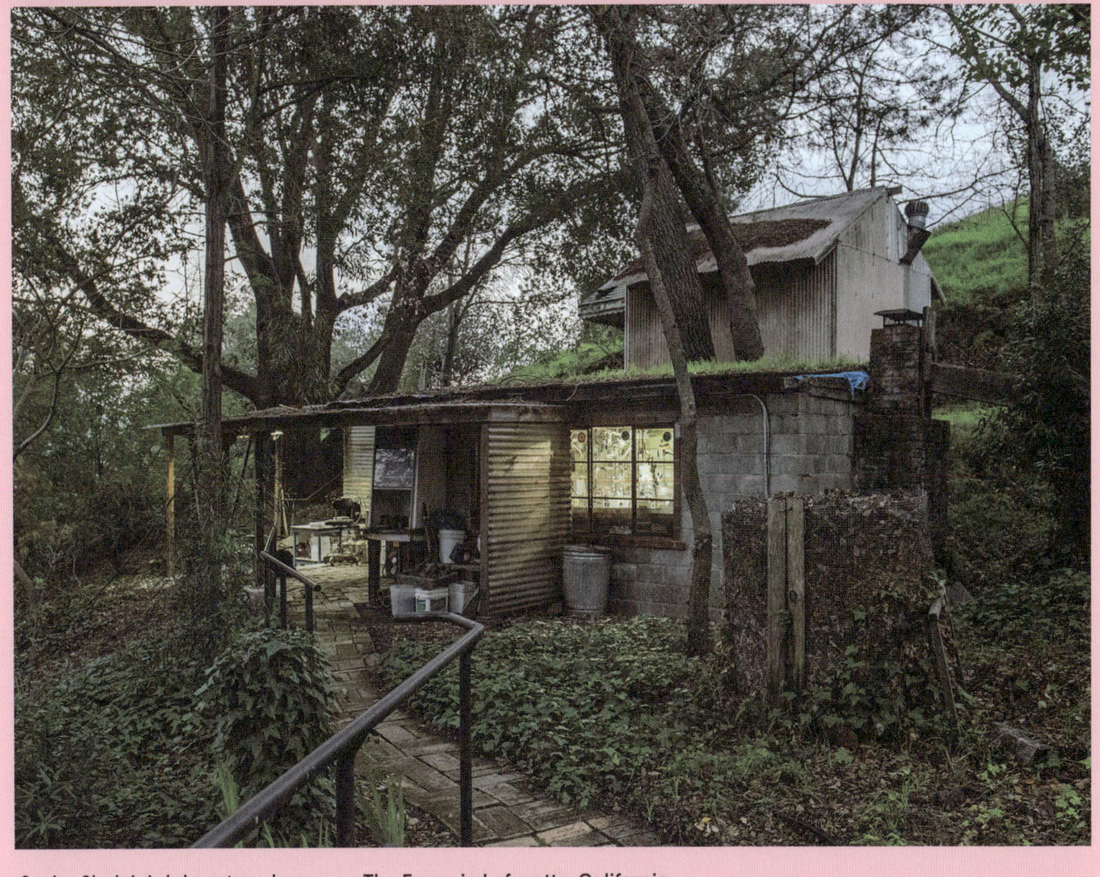

Sasha Shulgin's laboratory, known as The Farm, in Lafayette, California

Types of MDMA

MDMA comes in various forms, including as a white or brown powder (that may come in a capsule or a baggie, depending on how much you get); crystals that are often white, brown, or sometimes purple (also in capsule form or baggies); and as pressed pills that come in different colors and may feature designs. Pure MDMA, also known as molly, comes in the form of raw crystal or powder, although sometimes dealers will say something is "molly" to imply it's pure when it's not. Ecstasy is MDMA mixed with whatever other ingredients are needed to allow it to be pressed into tablet form; these tablets are more likely than other forms of MDMA to be cut with another substance, such as speed (amphetamine or methamphetamine), as well as caffeine, synthetic cathinones ("bath salts"), or other drugs that mimic or modify MDMA's effects. Be careful. Just because someone tells you you're getting high-quality MDMA doesn't mean that you are. That's where testing comes in.

One of the easiest and most straightforward ways to ensure that you have a positive MDMA experience is to make sure that your supply is pure. Although there are many testing kits on the market, we recommend those from the harm reduction nonprofit DanceSafe, as they're trusted and affordable. DanceSafe, a leader in the drug testing world, has been popping up at festivals and selling its kits for decades. Once the testing kit is in your hands, you'll find that it comes with various liquid reagents that enable you to identify whether your substance is actually MDMA and/or whether it contains certain other compounds, such as amphetamines, methamphetamine, and cathinones. You must test for fentanyl separately, but DanceSafe's MDMA testing kit comes with a fentanyl test strip.

What's an MDMA Trip Like?

Taking MDMA can feel a bit like riding a wave. In one moment, you might want to curl up with a loved one and get cozy, while in the next you may want to get up and dance; you might face a flood of emotions or a burst of energy. The effects of the MDMA might come and go, feel up and down, or hot and cold, and you may even want to swivel your head around in a circle. For all these reasons, the experience of taking MDMA is sometimes called "rolling."

Although its effects vary among individuals, MDMA is generally more reliable and consistent than other more classic psychedelics like LSD or mushrooms. It's somewhat common for MDMA to bring on feelings of empathy, compassion, euphoria, self-acceptance, and social connection.

On a physical level, MDMA can help you feel more in your body and sensitive to tactile sensations or stimulation. It can also feel like a wave of energy and calm, though in some cases you may also feel agitated, with effects like locked jaw, teeth grinding, and increased blood pressure or heart rate. It's also not uncommon to experience dry mouth. More on these side effects on page 161.

MDMA generally lasts about five hours. It usually begins to take effect within the first forty minutes of dosing and peaks at around ninety minutes to two hours. Note, however, that everyone is affected differently, and some people may have a longer roll and stronger effects or a delayed peak. Keep in mind that as you're coming down from molly, after the peak, you might feel jittery, tweaky, or anxious. In some cases, on the way up or down, you might also feel dizzy.

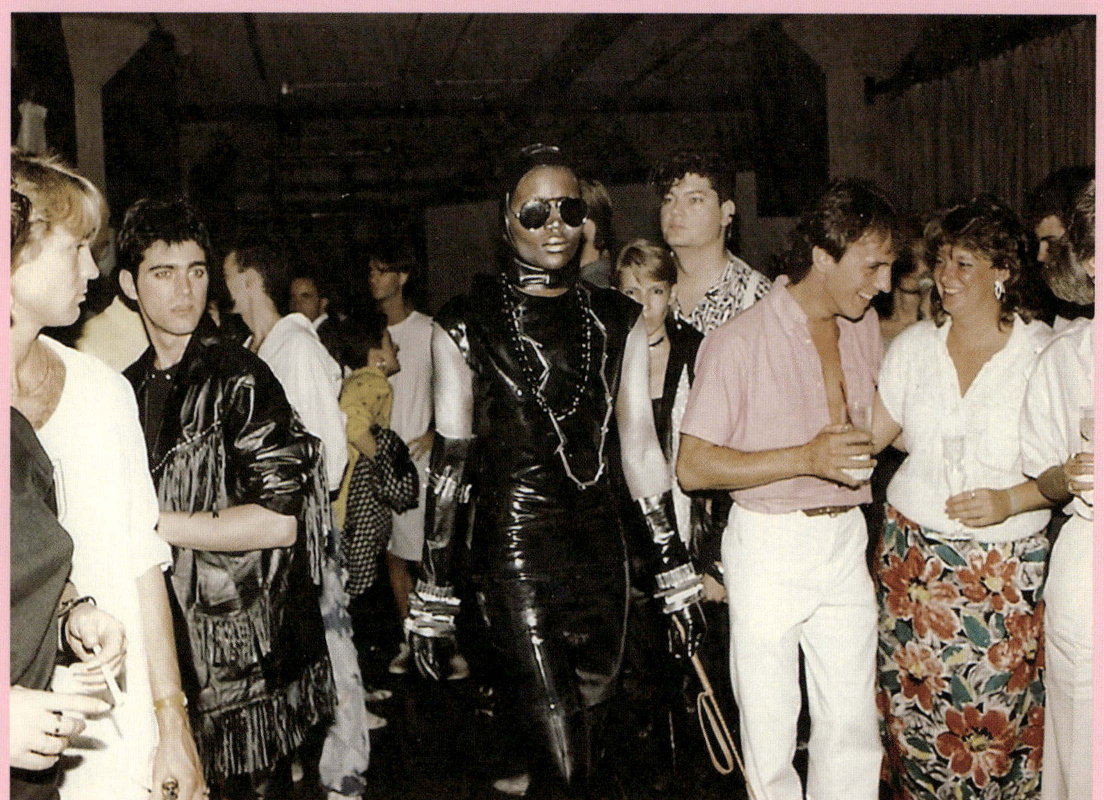

Grace Jones—the legendary Jamaican-born model, singer, and actress—was a frequent attendee at the Starck Club in the eighties and performed there multiple times. Her presence and performances became a defining part of the club's history and lore.

BEYOND THE JOURNEY

THE STARCK CLUB

If we could be transported back in time to any party, we'd probably choose the Starck Club in Dallas, Texas, circa 1984. Designed by French designer Philippe Starck, the club was a hub for avant-garde culture, attracting glittery tastemakers and playing a pivotal role in the emergence of rave culture and the evolution of LGBTQIA+ nightlife. MDMA, then still legal, was widely used at the club, fueling the birth of electronic music as a genre and the inclusive energy that continues to define the underground. The Starck was ultimately shut down after a DEA raid in 1986, but its legacy lives on on dance floors around the world. Beyond the hedonism, club parties continue to serve as meaningful gathering places for queer folks, many of whom, having faced rejection elsewhere, find deep catharsis in nightlife.

MDMA Dosage

A standard dose of MDMA ranges between 80 and 125 milligrams. Sometimes a person may start off on the lower end of that spectrum and take a booster (see page 58) of 30 to 40 milligrams about an hour (or a maximum of two hours) in. If your MDMA comes in the form of a powder or crystal, it's easy to measure the dose with a milligram-accurate drug scale. If you're taking it in the form of a pressed pill, dosage can vary widely, with some pills testing at over 200 milligrams of MDMA—significantly more than a standard dose—so it is recommended to start with a quarter or half of a pill and wait to feel the effects before considering more.

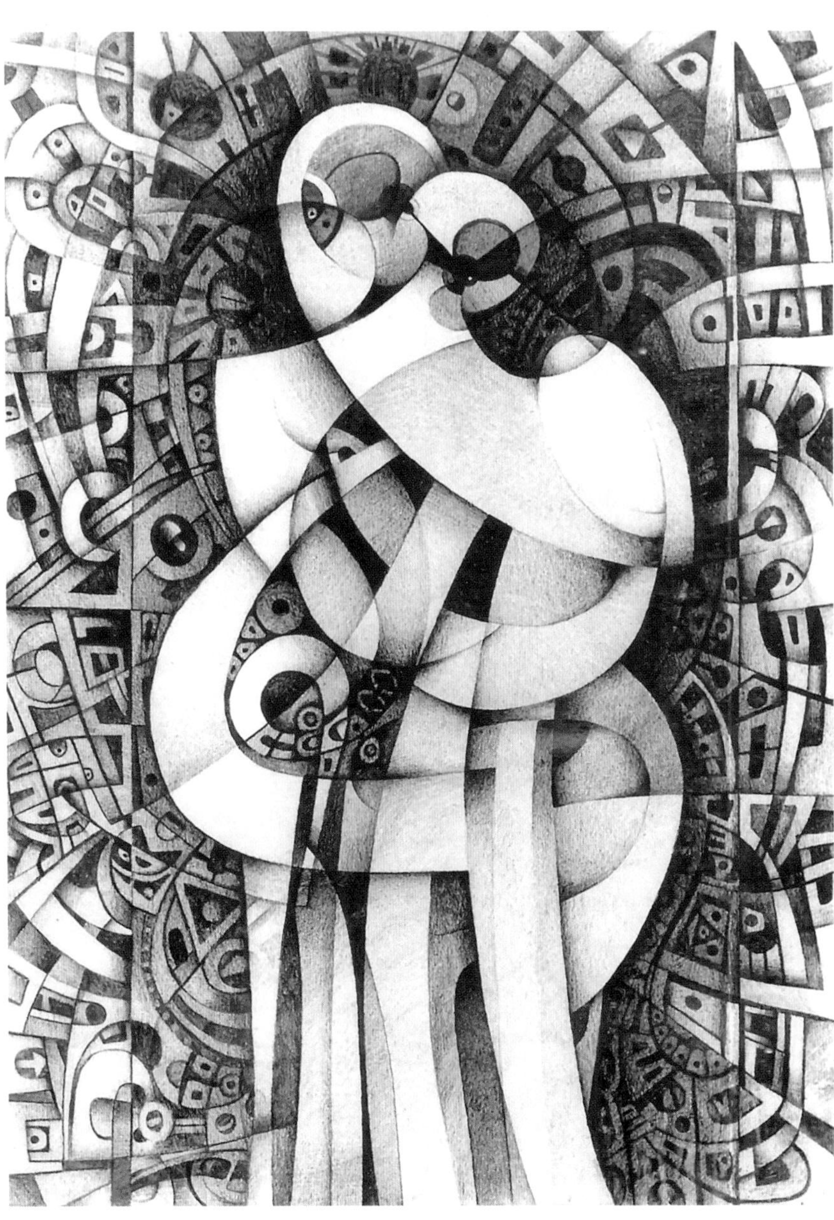

Side Effects of MDMA

While MDMA is more reliably a feel-good substance than psychedelics like shrooms and LSD, it nonetheless comes with its own side effects, such as dry mouth, anxiety, oscillating feelings of coldness and warmth, lack of appetite, clenched jaw, thirst, and high energy. Because MDMA can impact your body's ability to regulate its temperature, be sure to take dancing breaks and stay hydrated in scenarios like hot and sweaty clubs, where in rare cases it's possible to overheat.

While it's important to stay hydrated during your roll (and, ideally, to be hydrated before going into it), be sure not to *over*hydrate, thinking that the dry mouth indicates dehydration. Both dehydration and water toxicity are not unheard-of risks accompanying the MDMA experience. The best way to monitor your intake is to make sure you're drinking roughly eight to sixteen fluid ounces of water per hour; adding electrolytes is a plus. If you're feeling really thirsty, your mouth is dry, or you find yourself biting down on your teeth and you don't want to drink more water, it's good to have throat lozenges on hand. While many people drink alcohol while on MDMA, we don't recommend it—and if you're going to be in a recreational setting where alcohol may be more abundant than water, consider bringing water, or even an iced herbal tea or coconut water, with you.

In the days following an MDMA experience, it's not uncommon to feel a little down or lethargic or to have decreased appetite or slight changes to your immunity. This doesn't happen to everyone, however, and for some people, the day after MDMA feels light and joyful, and they're able to revel in the positive memories of the experience.

The quality of the MDMA and how you take it might affect how you feel the following day. While pure MDMA doesn't often cause an intense come-down, if your stash is impure, the adulterants might influence your recovery. If you took too high of a dose, or if you didn't wait long enough in between rolls, it's also possible to feel a little fried or blue in the aftermath.

Because MDMA causes the brain to release more serotonin, a neurotransmitter that regulates mood, emotion, and sleep, it may be risky to roll too often. The brain needs time to restore serotonin levels naturally. Using MDMA too frequently may lead to long-term serotonin depletion, which may result in depression, anxiety, and memory problems. This is why the general recommendation is to wait about three months in between each time you take MDMA, but not everyone follows this standard, and even people in clinical trials that include multiple dosing sessions are scheduled to ingest it more frequently.

In the psychedelic community, it's common for people to take supplements such as 5-HTP and magnesium following an MDMA experience to try to combat the serotonin depletion and aid in recovery. There's no harm in doing this and there's some scientific rationale behind it, but it's worth noting that there isn't any real data to support this practice.

Risks and Contraindications

As noted, MDMA can be adulterated with other substances, some of which may be dangerous, but this risk is easy to avoid by simply using a drug testing kit.

MDMA is different from classic psychedelics like LSD and psilocybin in that it can be physiologically toxic in high doses and for people with compromised health. The deaths attributed to MDMA have all been caused by hyperthermia and cardiovascular collapse, generally due to very high doses or repeated high doses. MDMA is contraindicated for people with high blood pressure. Other risks to be aware of include overexertion during the MDMA experience and drinking too much or too little water (see page 161). MDMA might also make you more impulsive, so be sure that you're in a relatively safe place and in safe company when you roll.

While it's not recommended that anyone do any psychedelic while pregnant, it's particularly risky to do MDMA.

It remains up for debate as to whether it's best to wean off an SSRI or SNRI prior to taking a classic psychedelic, but a facilitator is more likely to recommend it for MDMA due to the risk of serotonin syndrome. Common wisdom is, if you're on such meds, abstain from MDMA and definitely do not take "extra" to compensate for the reduced effect.

Most important, do not take too much MDMA. While it's rare, it is possible to overdose on MDMA. That said, as with the other psychedelics, MDMA is relatively safe so long as you do your homework and prepare properly. And the upside is that, for people who are afraid of a "bad trip," it can be a gentler way into exploring consciousness-shifting experiences.

Final Thoughts

While research on MDMA-assisted therapy has made strides, legal access remains fragmented. Unlike some other psychedelics, MDMA has been largely excluded from decriminalization measures, with progress confined to patchwork legislation being introduced at the state level around lifting barriers to research and access ahead of FDA approval. Veterans' groups, recognizing the urgent need for solutions to address PTSD, have been at the forefront of advocacy, working to influence policy at both state and federal levels. You can support this effort by calling your legislators, urging them to review the promising research, advocate for federal funding of MDMA and psychedelic research, and ensure veterans and others in need gain access to these therapies.

Reciprocity in the context of MDMA means taking care of the people around you. MDMA is among the psychedelics most often linked to hospitalizations, frequently because of preventable harm—such as drinking alcohol, consuming unsafe substances, or overhydrating while on MDMA. One of the simplest but most impactful ways to engage in reciprocity is by educating others about harm reduction. Encourage people to test their drugs using kits from organizations like DanceSafe, share information about safe practices, and watch out for one another. Helping someone stay safe during an MDMA experience, whether through education or practical support, is an act of care that strengthens the communal spirit inherent to this medicine. It also decreases the chances of incidents that could derail the progress we're making in getting MDMA on the market as a federally legal therapeutic treatment.

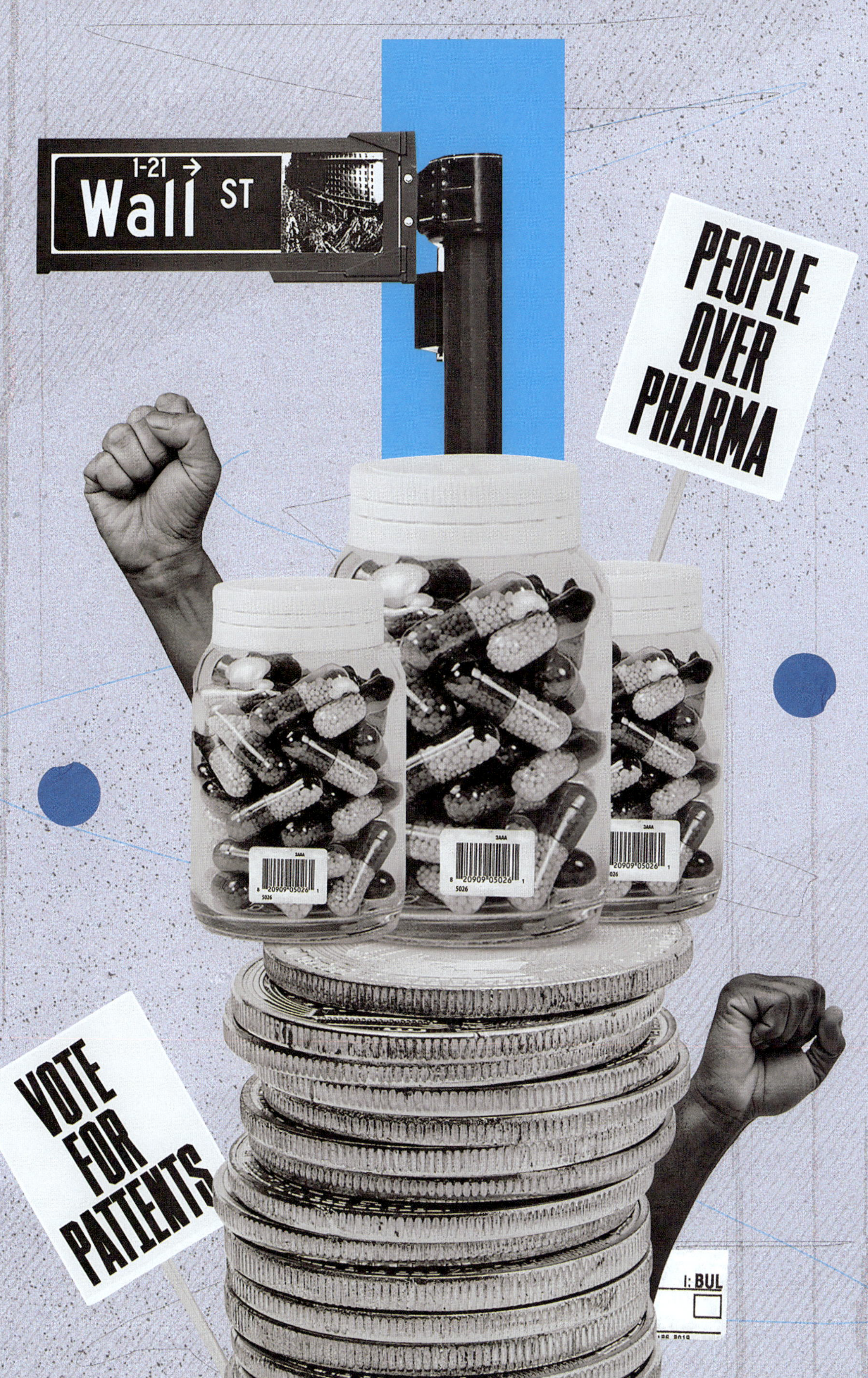
1-21 →
Wall ST
PEOPLE OVER PHARMA
VOTE FOR PATIENTS

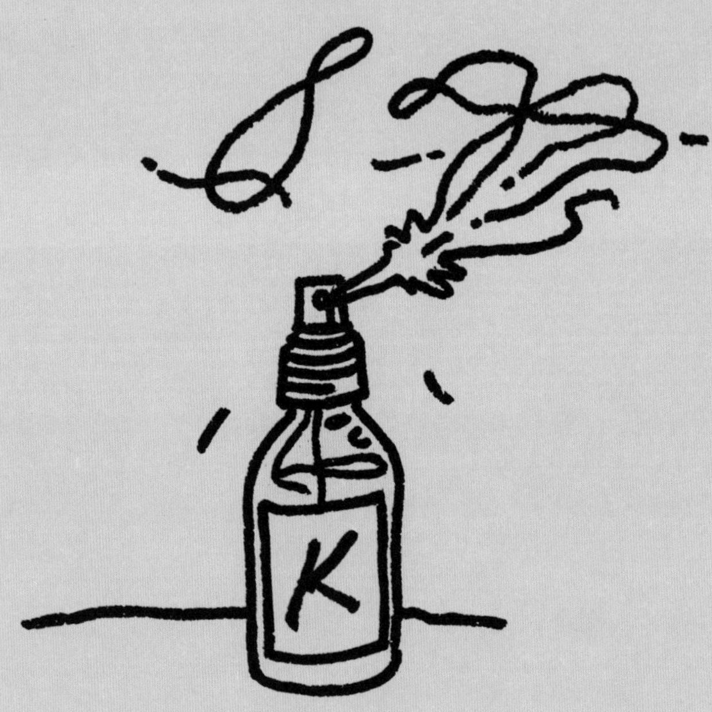
K

CHAPTER 10

KETAMINE

Perhaps you've heard of ketamine already, whether from the party scene, where it's akin to what cocaine was in the 1980s, or from talk among clinicians and their patients, as ketamine clinics proliferate across the country.

While ketamine does carry profound psychoactive potential, whether it can be called "psychedelic" is up for debate. Officially, ketamine is a dissociative anesthetic that can produce out-of-body effects that may offer the user insights from a fresh perspective. Unlike most classic psychedelic substances, ketamine is legal, though it must be prescribed, and it is used throughout the world to treat mental health conditions like depression and trauma.

Ketamine can be a transformative experience, especially for psychedelic newbies who are afraid of a more traditional trip, want to have a legal experience, and/or want to ensure that their vitals are being monitored in a clinic while they are journeying. The beauty of ketamine is that, due to its legality, folks who are elderly, have a history of trauma, or just feel they need more support can have this experience in a supervised environment. It can also be a great way to dip your toe into the psychedelic universe without diving fully in.

A fairly novel substance, ketamine was developed in 1962 by Calvin Stevens, a chemist who was working for Parke-Davis & Company (today a subsidiary of Pfizer). The idea was to create a somewhat less hallucinogenic and faster-acting agent than its chemical cousin phencyclidine (PCP). While both ketamine and PCP were originally developed as pharmaceutical anesthetics, PCP has since become subject to harsh stigma due to its popularity as a street drug, while ketamine (despite also being used in underground settings) benefits from its association with high-end clinics.

Less than a decade after it was first synthesized, ketamine gained FDA approval as an anesthetic to treat soldiers wounded in the Vietnam War. Today, it is one of the most widely used medications for pediatric surgery, emergency sedation, and acute pain management. It's also administered for mental health as an "off label" treatment. (This means that the FDA approved it for one purpose—as an anesthetic—but it's shown promise for another, mental health.) Its off-label use is not covered by insurance, and a round of infusions in a clinic typically costs several thousands of dollars. The one exception is Spravato, a ketamine nasal spray that was approved by the FDA for use in treating depression in 2019 (more on that on pages 170 and 171).

Because low doses of ketamine can give the user feelings of euphoria and social ease, it's also a recreational favorite in clubs, on the dance floor, and at festivals like Burning Man and Lightning in a Bottle. From the 1970s through the 1990s, ketamine grew in popularity as a party drug, becoming a central part of rave culture. By 1999, due to its ubiquity in the underground, it became a Schedule III controlled substance. Nonetheless, nowadays more people than ever before are using it in a variety of forms, from nasal sprays to lozenges.

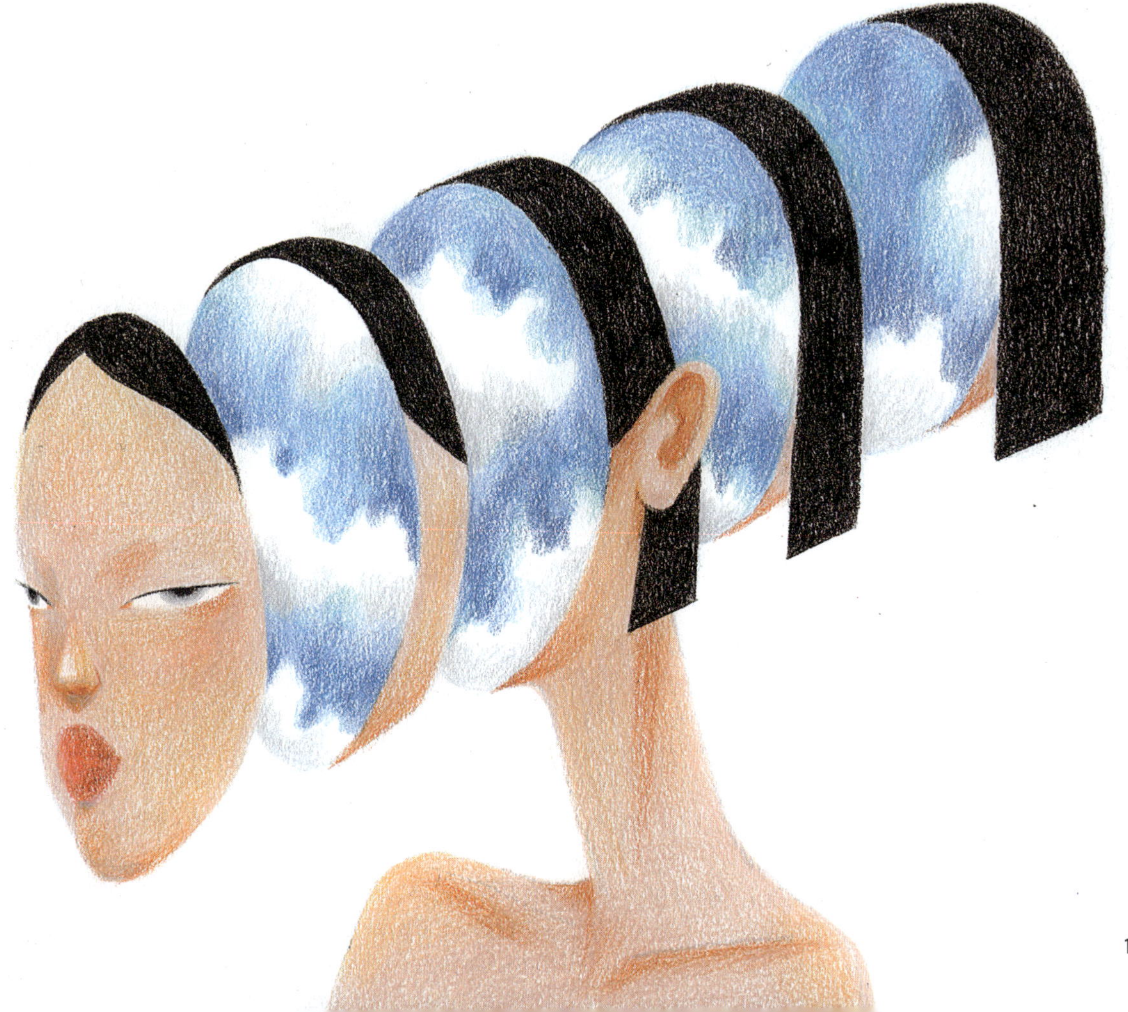

THE KETA-VERSE AND DOLPHINS ON PSYCHEDELICS

Both a controversial and celebrated figure, dismissed as a madman and revered as a genius, John Cunningham Lilly was perhaps one of the most far-out researchers to experiment with psychedelics. Impelled by an ever-burning desire to push the frontiers of human knowledge, Lilly built a career spanning eclectic heights: He was a physician, neuroscientist, psychoanalyst, consciousness researcher, and inventor all in one.

In 1954, Lilly invented the isolation tank, sometimes referred to as a flotation tank, as a means of sensory deprivation. Far from sensory deprivation, he reported that the isolation tank was able to induce a multiplicity of altered states of consciousness, ranging from waking dreams to out-of-body experiences to encounters with alternate dimensions. It was during Lilly's long periods spent in isolation tanks that he began to wonder if there were any intelligent beings that, like humans, demonstrated complex cognition and social behavior, but spent their entire lives in water, experiencing a state of weightless immersion. Lilly shared this reflection with his friend Pete Shoreliner, who suggested dolphins.

Lilly began to study them, becoming mesmerized by their large brain size and coming to believe they were a superior form of intelligence that represented exciting possibilities for interspecies communication. His theories around interspecies communication had special significance for astronomers like Carl Sagan, who felt that such research could help set a precedent for establishing communication with extraterrestrial life forms. This helped Lilly secure financial backing from NASA and other government agencies to build a lab in the Caribbean in 1963.

Eventually, amidst controversy around his unorthodox research methods, funding for Lilly's dolphin research dried up. Upon returning to the States, Lilly decided to focus on his own writings and experimentations in consciousness. In the early 1970s, his writings and interests became increasingly opaque when he began combining his sessions in the sensory deprivation tank with ketamine.

Perhaps overcommitted to understanding the inner realities opened up by ketamine, there was a point at which he ingested 50 milligrams every hour on the hour for twenty-two hours a day for three weeks. It was in a ketamine vision that he came to believe in the "Solid State Intelligence," a malevolent entity that would arise from human computational systems and evolve into an autonomous bioform bent on destroying humanity. He also became convinced of the existence of a hierarchical group of cosmic entities, which he referred to as the "Earth Coincidence Control Office," or E.C.C.O., part of a much larger cosmic institution, steering the long-term coincidences of his life, fatefully guiding him in specific directions.

Lilly passed away in 2001, at the age of eighty-six, from heart failure. In spite of his mishaps and unorthodox research methods, Lilly's contributions to both science and psychedelics have left a permanent imprint on modern culture. His prolonged sessions in his sensory deprivation tank with psychedelics served to shape the narrative of the 1980 film *Altered States*, and he was also likely the inspiration behind the Sega Genesis game *Ecco the Dolphin* and the *Flipper* [TV] series. Perhaps more importantly, his work with dolphins changed the public perception of marine creatures, laying the foundation for the Marine Mammal Protection Act of 1972, the first act of the United States Congress to call specifically for an ecosystem approach to wildlife management.

This excerpt comes from a story reported for DoubleBlind's print magazine by Jasmine Virdi.

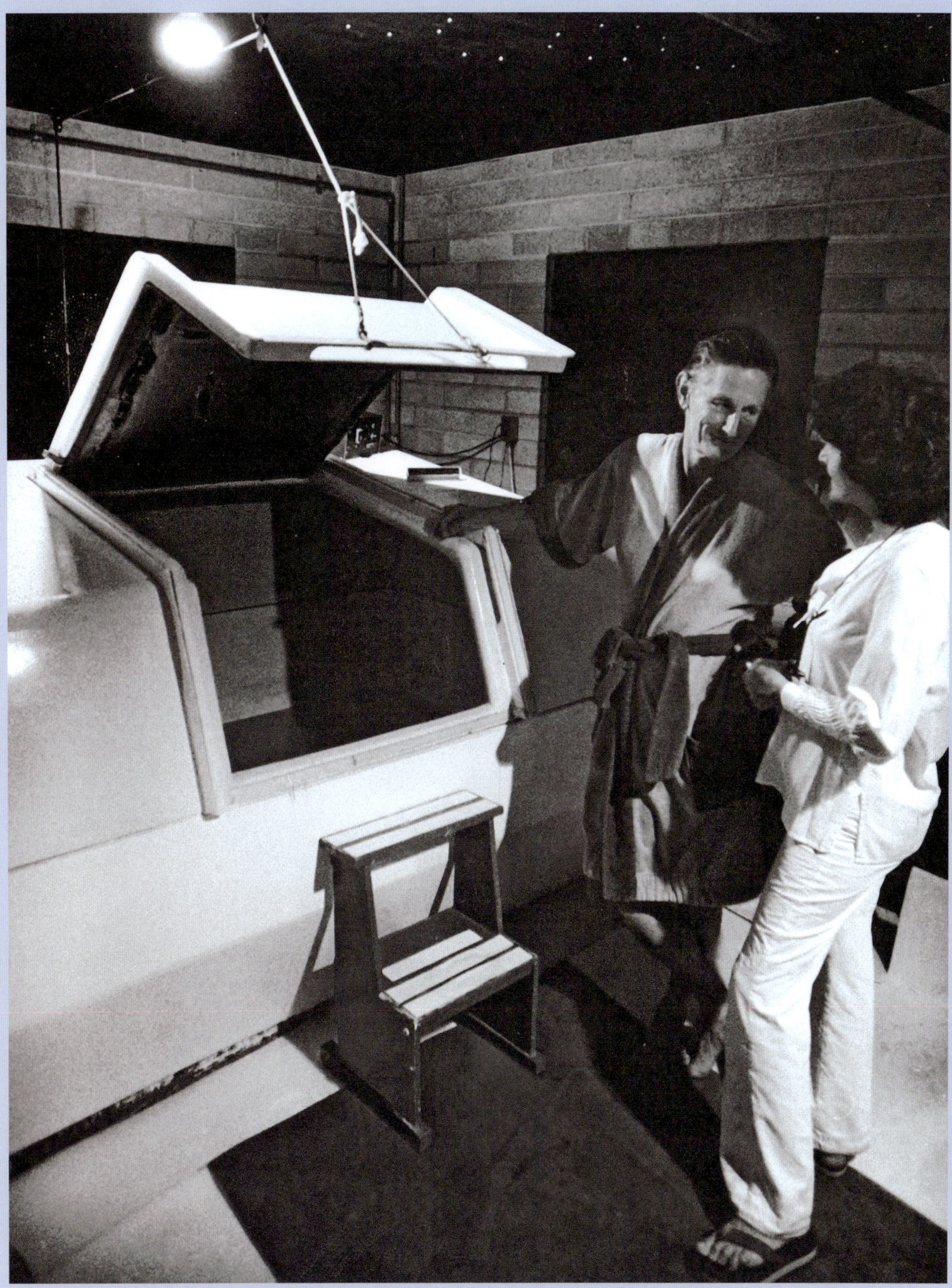

Physician and psychoanalyst Dr. John Lilly decompressing with his wife, Toni, after being in an isolation tank for an hour

Types of Ketamine

To understand the types of ketamine, it helps to start with basic chemistry. Many molecules, including ketamine, exist in two forms, called enantiomers. These are like mirror-image versions of the same molecule—but because of their opposite orientations, they're not *exactly* the same (similar to how your right and left hands are mirror images but don't match if you try to place them on top of each other). These mirrored forms can have slightly different effects in the body.

In ketamine's case, the two enantiomers are S-ketamine (also called esketamine, which is the "left-handed" version) and R-ketamine (also called arketamine, the "right-handed" version). Most generic ketamine is a mix of both types, known as a "racemic" solution. Spravato, the ketamine nasal spray brought to market by Johnson & Johnson Innovative Medicine, is an exception; it consists only of S-ketamine.

According to the FDA, S-ketamine is different from racemic ketamine, although both are used in mental health treatment (albeit off-label in the case of the latter).

Some say that R-ketamine, which doesn't have official FDA approval for depression, has fewer hallucinogenic, dissociative, and dopaminergic effects. While there isn't much research on R-ketamine for depression, some research does point to its efficacy in forming new neural connections, which may enable it to have greater potency and longevity in the integration period, while producing fewer side effects than S-ketamine. Currently, no R-ketamine products are commercially available, but several pharmaceutical companies and researchers are actively exploring its development for clinical use.

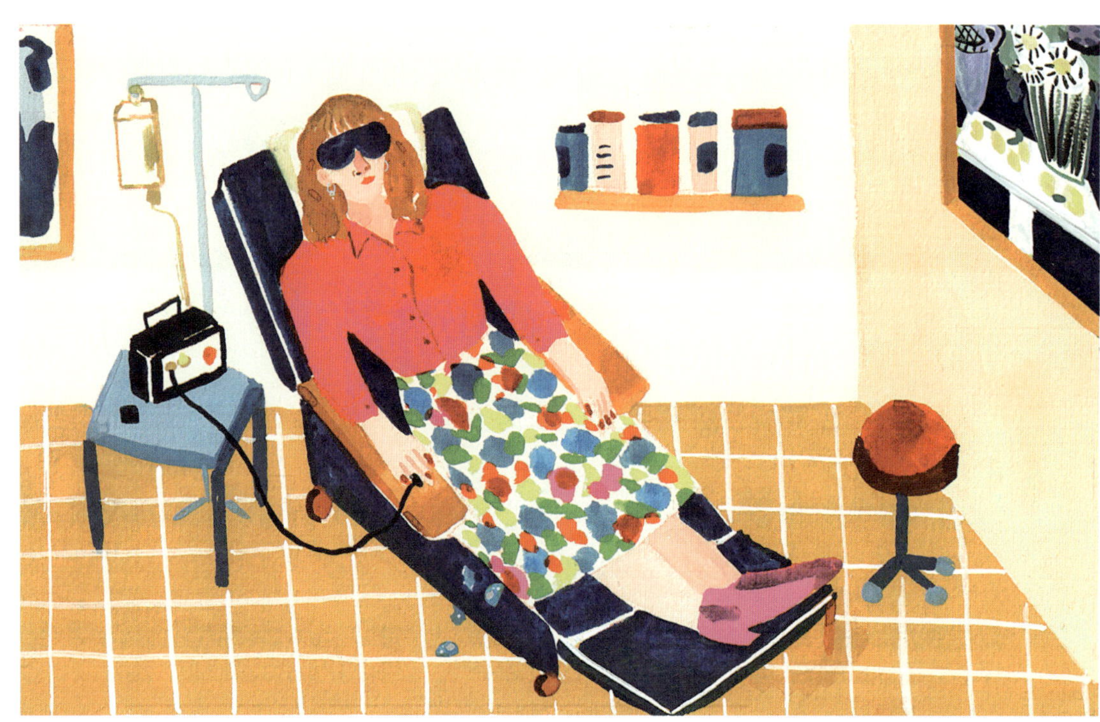

The Price of Healing

One of the biggest arguments for getting psychedelics approved by the FDA is that they may then be covered by insurance. Ketamine reveals the complexities of that issue. When a drug is approved by the FDA, it is approved for a particular condition, such as major depressive disorder or post-traumatic stress disorder. If a doctor prescribes the drug for something else (called "off label" treatment), insurance likely won't cover that treatment. This is why ketamine infusions are so expensive, and the same will be true if doctors are prescribing any psychedelic for conditions it wasn't approved for. At the time of writing, for example, the ketamine nasal spray Spravato costs around $590 per session. If a patient qualifies for it through their insurance and a savings program operated by Spravato, however, the cost can be as low as $10.

---

ketatation
noun

a meditation that involves ketamine, typically in a light dose that enables a person to sink more deeply into the present without disassociating

---

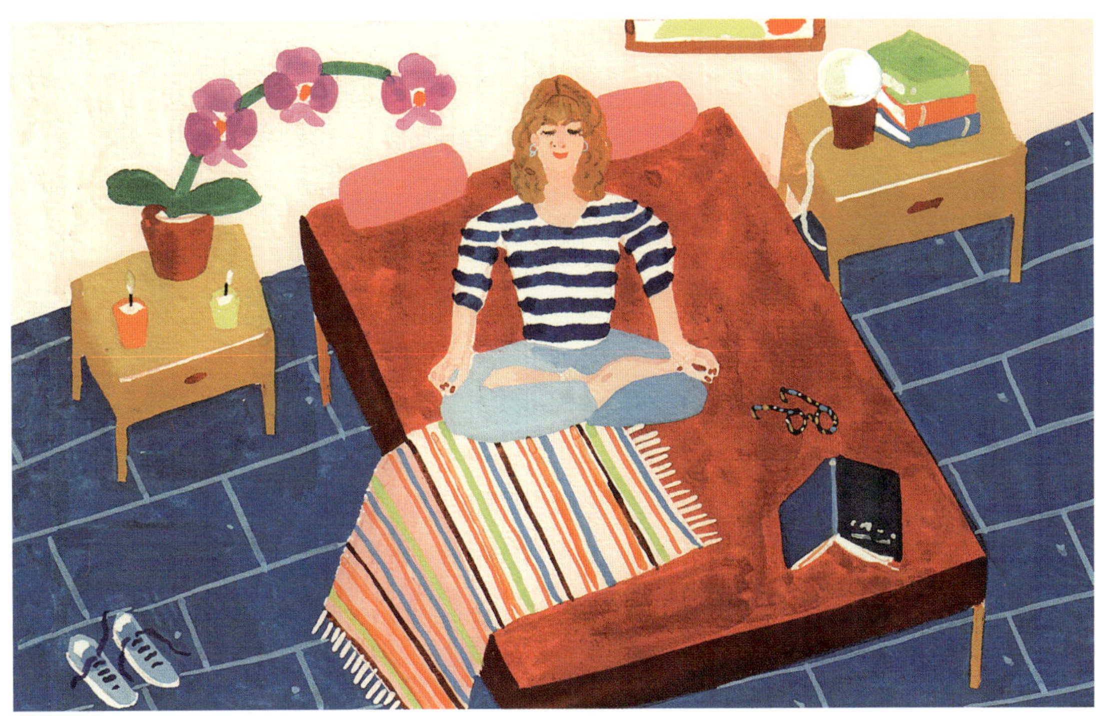

Delivery Methods

Ketamine comes in many different shapes and sizes, literally. If you're obtaining ketamine underground, you're likely going to snort it. You'll often get it as a fine powder, which is ready for insufflation, or larger crystals or clumps that need to be crushed. If you get the latter, first you must grind it up into a fine powder. If you do not grind it, the salt-like crystals can damage your nasal passages.

If you're doing ketamine aboveground, your choices will likely be insufflation, intravenous, intramuscular, sublingual, and oral. Note that if you go to a clinic for ketamine treatment, even after the experience ends, you may feel a little woozy and should exercise caution. Do not drive and make sure to have a loved one available to take you home and get you settled.

Now, let's go over some of the basics of delivery methods.

INSUFFLATION

Ketamine can be snorted as a powder or sniffed in the form of a nasal spray. Ketamine is processed by intramucosal tissue, not by your stomach, so when snorting, make sure to avoid swallowing the "drip" that will occur. It is best not to snort as hard with ketamine as you would with cocaine so as to allow the most intramucosal absorption possible. Swallowing ketamine reduces its bioavailability and can result in a less predictable or less effective experience, as it is metabolized differently when absorbed through the stomach. Some people put their powder or crystal ketamine into a nasal spray bottle to make intranasal ingestion easier, which is a great practice for nose health.

The onset of effects for nasal ketamine is rapid, within minutes. The peak of the experience occurs around twenty to thirty minutes after use. Overall, the main effects last approximately forty-five minutes to one hour, though residual effects, such as mild dissociation or an afterglow, may linger for one to two hours. Nasal methods have lower bioavailability than IV (intravenous) and IM (intramuscular) methods, meaning that a smaller percentage of the drug is absorbed into the bloodstream and reaches the brain compared to these other delivery methods.

INTRAVENOUS (IV)

Ketamine can be administered through an IV drip stationed in a vein for the duration of the experience. This is one of the most popular methods of administration within clinical settings. The onset is rapid, and the sessions usually last about an hour to an hour and a half, with the effects ending shortly after the IV drip is removed. Unlike with insufflation, the IV method allows for precise dosing and 100 percent bioavailability. One downside is that you won't have as much freedom to move around, because the IV needs to remain in place.

INTRAMUSCULAR (IM)

Alternately, ketamine may be delivered through a shot in the arm as an intramuscular injection. This is also a popular clinical method of administration. The onset and duration of IM ketamine might be slower than IV or nasal administration, but it may last longer, with the effects typically persisting for 90 minutes to two hours. IM ketamine might be among the more intense forms of the drug, with high bioavailability (almost at the level of IV ketamine). Note, however, that the dosage is fixed. Think of it like a shot. It's administered once and typically no more is given after that, as opposed to an IV drip that is consistently delivering ketamine into the bloodstream throughout the session.

SUBLINGUAL

Sublingual ketamine is typically administered via lozenges or troches that are held in the mouth—either under the tongue or between the cheek and gum—to allow the drug to be absorbed through the mucous membranes. This method enables ketamine to enter the bloodstream through the oral venous system, which can partially bypass the liver's first-pass metabolism. However, this bypass is only partial. Many users unintentionally or intentionally swallow some portion of the dose, especially as the lozenge dissolves, which means a portion of the drug is still absorbed through the gastrointestinal tract and processed by the liver. As a result, both unmetabolized ketamine and its primary metabolite, norketamine, can enter systemic circulation, potentially leading to a two-phase experience—with an initial peak from mucosal absorption and a second wave of effects once the swallowed portion is metabolized.

The onset of effects is relatively slow, usually occurring after fifteen to thirty minutes, and the experience can last several hours. While the bioavailability of sublingual ketamine is still lower than that of IV or IM routes, it is higher than that of swallowing a pill because it avoids first-pass metabolism—at least in part. Sublingual bioavailability is estimated to be between 24 and 30 percent, though this can vary based on how long the lozenge is held in the mouth and how much is swallowed.

Doses vary widely. Lozenges typically range from 100 to 300 milligrams, but some are as high as 400 milligrams. In some cases, patients are instructed to take multiple lozenges in one session, with total dosages reaching 500 to 600 milligrams or more. While lower doses (100 to 200 milligrams) tend to produce a mild, floaty dissociation, doses above 300 milligrams can become deeply psychedelic, especially with eyes closed.

ORAL (SWALLOWED)

In medical terminology, *oral administration* refers specifically to swallowing a capsule or tablet, in which case the drug is absorbed through the gastrointestinal (GI) tract. Swallowed ketamine typically has lower bioavailability—around 17 to 20 percent—compared to other delivery methods, and it has a longer onset and duration due to digestion and liver processing. While this method is considered less efficient for delivering ketamine, some research suggests that the metabolites may still contribute meaningfully to antidepressant effects. The onset of swallowed ketamine usually occurs within twenty to sixty minutes, and the experience tends to last for three to six hours. Typical oral doses in clinical or experimental settings range from 1 to 3 milligrams per kilogram of body weight, which is approximately 70 to 200 milligrams for most adults, though higher doses of up to 5 to 7 milligrams per kilogram are sometimes used in palliative care or investigational protocols. This route is rarely used in clinical practice due to its unpredictability and inefficiency, but it's occasionally employed in specific at-home protocols or experimental contexts.

QUESTIONS TO ASK YOUR KETAMINE PROVIDER

When considering ketamine therapy, it's essential to research and vet your provider thoroughly, as clinics can vary significantly in their level of integrity and approach. Just as you would evaluate a psychedelic retreat, understanding how the session will be structured, who will be present, and the type of support offered is crucial to ensuring a safe and meaningful experience. Below are some key questions to guide your evaluation and help you make an informed decision, ensuring that the clinic or provider aligns with your needs and offers not only safety but also the emotional and therapeutic support to make your ketamine experience as effective and meaningful as possible:

- What does the entire session look like, from beginning to end?
- What is the environment like during the session? What sort of music and lighting will be present? Where will you be seated?
- Who will be present if you need support? Will this person offer just medical support (like a nurse practitioner), or are they trained to provide emotional support as well?
- If the clinic's supervisory person leaves the room, how will you be monitored, and will there be a way to call for assistance if needed?
- What are the clinic's success rates? How do they measure their success?
- Is the clinic's approach rooted in a therapeutic model? Will someone work with you to establish a rapport ahead of time, discuss your intentions, and help you integrate the experience afterward?
- How does the clinic ensure your physical safety during the experience?
- Are post-session integration or follow-up sessions offered as part of the care model?
- What does the clinic typically recommend to patients after the first batch of sessions? Do patients typically come in for "tune-ups," and, if so, how often?

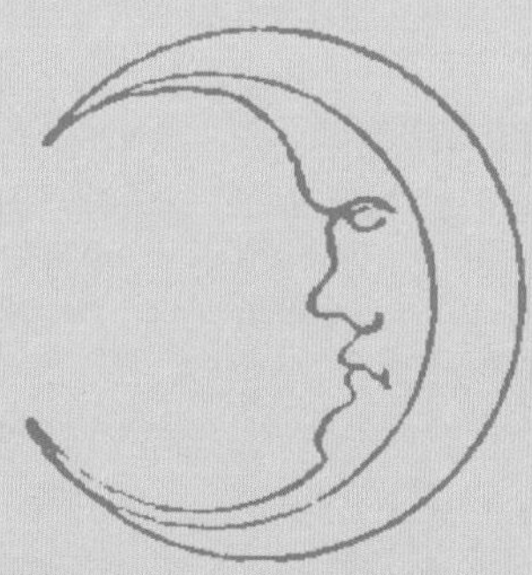

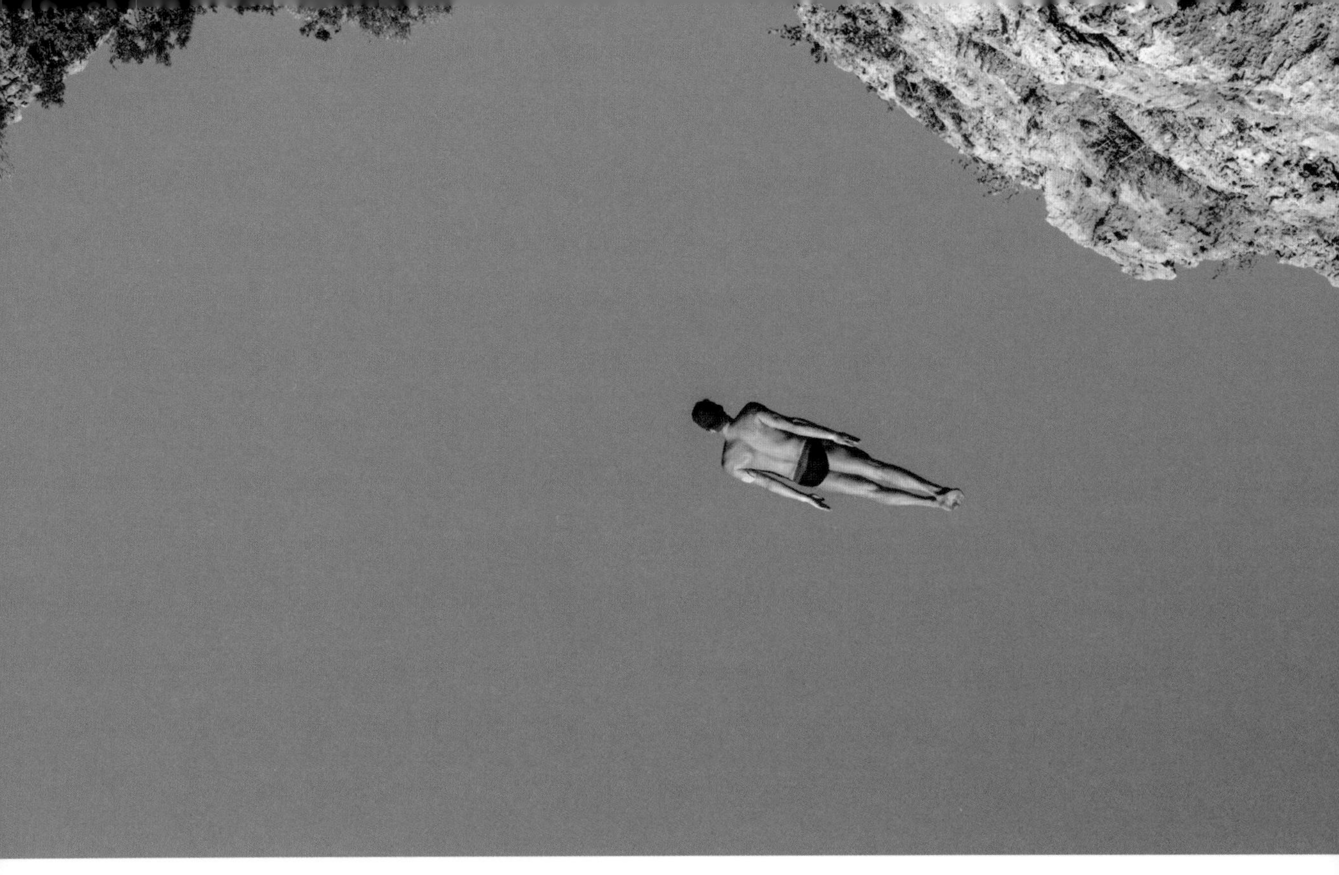

Mail-Order Ketamine

If you're interested in psychedelics and have been researching them online, those pesky pixels that track our web activity may have picked up on it and started advertising ketamine lozenges to you. It's hard for even us to believe, but a growing number of telehealth companies are now running targeted ads on social media platforms with text like "Want to try psychedelics right at home? What are you waiting for? Start now for $299."

Believe it or not, what these companies are doing is legal. During the COVID-19 pandemic, Congress passed provisions that allow clinicians to prescribe medications virtually, a legal shift that transformed both the ketamine industry and health care at large. Perhaps the most well-known company in this field is Mindbloom, but several others have followed. You basically fill out a form and have a Zoom call with a licensed health professional about your intentions for wanting to journey, and then, assuming there aren't any red flags, they send you ketamine in the mail.

The ketamine, which looks like a throat lozenge and typically tastes bitter, comes with goodies such as an eye mask, a journal, and a digital portal with videos on how to take the ketamine, meditations for the session, and more. The upside is that the ketamine is much more accessible financially and comes right to your home. Some people just prefer the convenience and comfort of journeying in their home, as opposed to in a clinic. Many have reported transformative experiences from doing lozenges at home, but others are concerned that this model doesn't come with enough oversight. These companies ask you to agree that you'll have a sitter present, but there's no one making sure that you do, and these experiences, just like classic psychedelic trips, can bring unconscious material to the fore. This model is a reminder to be critical. Whether it's a telehealth company, a retreat center, or a facilitator, be sure you always trust your source of information.

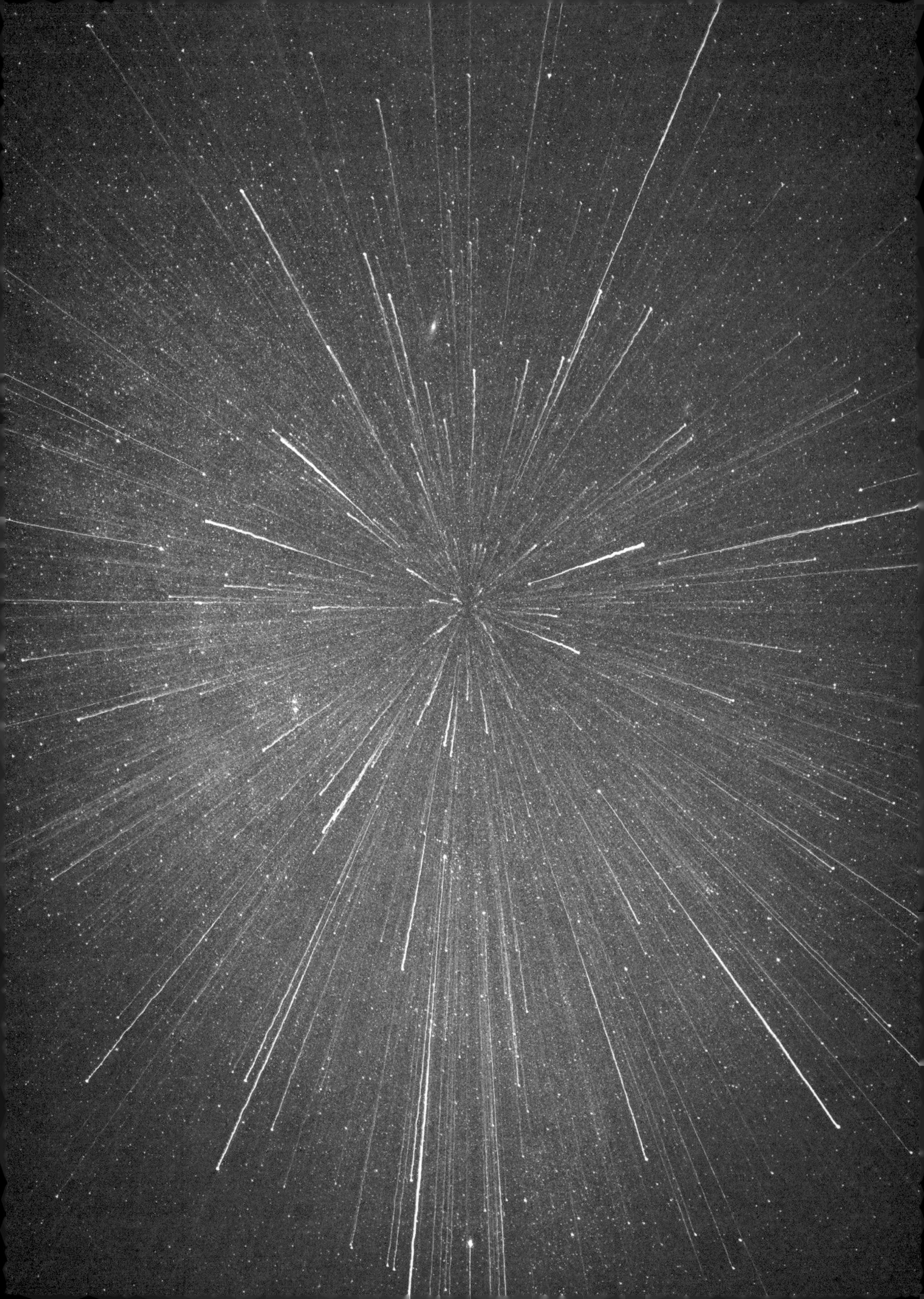

What's a Ketamine Trip Like?

At lower doses, ketamine can feel like something of a "clean drunk," producing floaty, dreamy, or trancelike effects. At higher doses, it might cause feelings of dissociation or being out of body, making it hard to physically move around. (It's important to ensure that someone under the influence of ketamine has somewhere to sit or lie down if the effects become more intense.) At higher doses, some people enter what is often referred to as a "K-hole." This intense, out-of-body experience can feel near-death-like, with sensations such as rising above your own body or being teleported to another world. A true K-hole occurs when someone ingests an anesthetic-level dose of ketamine. While some intentionally seek out this state, others can land there accidentally, which can be disorienting or frightening. If you're trying to intentionally enter a K-hole, it's generally recommended to start slow and steady, gradually increasing the dosage.

Many people assume ketamine isn't as psychedelic as substances like shrooms or LSD, but that's not true. With a blindfold and at high doses, people can enter other dimensions and lose their sense of reality and self entirely. They may experience colorful, vivid visions, distortions of space and time, and full-blown emotional releases, ranging from laughter to tears. People also describe the ketamine universe as having its own unique qualities, sometimes referred to as "astral" or "galactic." Others report feeling weightless, floating, or traveling through space, often accompanied by vivid imagery of stars, galaxies, or vast open landscapes.

It remains up for debate whether these psychedelic experiences are therapeutic in themselves or whether ketamine's benefits, such as combating depression, are due to its ability to help the brain form new connections. Many clinics and telehealth companies mailing ketamine lozenges for at-home use do not provide integration support, which some researchers and therapists view as unethical. These professionals believe that insights gained from ketamine journeys are just as valuable as those achieved through other types of psychedelic experiences. Whether you are pursuing ketamine therapeutically or recreationally, it's strongly recommended to have proper integration support to help you process the journey.

Ketamine Dosage

When doing ketamine for personal use in a nonclinical environment, most people snort "bumps," or small lines of ketamine of about 30 to 60 milligrams. The effects come on within five to fifteen minutes, and 100 milligrams is usually enough to enter a full dissociative state, or K-hole. The effects last for forty-five minutes to one hour, with most people returning to a complete baseline within one and a half to two hours.

Whether you make it yourself or purchase it underground, a ketamine nasal spray often comes in a 10-milliliter bottle containing around 100 milligrams of ketamine in total, which works out to a concentration of 10 milligrams per milliliter—or roughly 10 milligrams per spray, depending on the sprayer mechanism. But some bottles may contain significantly more ketamine—as much as 1,500 milligrams—so it's important to start slowly and understand what you're working with.

A cautious starting dose is one spray per nostril, or about 20 milligrams total, then waiting five to fifteen minutes to gauge the effects. Most people will need around 30 milligrams or more to feel noticeable effects. The K-hole threshold—a dissociative, out-of-body state—typically begins around 60 to 125 milligrams, or six to twelve sprays if your bottle delivers 10 milligrams per spray. The entire experience generally lasts forty-five to sixty minutes.

A therapeutic dose of ketamine generally starts at around 25 milligrams, though this can vary significantly depending on the route of administration and the individual's body weight and sensitivity. For IV use, a dose of 25 milligrams or higher may be appropriate for a person weighing around 110 pounds, with 100 milligrams representing a higher-end or dissociative threshold for someone of that weight.

The so-called "K-hole" state can potentially occur at much lower doses, especially when the drug is administered all at once intramuscularly rather than slowly via IV infusion. For example, 60 milligrams given intramuscularly may be sufficient to induce this state in some individuals. Much depends on the person's sensitivity and how rapidly the ketamine enters the system.

In clinical settings, IV protocols typically begin at around 0.5 milligram per kilogram of body weight, administered over forty minutes. If a patient is particularly sensitive, the infusion rate may be slowed. Following the initial session, the dose is often gradually increased over subsequent treatments to help the patient reach a more immersive dissociative state. Many practitioners consider this deeper level of dissociation to be correlated with greater therapeutic benefit. If the dose is too light and the experience remains too shallow, it is common for patients not to experience the same sustained relief from depressive symptoms in the days following treatment. While these practices represent widely adopted clinical standards of care, they are not always easy to find in published research.

If you're doing ketamine lozenges at home through a legal telehealth company, dosages range from about 100 to 300 milligrams or more. Note that some companies will recommend two lozenges with a dosage of as high as 800 milligrams. This is an incredibly powerful dose and some psychedelic advocates think this is a negligent practice, so just be careful and be sure to have proper supervision if you're going that high.

Testing Your Ketamine

Unless you're taking ketamine in a trusted clinic, you can never be sure that the stuff you get through the underground market is pure. Unfortunately, other adulterants, including and especially the opiate fentanyl, are making their way into what's sold as ketamine powder. A good rule of thumb is that if the ketamine comes in large crystals and not small crystal-like shards, there is a higher chance it has been cut with an adulterant.

Therefore, it's important to use a drug testing kit in order to make sure that your ketamine is what you think it is. There are many bunk drug testing kits on the market, so be sure to get one from a reliable source, such as the nonprofit DanceSafe, and follow the instructions that come with it.

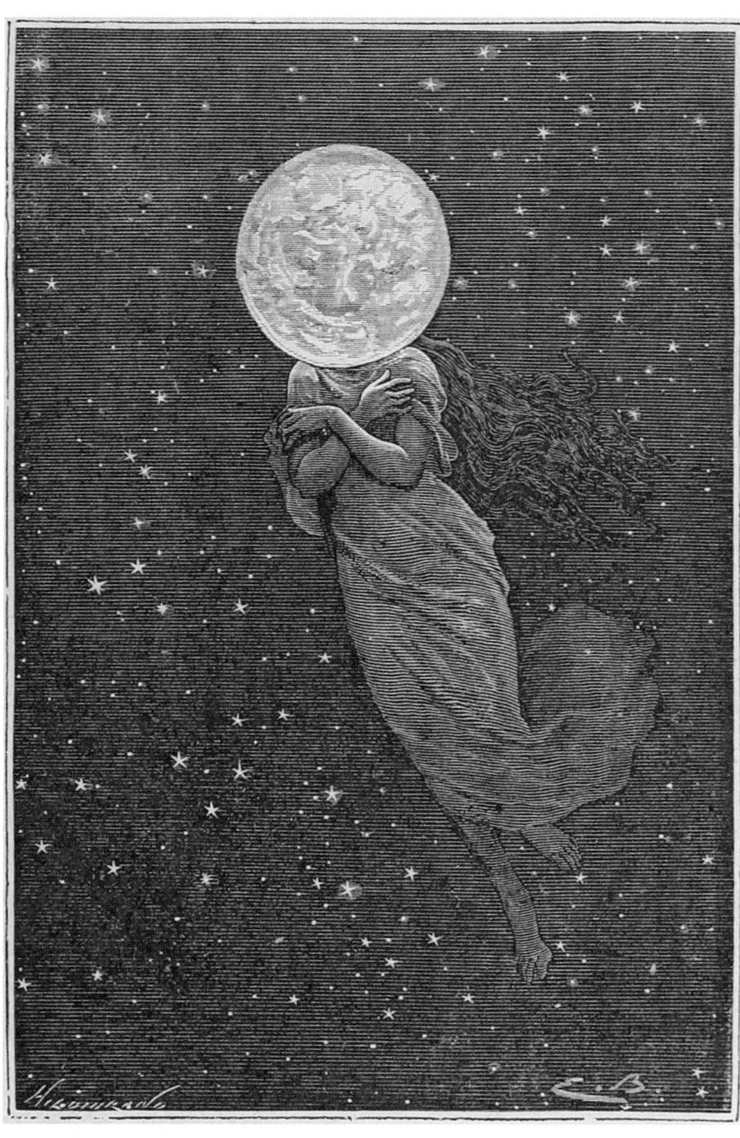

Risks and Contraindications

Ketamine comes with additional considerations compared to LSD, psilocybin, or cannabis. It can be risky to combine ketamine with depressant compounds like alcohol, benzodiazepines, or GHB, which can lead to blackouts, spins, vomiting, loss of consciousness, and erratic body temperature. Like with other psychedelics, it increases heart rate and blood pressure, so it's not recommended for people with hypertension, cardiovascular disease, or a history of stroke except under the close supervision of a medical professional. Long-term use of ketamine can lead to a condition called ketamine cystitis, otherwise known as damage to the lining of the bladder.

As a general rule, do not take ketamine alone, as there have been reports of people dying from high doses of ketamine and of ketamine causing people to choke on their vomit or fall forward into a mode of suffocation on their pillows. And please, please do not get into a body of water, even a bathtub, while on ketamine, as drowning can be a real risk.

Ketamine does have the potential for addiction, and abuse of ketamine in recreational environments is becoming a significant problem in nightlife. This is all to say: If you start to cultivate a relationship with ketamine, be conscious of how often you're using it—and why.

Final Thoughts

Much like with MDMA, practicing reciprocity when it comes to ketamine can look like caring for people within your immediate vicinity. Given its addictive potential, be mindful of not only how you're using it, but how the people close to you are, including the amount, the frequency, and their stated intentions. It's a substance that can easily be abused.

If someone you care about wants to try ketamine for therapeutic reasons, then reciprocity can also take the form of helping them do that. If they want to do ketamine in a clinical context, they're going to need someone to drive them to and from their appointments, as well as to check in with them afterward. They may also need help paying for the treatments, so you could start a GoFundMe or try to raise money among their friends. If they would like to try the lozenge route instead, you can offer to hold space for them, in case they need help getting to the bathroom, drinking water, or anything else.

Ketamine offers profound potential for healing, but with its accessibility and legality come risks. By being a steward of responsible use, you can help ensure that this substance remains accessible to those who are seeking to heal.

CHAPTER 11

OTHER PSYCHEDELICS

While major players like magic mushrooms and ayahuasca may hog the limelight in the psychedelic discourse, there are in fact dozens of lesser-known, paradigm-shifting plant and chemical compounds used to alter consciousness and to heal. We could never possibly write the definitive guide, but in the pages that follow we'll outline a few noteworthy ones. The substances in this chapter vary widely in their legal status, with some being federally legal but restricted at the state or local level, while others are outright prohibited or subject to strict regulation internationally. The patchwork legality is due to the fact that many of these substances are lesser known and have slid under the radar of officials domestically and abroad.

2C Compounds

The 2C family of substances represents a series of phenethylamines synthesized by Alexander Shulgin, the godfather of MDMA (see page 156). These compounds—2C-B, 2C-I, 2C-E, and others—function as both stimulants and psychedelics, offering unique sensory experiences that can be described as a cross between MDMA and LSD highs. The 2C series can be characterized by visual enhancements, altered cognitive perception, increased creativity, emotional depth, and a generally lighter, more playful quality than their more classic psychedelic counterparts.

The 2C compounds are usually taken orally, either in pressed pill form or as a powder measured and dissolved in liquid, with effects typically lasting four to eight hours, depending on the dose and specific compound. When snorted (insufflated), the effects are more rapid, often beginning within five to fifteen minutes, but the overall experience tends to be shorter, lasting approximately two to four hours. Snorting also increases the intensity of the effects and can lead to significant nasal discomfort due to the caustic nature of the powder. The powders are typically white or off-white, and the pills may come in various shapes and colors, similar to MDMA tablets.

Most 2C compounds, including 2C-B and 2C-I, are classified as Schedule I controlled substances in the United States, making them illegal to possess, use, or distribute. In some other countries, they remain unscheduled or in a legal gray area, though this is changing as governments become more aware of these substances.

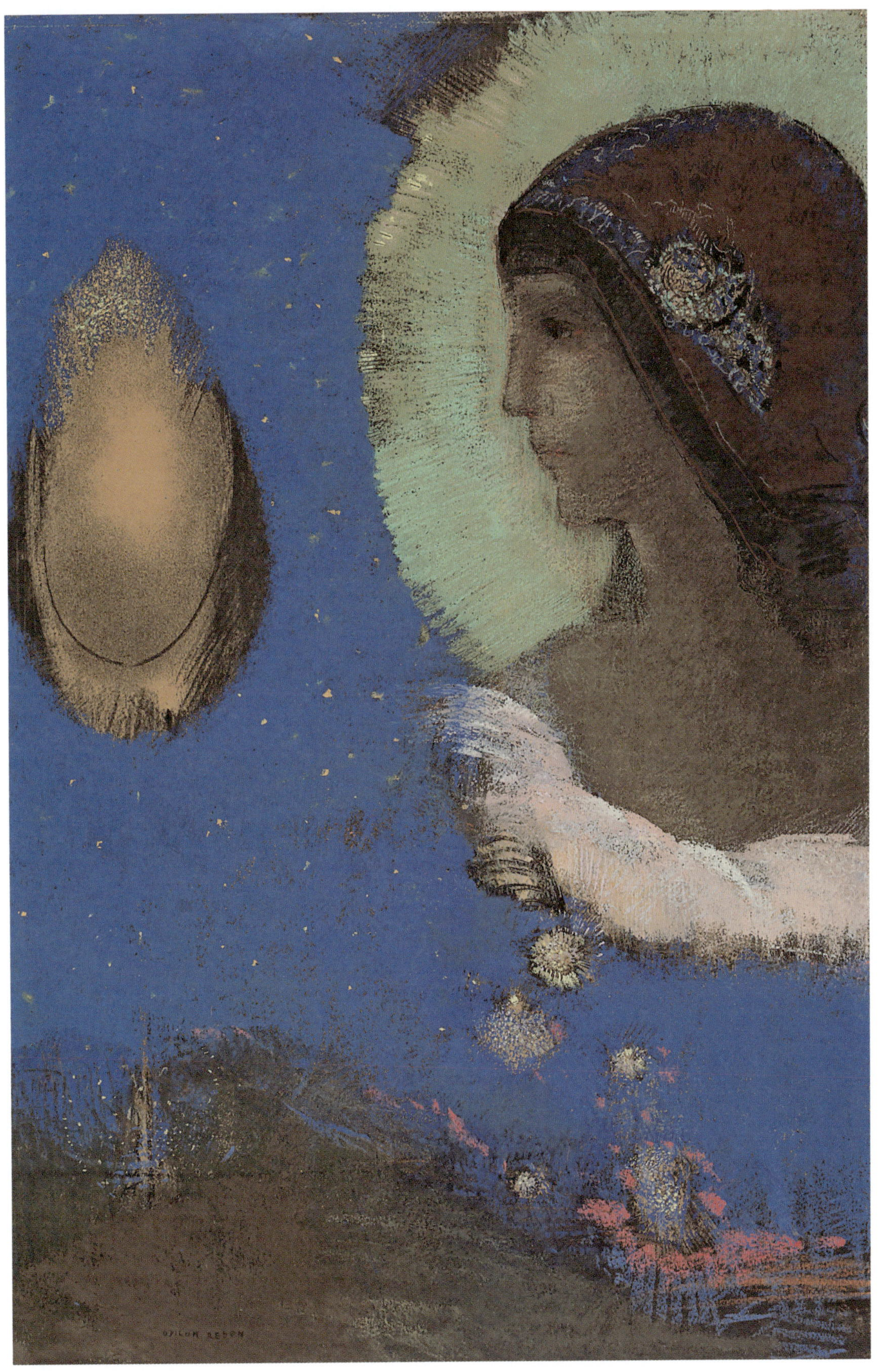

5-MeO-DMT

5-MeO-DMT, a.k.a. "the God molecule," is a highly potent, dissociative, and short-acting psychedelic that can be synthesized in a lab, found in many plants and at least one type of fungus, or extracted from the secretion of the Sonoran Desert toad (*Incilius alvarius*). Unlike N,N-DMT, 5-MeO-DMT can lead to a "whiteout" and total ego dissolution, and it is known for its intense and often mystical experiences. Its effects come on rapidly and often last for only ten to thirty minutes, yet they can produce feelings of profound interconnectedness, love, and transcendence, as well as fear or panic.

5-MeO-DMT is typically vaporized or smoked, either in its natural form (toad secretion) or as a purified synthetic powder. The vaporized substance is usually inhaled through a pipe or vaporizer, leading to an almost immediate onset of effects. Alternatively, it can be administered sublingually (placed under the tongue) or intramuscularly in therapeutic settings, though these methods are less common. It's worth noting that sublingual administration is possible only when 5-MeO-DMT is in a salt form, such as hydrochloride, fumarate, or citrate. It cannot be effectively absorbed sublingually in the more common freebase form that most people encounter when acquiring synthetic 5-MeO-DMT. In addition to intramuscular use, the subcutaneous route (in which the compound is injected into the fat layer beneath the skin) is being increasingly adopted in therapeutic settings. Subcutaneous administration offers similar effects and comparable bioavailability but may carry fewer risks and allow for more controlled absorption than intramuscular injection.

While there's limited research on the compound, 5-MeO-DMT nonetheless has boasted promise in treating conditions like stubborn addictions, depression, and PTSD, in addition to having the potential to boost a person's mood and outlook on life. "In my opinion, 5-MeO-DMT holds more promise in terms of therapeutic potency than anything I've seen. That said, it also has more potential to harm or destabilize participants when administered by untrained facilitators," says Joel Brierre, founder of Tandava Retreats, a retreat center offering 5-MeO-DMT in Mexico, and cofounder of F.I.V.E., a resource hub dedicated to safe and ethical 5-MeO-DMT use.

5-MeO-DMT is a Schedule I controlled substance in the United States, making its possession, use, and distribution illegal. In Mexico, 5-MeO-DMT occupies a legal gray area. While it is not explicitly banned under Mexican law, its use is not formally regulated, and possession may still lead to legal consequences depending on interpretation and local enforcement. This gray area has contributed to its growing popularity in retreat centers and therapeutic contexts in Mexico, though its unregulated status also raises ethical concerns about safety and sustainability, particularly regarding the extraction of toad venom (see below).

UM, SO WHAT ABOUT THE TOADS?

Some people are concerned about the Sonoran Desert toad's well-being and risk of extinction, claiming that catch-and-release methods of extracting the venom for its 5-MeO-DMT may endanger the toad populations. However, others argue that unlike a synthetic extract, the organic material contains other compounds that contribute to what's known as the "entourage effect"—a synergistic relationship among all the compounds that play off and enhance each other. While scientists in the know argue that the differences in consuming synthetic versus natural 5-MeO-DMT are likely insignificant, not everyone with experience administering it agrees.

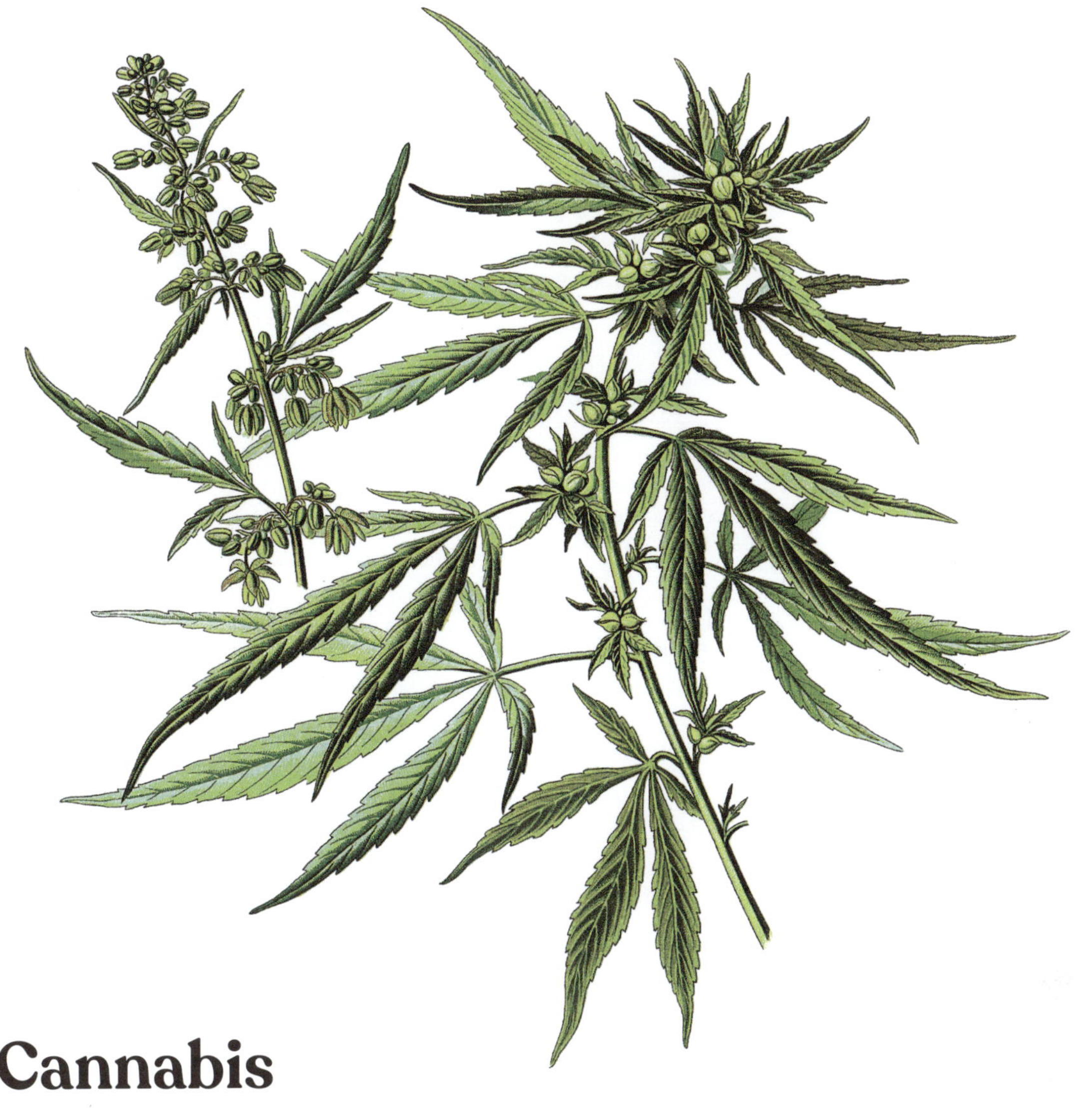

Cannabis

While cannabis, and in particular its most well-known compound, THC, is without a doubt viewed as a psychoactive substance, it also carries psychedelic potential. Yes, it's possible to trip on weed, and even to see visuals and experience sensations reminiscent of other more classic psychedelics like psilocybin. Cannabis can induce profound shifts in perception, creativity, spirituality, and connection with self, others, and nature. For that reason, the more you put into your cannabis journey ahead of time, with regard to preparing your set and setting, the more you will get out of it during the experience and afterward in the integration phase.

Generally speaking, it's more likely that you'll have a "psychedelic" experience with cannabis through consumption methods like edibles or concentrates. That said, while some people might feel a sense of euphoria and have a heightened sensory experience, others might feel a sense of fear, paranoia, or anxiety (again, not dissimilar from a more classic psychedelic experience). As the legality and societal acceptance of cannabis shifts, it's gaining its own place within the psychedelic canon, with an increase in cannabis-fueled rituals, ceremonies, and other sorts of intentional gatherings. Whether you've enjoyed cannabis in the past or not, it's worth trying it in a meditative setting as opposed to a social one. The experience can be vastly different.

Iboga and Ibogaine

Iboga (*Tabernanthe iboga*) is a plant native to West Africa and traditionally used in rituals by the Bwiti people. The root bark contains ibogaine, a powerful psychoactive alkaloid known for inducing intense visionary experiences and deep introspection. While it's less common, ibogaine can also be extracted from the voacanga tree (*Voacanga africana*). Ibogaine may in fact be the strongest known psychedelic because the experience can last twenty-four hours or longer. We know—*intense.*

In traditional Gabonese ceremonies, which have been growing in popularity among psychedelic tourists over the past decade, iboga is typically prepared by grinding or shredding the root bark into a powder, which is then consumed orally. The ceremonies, which are deeply spiritual, are often guided by an experienced shaman or elder known as a nganga. Participants may consume the iboga bark powder directly or mix it with water to form a paste for easier ingestion. These ceremonies are highly structured and involve prayer, music, and rituals designed to support the spiritual journey and healing process. The amount consumed is carefully monitored, as the experience is not only physically intense but also profoundly psychological, often involving vivid visions that participants are guided to interpret within a spiritual framework.

In the psychedelic community, iboga has gained attention in the West largely due to the extraction of ibogaine, its active compound, which has shown promise in treating severe addiction, particularly to opioids, by reducing withdrawal symptoms and cravings. In a clinical context, ibogaine is typically administered as a purified substance, often in capsule or liquid form, to allow for more precise dosing compared to the traditional consumption of iboga root bark.

Unlike classic psychedelics, ibogaine has been linked to several dozen fatalities at clinics. Ibogaine is generally safe for a person who has been properly vetted ahead of time and is monitored during the session, but there is a serious risk for people with a history of cardiac issues, and ibogaine clinics abroad are not properly regulated. That's why it's particularly important to work with a trusted, reputable clinic if you decide to try ibogaine. Conservation activists are calling on the international community to source ibogaine from the voacanga tree instead of the iboga plant—and we recommend you look for a clinic that is doing this. Ibogaine is a Schedule I controlled substance in the United States, though it remains legal or unregulated in other countries, including Mexico, New Zealand, and Canada, where some clinics operate.

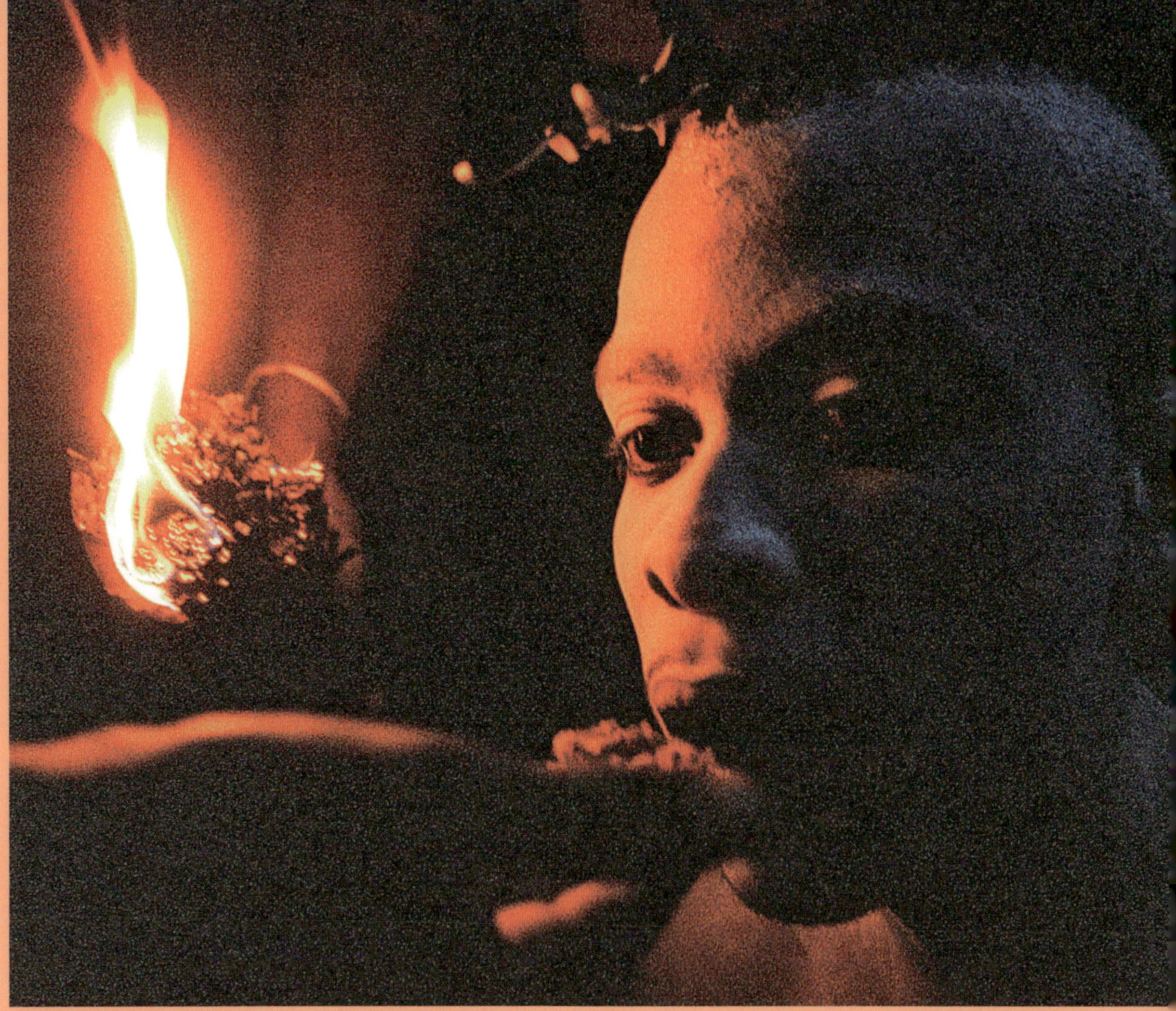

A man ingests a dose of iboga during his initiation.

INDIGENOUS WISDOM AND STEWARDSHIP

THE BWITI

If you or someone you know has undergone an ibogaine treatment, the medicine was likely sourced from an illegal harvest taken in Gabon by poachers from neighboring Cameroon and sent to Mexico or Costa Rica through illegal channels. The Bwiti spiritual tradition, practiced by various ethnic groups in Gabon, has utilized the iboga plant for centuries in initiation rites and healing ceremonies. Iboga's psychoactive root bark induces profound visions and introspection, serving as a cornerstone of Bwiti religious practices. However, the increasing global demand for ibogaine has led to significant overharvesting of iboga in Gabon's forests. "Ninety-five percent of the iboga [or ibogaine] sold online is from trees that have been poached from the Gabonese public domain, reserved for local traditional Bwiti practitioners, and from the protected national parks of Gabon," says Yann Guignon, cofounder of Blessings of the Forest, a nonprofit devoted to preservation of iboga. This unsustainable exploitation threatens both the survival of the iboga plant and the cultural heritage of the Bwiti people. In response, organizations like Blessings of the Forest are collaborating with Gabonese authorities to develop a fair and sustainable iboga industry, aiming to protect the plant and support Bwiti communities.

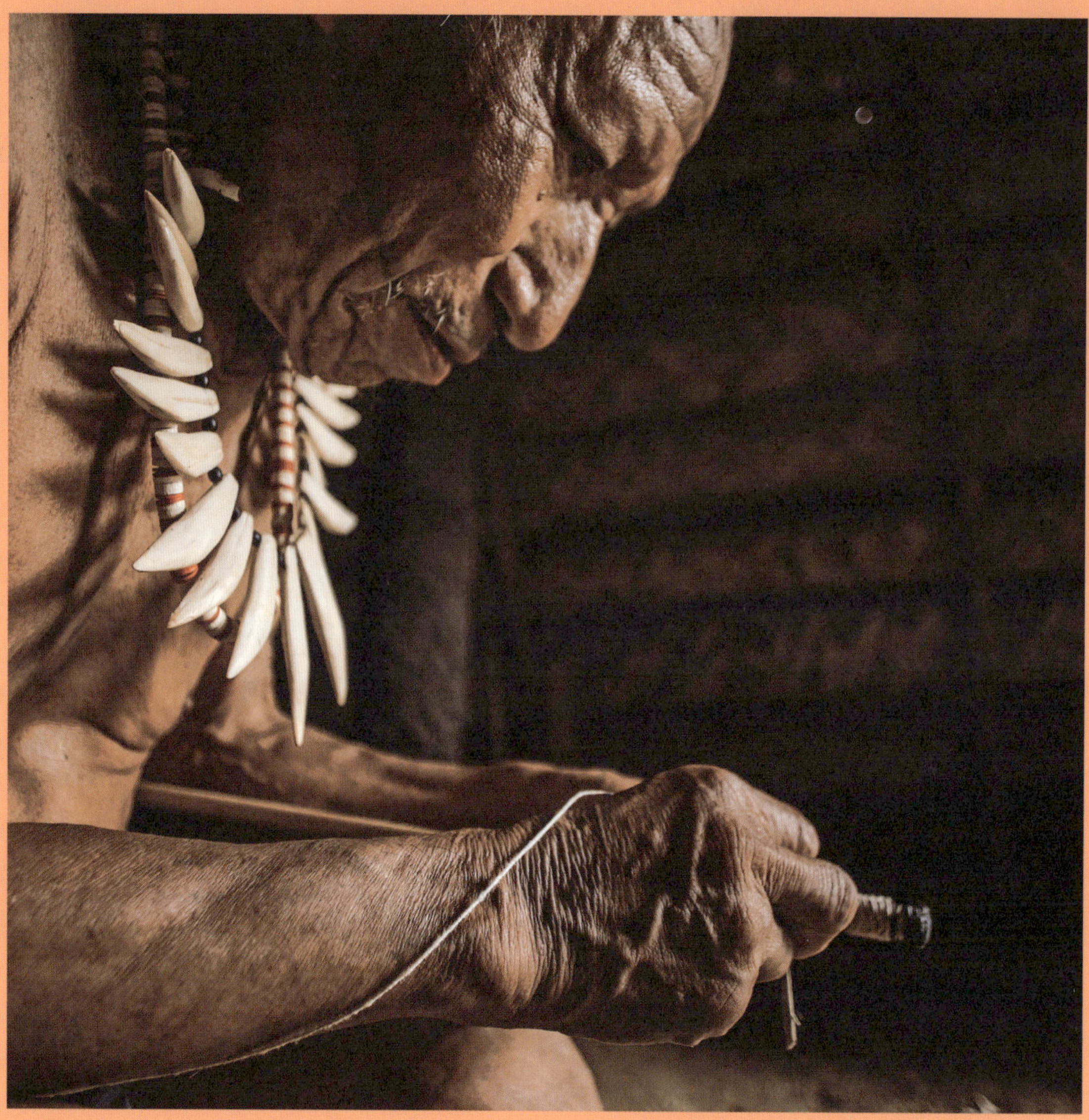

Nestor Matsés crafting an arrow.

INDIGENOUS STEWARDSHIP AND RECIPROCITY

THE MATSÉS

The Matsés preserve an extraordinary amount of ecological knowledge given the size of their population. There are approximately 2,500 Matsés in the Peruvian Amazon, and 1,300 across the Javari River in Brazil, but their territory is more than 3,800 square miles. Like many Indigenous communities throughout the jungle, their very existence—not to mention their elders' wisdom of more than 1,000 plants in their territories and their medical value—has been at risk of getting lost for decades as they've assimilated into Peruvian culture amid limited economic opportunity in their territory. The *Phyllomedusa bicolor* frog, which creates a secretion used to make kambo—a medicine often used in nonindigenous communities who also drink ayahuasca, snuff rapeh, and use other traditional psychoactives from the Amazon—has also come under threat as it grows in popularity as a treatment for everything from autoimmune conditions to depression.

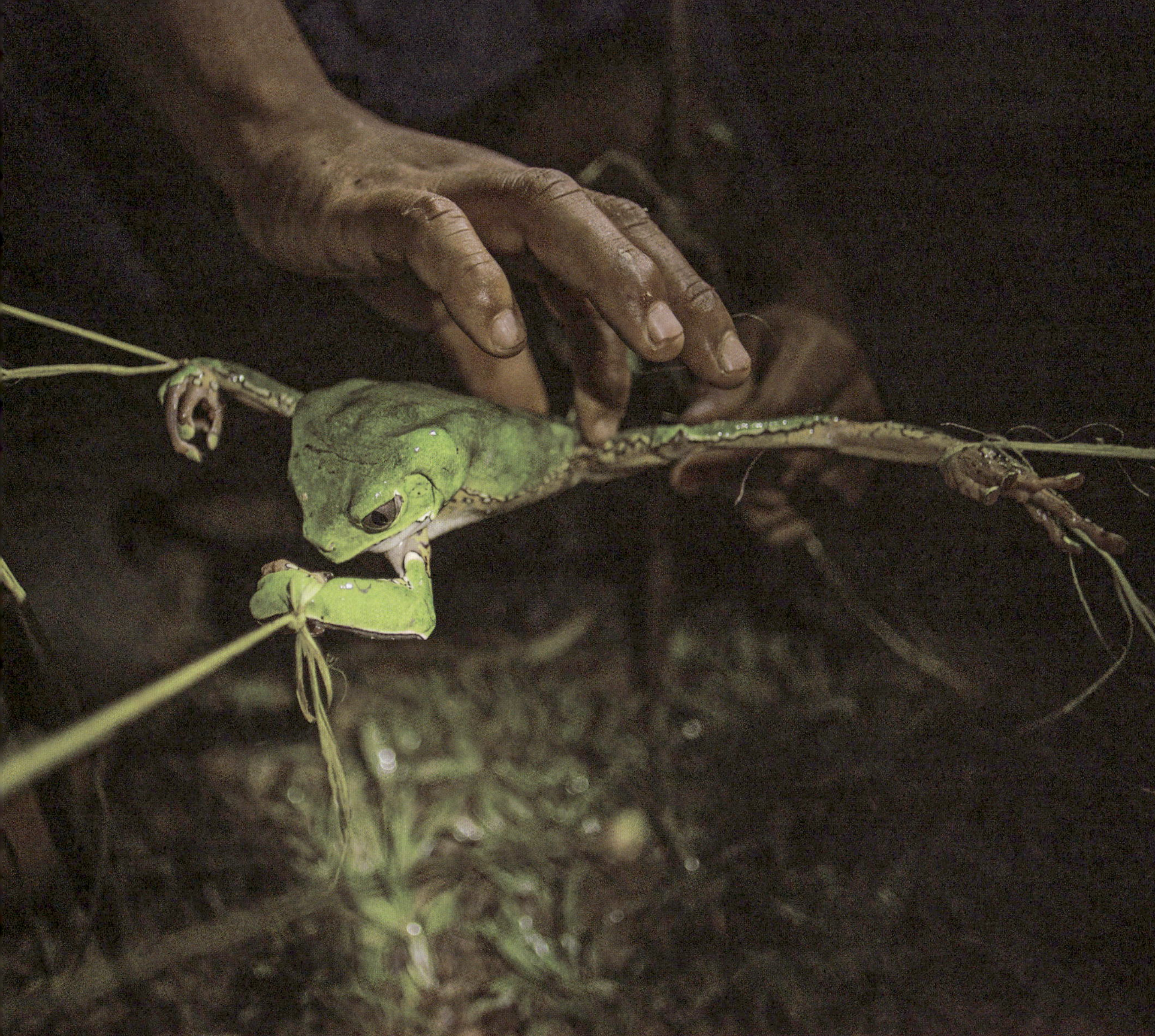

The secretion of a *Phyllomedusa bicolor* frog is extracted in Matsés territory, Javari Valley, 2018.

At this time, the frog is not currently classified as endangered by the International Union for Conservation of Nature, though localized pressures—such as deforestation, overharvesting, and the commercialization of kambo for Western markets—have increased the risk of exploitation. "I do not agree with Acate [kambo] leaving our lands," says Matsés Elder Antonio Manquid. "The outside people [involved in the commercial trade of frog secretions] are misappropriating our traditional practices."

It's important to note that the Matsés are not the only Indigenous group who use kambo. The Katukina, Yawanawá, and Cashinahua (Huni Kuin), among others, also administer it as part of their healing practices. Some of these groups have expressed concern that the rising demand from foreigners could deplete frog populations or dilute the cultural significance of the medicine. At the same time, other Indigenous practitioners administer kambo to Western visitors, sometimes as part of structured retreats, seeing it as a way to generate income while sharing their traditions. This tension reflects a broader debate in the Amazon: how to safeguard biocultural knowledge and species while navigating the economic realities of globalization and the interest of outsiders in Indigenous medicines.

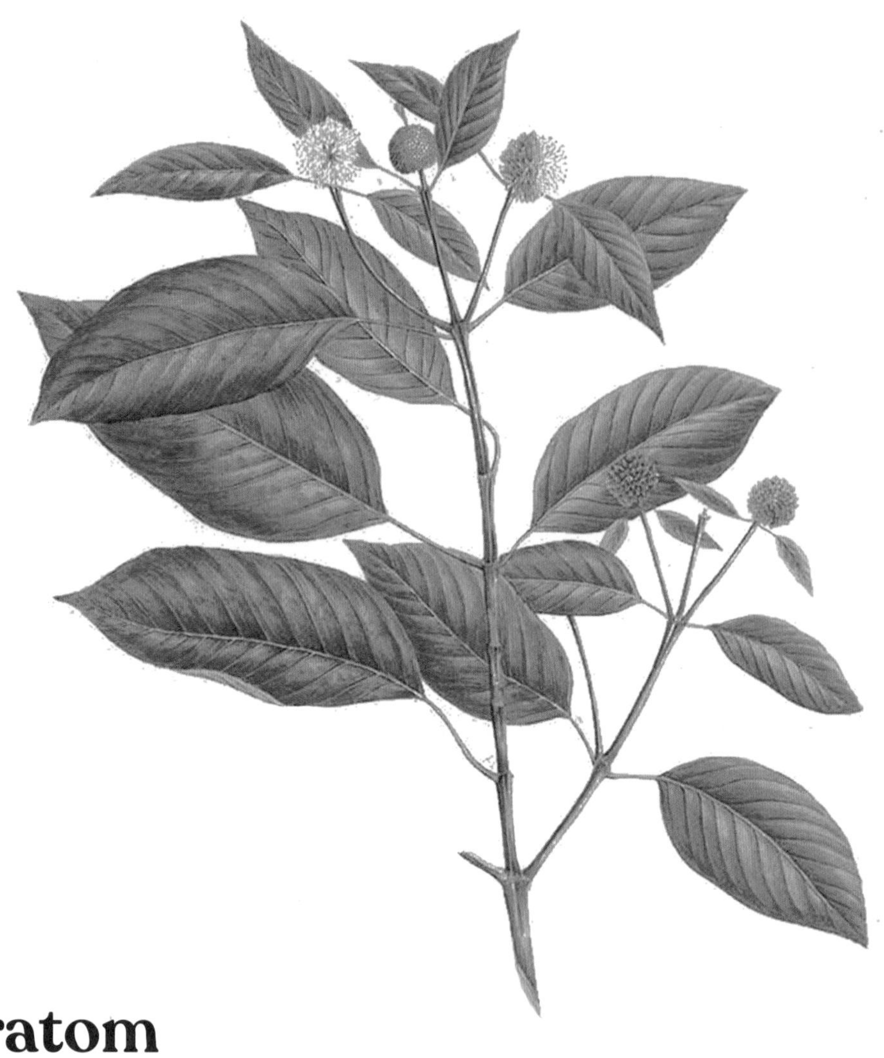

Kratom

Kratom (*Mitragyna speciosa*) is a tropical tree native to Southeast Asia. Generally used for its analgesic effects, kratom also has the capacity to bring about psychedelic qualities. At lower doses, kratom can be a stimulant, offering greater energy and sociability, while at higher doses it can foster a relaxed, dreamy, maybe even euphoric state.

Kratom is most commonly consumed as a powdered leaf, either mixed with water or brewed into a tea. A few kratom beverages are now being marketed as alcohol alternatives and are available in some grocery stores and bodegas. Kratom is also available in capsule form for easier dosing or as a concentrated extract for stronger effects. The duration of its effects varies depending on the dose and method of ingestion but typically lasts for between two and six hours. Lower doses tend to have a shorter duration, while higher doses produce longer-lasting effects.

It's worth noting that there's been controversy over kratom's legality for quite some time because it can be addictive, so be mindful of how often you're using it—and why. Kratom is legal in many US states, but a few have banned it. Efforts to regulate kratom federally in the United States continue to evolve, with advocates pushing for responsible use and access.

BEYOND THE JOURNEY

THE COMMODIFICATION OF TOBACCO

Tobacco is the first shamanic plant. Archaeological evidence for the human use of tobacco in the Americas stretches back at least 12,300 years. According to distinguished botanist Dr. Thomas Harper Goodspeed, among other experts, people indigenous to the Americas first domesticated tobacco roughly eight thousand years ago—on par with the domestication of the first food plants in the Americas.

At the time of European contact, it was cultivated from southern Alaska to modern-day Chile. Among the diversity of cultures and spiritual traditions of the Indigenous Americans, the use of tobacco as a sacred medicine is universal.

Even today, peyote, ayahuasca, San Pedro, coca, yopo, and other sacred plants are all used along with tobacco. Among these Indigenous traditions, tobacco is not considered an addictive poison. Instead, tobacco is considered the most sacred plant: It's the connection to the creator, and what one does with smoked tobacco is made true.

Yet tobacco, as a globalized commodity, is not sacred. It is instead adulterated with chemicals to make it more addictive and give it a branded flavor. The World Health Organization estimates the worldwide use of tobacco is responsible for eight million deaths per year. Indigenous peoples use the journey of tobacco, from sacrament to commodity, as a warning for what could happen to other sacred plants and fungi if profit is prioritized over healing.

The first slaves were brought to the American colonies in 1619 to work the tobacco fields at the Jamestown colony. The new industry was the backbone of the Southern colonial economy, driving the expansion of the African slave trade across the Atlantic and of the tobacco plantations westward from the coast, expelling, if not outright exterminating, Indigenous peoples as they ate deeper into the continent.

Wrested away from prayer and ceremony, tobacco has been a powerful source of wealth and political control for more than five hundred years, since Columbus first encountered Taíno tribe members smoking cigars on Hispaniola. Twenty-five percent of the signees of the Declaration of Independence, the first American aristocratic families, were tobacco farmers. Wealth generation through the control of tobacco has been exponential ever since. By 2030, the global tobacco market is expected to exceed $1 trillion, according to a report by Grand View Research.

There are now dozens of companies seeking to take the active alkaloids of sacred medicines and commercialize them. Filament Health and their chemically synthesized "ayahuasca" pill—what people often refer to as "pharmahuasca"—aim to make the "trip" more predictable and manageable for a psychiatrist or therapeutic facilitator who's never set foot in the Amazon. Meanwhile, Compass Pathways has been granted a patent for their synthetic psilocybin, the primary psychoactive compound in sacred mushrooms.

The websites and investor pitches demonstrate that these are businesses first and note their commitment to creating and protecting their intellectual property around chemical extractions or "novel" uses of Indigenous intellectual property. Whatever commitment they make to reciprocity or access is secondary to the protection of their ability to turn a profit from these medicines.

However, there are risks in deviating from the sacred and traditional practice of the Indigenous peoples who have introduced us to these medicines. They carry the power to heal—and also to harm, even if that harm is self-inflicted. Is that not what happened with tobacco, opium, and coca, all in the name of profit?

This excerpt comes from a story reported for DoubleBlind's print magazine by Matthew Stoltz.

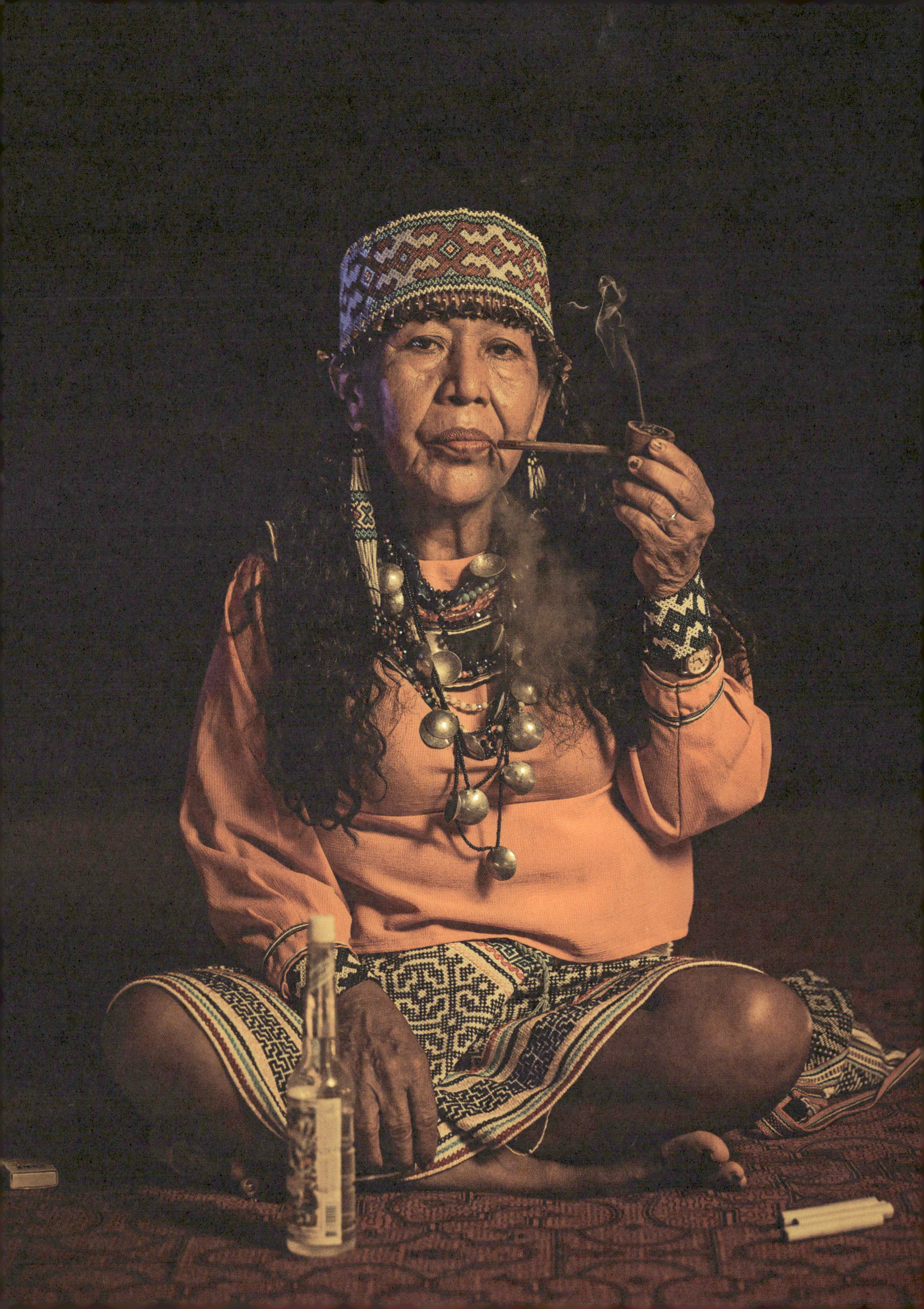

Mapacho

Mapacho (*Nicotiana rustica*), a type of wild tobacco native to the Amazon rainforest, has been used for generations by some Indigenous tribes for cleansing and protection. It will be smoked throughout some Indigenous ceremonies, filling the room with a sweet, cigar-like smell. If a person is struggling during a ceremony, a shaman might approach the person with the mapacho and do a blessing. Mapacho is legal worldwide but subject to tobacco regulations. Unlike commercial tobacco, it is not typically adulterated with additives or preservatives.

Maestra Laura, an advanced-level Shipibo Onanya (wisdom keeper/ plant-spirit shamanic healer), is shown smoking her shinatapon—a special pipe used for mapacho and imbued with the energetic essence of her plant-spirit dietas. All genuine Onanya healers work closely with their pipes, which are used to connect to the plant spirits, cleanse negative energies, transmit positive energies, and provide spiritual protection.

Mescaline

While mescaline is commonly associated with both peyote and San Pedro, it is also available as a stand-alone psychedelic that can be synthesized in a lab. As a phenethylamine, like MDMA, mescaline offers somewhat of a stimulating, psychedelic effect, with the capacity to also trigger heightened emotions and reflections. It was perhaps made most famous as the substance that Aldous Huxley took when he wrote *The Doors of Perception.*

Mescaline can be taken in several forms, including as a synthetic powder, capsule, or liquid solution, as well as in its natural forms extracted from peyote or San Pedro. Synthetic mescaline typically appears as a fine white or off-white crystalline powder, though it can also be encapsulated for easier dosing. The synthetic form tends to have a bitter, chemical taste, which some people find unpleasant, though it is more neutral compared to the intensely bitter flavor of peyote or San Pedro preparations.

Typically, doses of synthetic mescaline range from 200 to 500 milligrams, depending on body weight and sensitivity, and it can take up to one to two hours for the effects to set in. The total experience usually lasts for between ten and twelve hours, with a peak that can persist for four to six hours, followed by a gradual comedown. Mescaline is classified as a Schedule I controlled substance in the United States.

Morning Glory Seeds (LSA)

Morning glory seeds, particularly from the *Ipomoea purpurea* and *I. violacea* species, contain the psychoactive compound LSA (lysergic acid amide), a cousin of LSD. LSA can mirror LSD in its effects but is generally less intense; some people describe the experience as peaceful, introspective, and highly psychedelic. That said, consumers of the seeds should exercise caution, as it's not uncommon to feel nauseous or unwell after ingestion due to naturally occurring toxins or contaminants often present on seeds.

To prepare morning glory seeds for safe ingestion, it's essential to ensure that the seeds are free from harmful chemicals, as many commercially available seeds are coated with pesticides or antifungal agents to discourage consumption. Look for seeds labeled as "organic" or "untreated" from a reputable supplier. Before use, wash the seeds thoroughly and grind them into a fine powder to increase bioavailability. This powder can then be consumed directly, mixed with a liquid like water or juice, or used in a cold water extraction process to filter out some of the compounds that contribute to nausea. Cold water extraction involves soaking the ground seeds in distilled water for several hours, straining the liquid through a filter, and drinking the resulting solution.

While the effects of LSA are generally less intense than those of LSD, preparation and dosage play a significant role in the overall experience. Users often report that careful preparation can reduce physical discomfort and enhance the clarity of the experience.

LSA is not explicitly regulated in the United States, and the sale and possession of morning glory seeds are generally legal. However, extracting LSA for consumption may be considered illegal under the federal Controlled Substance Analogue Enforcement Act if authorities determine that it is being used as a substitute for or precursor to LSD, a Schedule I controlled substance.

ILLEGAL OR NOT? THE PSYCHEDELIC GRAY AREA

As of the time of writing, the federal Controlled Substance Analogue Enforcement Act, sometimes called simply the Analogue Act, allows substances that are chemically or pharmacologically similar to Schedule I or II drugs to be treated as illegal if intended for human consumption. This law was designed to prevent chemists and psychonauts from circumventing federal drug prohibitions by creating or extracting slightly altered compounds that mimic the effects of banned substances.

For example, LSA (lysergic acid amide) from morning glory seeds and synthetic compounds like 4-AcO-DMT, which is often compared to psilocybin found in magic mushrooms, might be deemed illegal under the act if they are deemed substantially similar to LSD or psilocybin, respectively. However, whether a substance officially falls under the act must be determined in court. Authorities would need to prove that the substance is chemically similar to a controlled drug, produces similar effects, and was intended for human consumption. Until such a ruling is made, many substances remain in a legal gray area, leaving their status ambiguous and subject to enforcement discretion.

Peyote

Peyote (*Lophophora williamsii*) is a cactus known for its psychoactive properties, which can be primarily attributed to its mescaline content. Used for millennia by Indigenous Americans, peyote can be eaten as dried chips, mixed with chocolate, or as a raw button and is traditionally taken in a ceremonial context. Peyote has been the topic of strong controversy because it takes a long time to cultivate and is at risk of endangerment. Because of this, the Native American Church has requested that non-Natives do not use peyote at this time and that it remain out of psychedelic decriminalization measures.

Peyote is classified as a Schedule I controlled substance in the United States, but there is an exemption for members of the Native American Church (NAC), who use it in religious ceremonies. In Mexico, peyote is protected as part of the cultural and religious heritage of Indigenous peoples, but its use is restricted to ceremonial practices and is illegal for recreational purposes. Internationally, it is banned in many countries.

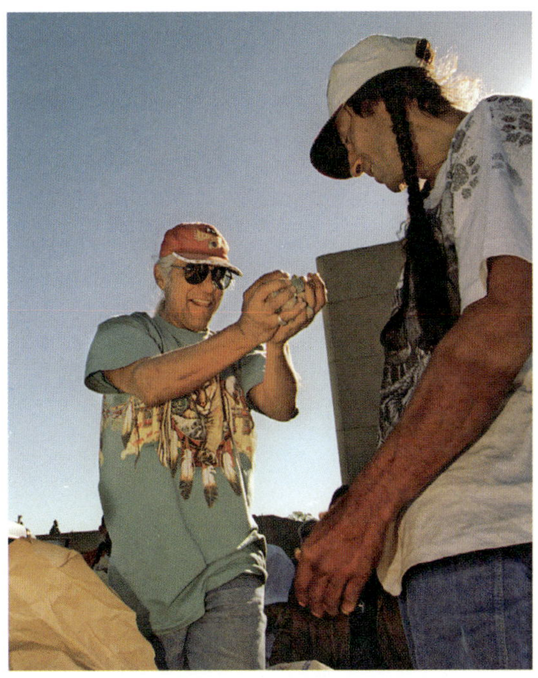

Paul Skyhorse Durant, left, holds peyote buttons in 1996, following a court ruling that they be returned

INDIGENOUS WISDOM AND STEWARDSHIP

THE NATIVE AMERICAN CHURCH

Few topics are more controversial in the psychedelic field than peyote. In June 2019, Oakland became the first city to decriminalize all natural psychedelic plants and fungi. Peyote was included in that initiative, adding fuel to an already fiery debate about whether non-Natives should take peyote, given the cactus's risk of becoming endangered.

The Native American Church (NAC), established around 1885, is the most widespread Indigenous religious movement in North America. Central to its practice is the ceremonial use of peyote, which has been used by Indigenous American people for generations. The NAC includes more than fifty tribes who view peyote as a sacrament—and they feel that Indigenous Americans should be given priority when it comes to access to the cactus.

There's legal precedent backing them. In 1990 the US Supreme Court ruled that states could deny unemployment benefits to individuals dismissed for using peyote, even when used in religious ceremonies. This decision led to the passage of the Religious Freedom Restoration Act (RFRA) in 1993, which broadly aimed to protect religious practices from government interference. The use of peyote by NAC members was then specifically protected under the 1994 amendments to the American Indian Religious Freedom Act (AIRFA), which legalized the ceremonial use of peyote by members of federally recognized tribes. "We as a people place explicit faith, hope and belief in Almighty GOD and declare full, competent and everlasting faith in our church, through which we worship for religion and protection of the sacramental use of Peyote," reads the NAC's mission statement.

INDIGENOUS WISDOM AND STEWARDSHIP

THE WIXÁRIKA

To the Wixárika people, Wirikuta—the Sierra de Catorce mountain range and the desert at its feet—is both a university and a temple of prayer. It's the destination of a pilgrimage made every year, when thousands of families travel—by bus, by pickup truck or van, and then by foot—from their homelands 400 miles east, to the desert to hunt for their sacramental peyote. According to carbon dating of the ashes from their ceremonial fireplaces, the Wixárika (often referred to as the Huichol, a name given to the group by outsiders) have been in this region for at least 15,000 years.

Despite its sacred significance, Wirikuta and the whole region have been a magnet for industrial megaprojects since the colonial era. In the 1700s, it was a silver mining area. Today, industrial activities, such as mining extraction and wide-scale farming, continue to expand into the region, damaging this biodiverse ecosystem and disrupting Indigenous communities' ability to access the peyote.

Susana Valadez, anthropologist and founder of the Huichol Center for Cultural Survival, married into the tribe in the 1990s, returning for the first time after many years with her family to discover that a chaos had emerged, with tourist buses pulling up alongside the sacred springs where Wixárika families gather to pray. "While the shamans and pilgrims sit around their ceremonial fire and chant the messages of the creators, the tourists roast hot dogs and drink beer at their adjacent campsites," says Valadez. "It's become a circus."

This excerpt and photos come from a story reported for DoubleBlind's print magazine by Tracy L. Barnett.

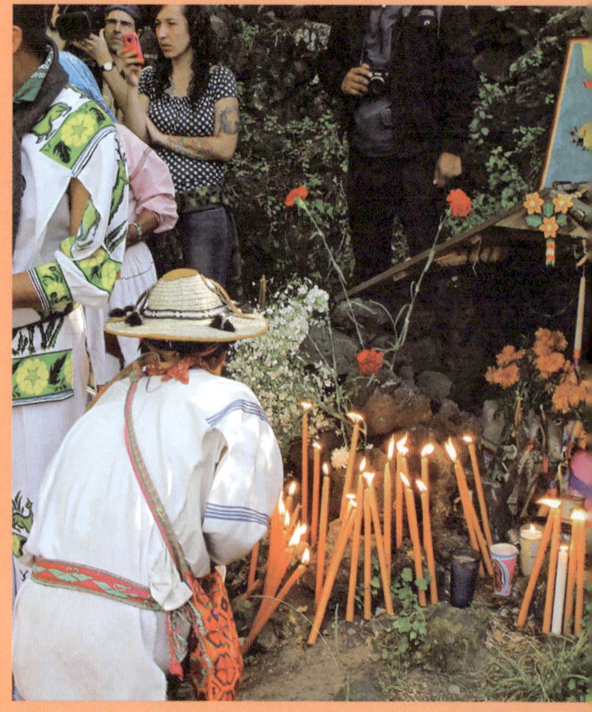

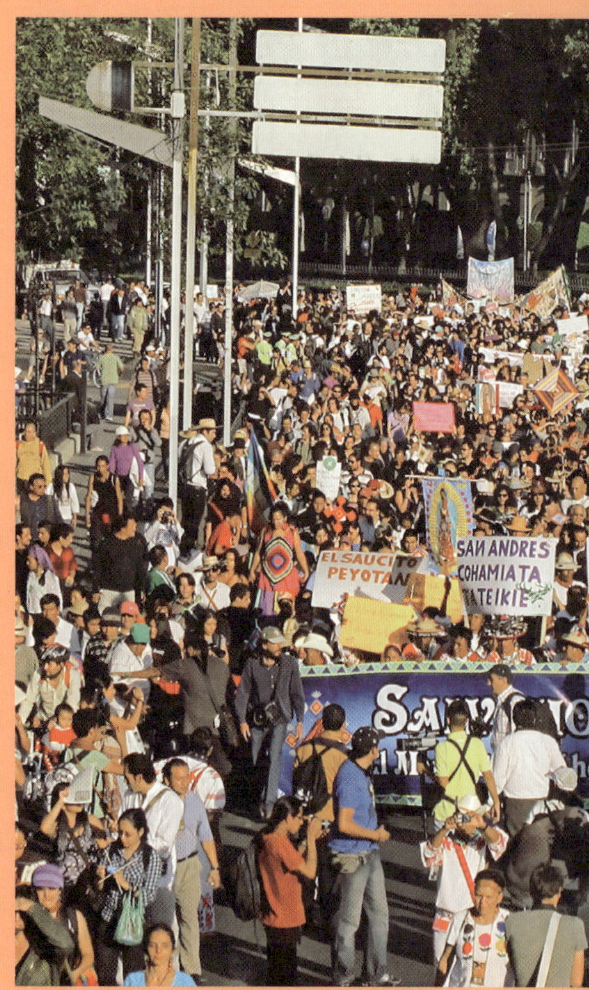

Clockwise from upper left: **One of a vast network of shrines spread across the Mexican countryside where Wixárika people leave their offerings; a Wixárika woman waters her crops; sunrise in Wirikuta, the sacred desert; 2012 mobilization in defense of Wirikuta, Mexico City.**

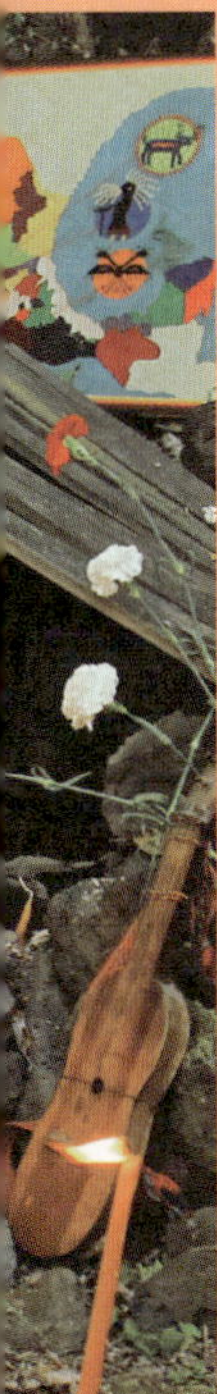

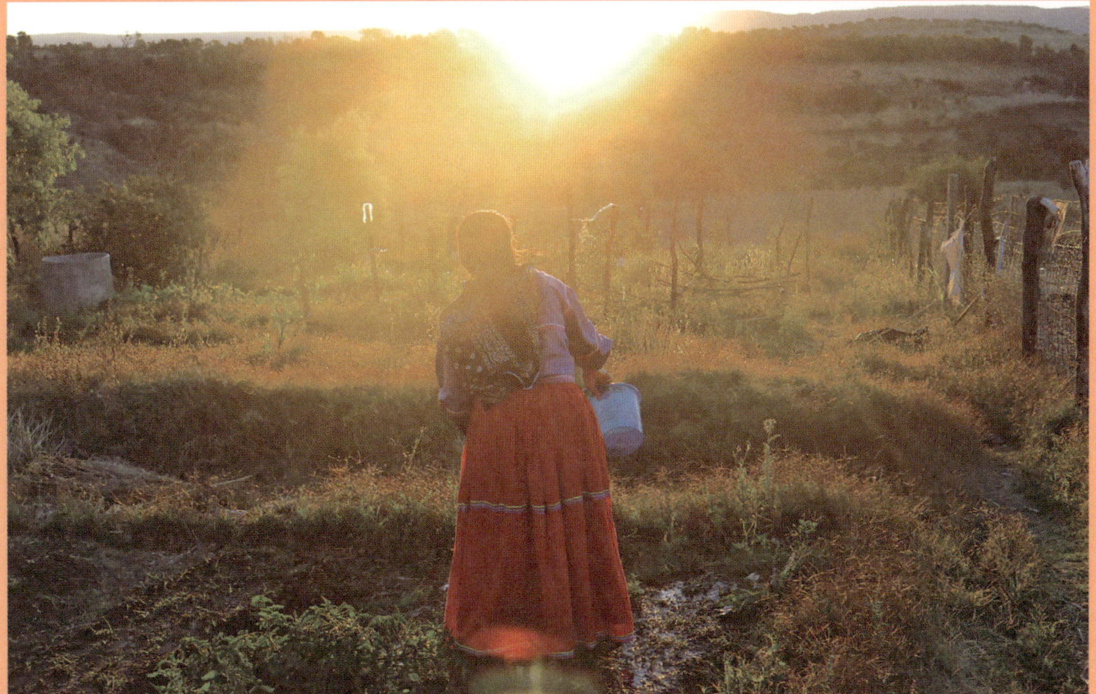

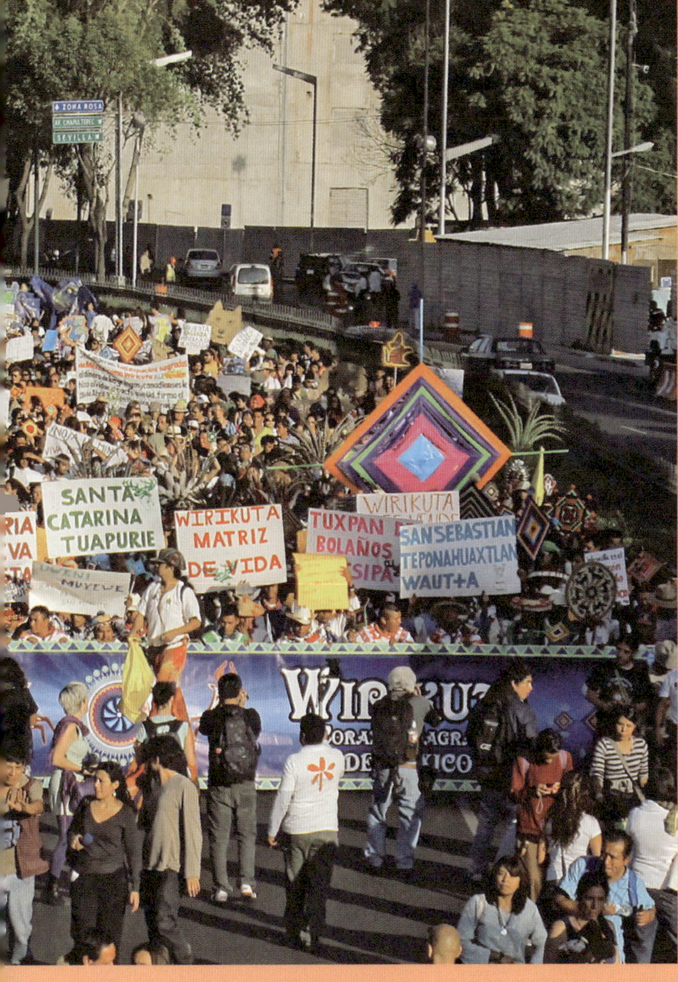
SANTA CATARINA TUAPURIE
WIRIKUTA MATRIZ DE VIDA
WIRIKUTA
SAN SEBASTIAN TEPONAHUAXTLAN WAUT+A

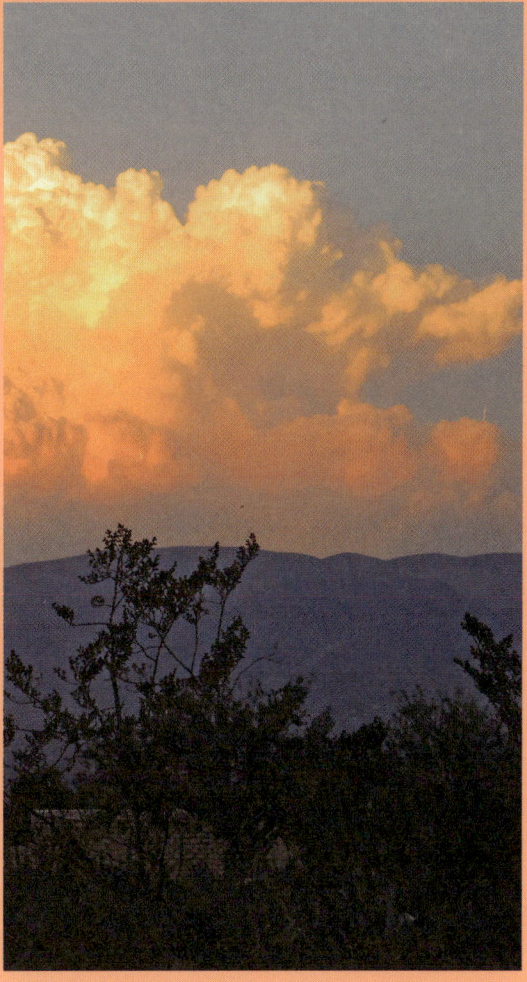

Rapé

Rapé (pronounced "ha-peh") is a traditional snuff made from tobacco that's been dried in the sun, ground, and sifted along with other plants that can vary depending on tradition and the person who prepares it. Used by several Indigenous tribes in the Amazon and most often associated with Brazilian Pano-speaking peoples, rapé is often used in ceremonial contexts to help with the release of negative thoughts or feelings or to reinforce positive ones. It is generally administered through an applicator—a traditional pipe called a curipe (for self-administration) or tipi (for administration from one person to another)—and blown up the nostrils. It is not psychedelic but is said to be grounding and can produce intense sensations in the head. It is not for the faint of heart.

Upon inhalation, users may experience a rush of clarity, energy, and sometimes purging. The effects, which typically last anywhere from fifteen to forty-five minutes, depending on the blend used and the individual's sensitivity, can include a heightened sense of awareness and spiritual connection, making rapé a popular tool for meditation and introspection. You may encounter it at a ceremony for another substance, such as ayahuasca, mushrooms, or kambo, where it's sometimes offered in conjunction. Users report that it can help clear emotional and psychological blockages that enable a person to go deeper into their psychedelic journey.

Rapé is generally legal in most countries, including the United States, as it does not typically contain controlled substances. However, its primary ingredient, mapacho tobacco (see page 193), is subject to the same regulations as other tobacco products.

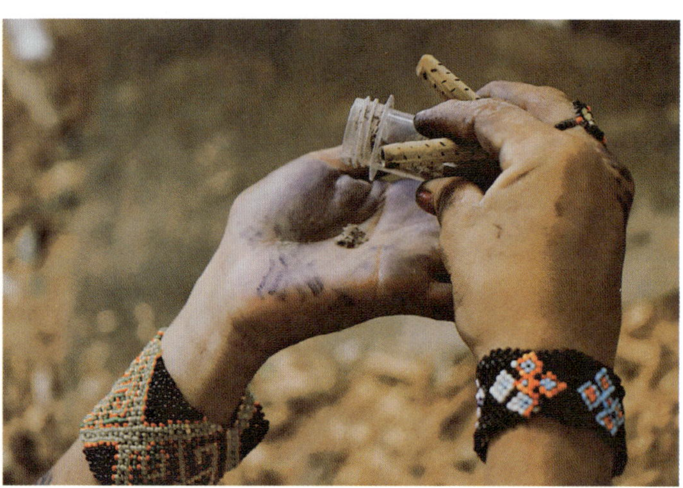

Rapé being scooped into a kuripe, a V-shaped self-applicator pipe used to blow the medicine into one's own nostrils

Salvia

You may or may not know salvia as the herb people were buying at smoke shops in the early to mid-2000s. At the time, the stuff was being sold alongside flip-flops on the Venice Beach boardwalk. A lot of teens filmed themselves flailing about and posted the videos to YouTube. It was not our generation's best moment—and now a lot of millennials, understandably so, just want to stay away from it. But salvia, more formally known as *Salvia divinorum*, is actually a sacred herb, native to the Sierra Madre Oriental of Oaxaca, Mexico, and used by the Mazatec (see page 94) for centuries.

Salvia induces short, intense experiences characterized by rapid shifts in perception, time distortion, and vivid hallucinations. Some have described the sensation of losing themselves, being transported to another reality, or merging into their surroundings, often with much fear attached. While the trip is short-lived, it is intense. When the herb is smoked or vaporized, the most powerful effects typically last for only five to fifteen minutes, though a return to baseline can take twenty to forty minutes. If it is chewed, the effects may be milder but can last for up to two hours. Salvia is legal in some US states but banned in others. Internationally, it is prohibited in several countries, including Australia and many European nations, though it remains legal in its native Mexico.

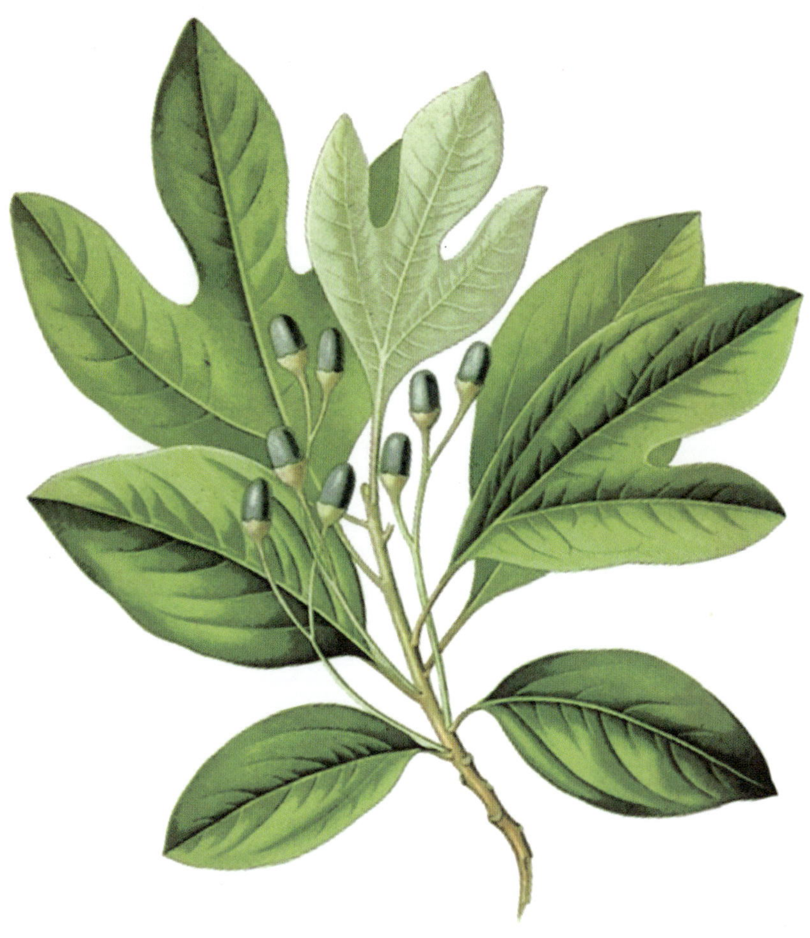

Sassafras and MDA

The sassafras tree (*Sassafras albidum*) and the compound MDA (3,4-methylenedioxyamphetamine) are often associated with MDMA, their better-known chemical cousin. The root bark of the sassafras tree is the source of safrole, an oily liquid compound that was first used to synthesize MDMA and MDA (which is sometimes interchangeably called sass). While MDA shares some characteristics with MDMA—such as its ability to increase sociability and emotional openness—it is often noted for its more psychedelic qualities, such as fostering enhanced visual perception and emotional complexity. The MDA experience tends to last a little longer than that of MDMA and can be both energetic and introspective.

Sassafras and MDA are typically consumed orally, often in capsule or pressed pill form, or less commonly as a powder. When sold illicitly, MDA may appear as white or off-white crystalline powder, pressed pills resembling those of MDMA, or capsules filled with powder. Sassafras oil, which contains safrole, has a distinct sweet, earthy aroma and is not typically consumed directly but serves as a precursor in the synthesis of MDMA and MDA.

MDA is classified as a Schedule I controlled substance in the United States, making its use, possession, and distribution illegal. Safrole, the precursor compound found in sassafras, is also heavily regulated due to its association with the synthesis of MDA and MDMA.

Wachuma (a.k.a. San Pedro)

Wachuma or San Pedro (*Trichocereus macrogonus* var. *pachanoi*) is a mescaline-containing cactus native to the Andes region of South America, and it has been used in Indigenous contexts for thousands of years. *Wachuma*, the traditional Andean name, is often preferred by practitioners who want to uphold reverence for the medicine's Indigenous history. While the depth and intensity of the experience depends on the dose, San Pedro offers users a connection with the natural world, deep understanding, and clarity. Some report heightened perception of colors, a shifted concept of time, and more intense or introspective emotional states.

Wachuma is one of the longer-lasting psychedelics. It's typically taken in a ceremony during the day, and the experience can last anywhere from six to twelve hours. It's possible to take wachuma on your own, as you should be relatively aware and able to navigate your surroundings. However, it's recommended to do it in a ceremony where you can be supported, especially your first time.

San Pedro is consumed in several ways, including raw, dried, or as a tea. Preparing it as a tea involves slicing the cactus and boiling it for several hours to extract the active compounds into a liquid. This process often results in a bitter, slimy brew that can be challenging to drink. Compared to eating it raw or dried, drinking it as a tea typically leads to a faster onset of effects, which usually emerge over the course of one to two hours.

Eaten raw or dried, the cactus has a different texture and taste. The raw cactus can be slimy and fibrous, with an extremely bitter flavor that some people find hard to tolerate. When dried, it may be chewed or ground into powder, which is sometimes mixed with other substances to make it more palatable. Consuming it raw or dried often requires ingesting a larger volume to achieve the same effects as drinking the tea, and the onset may be slightly slower.

While San Pedro can cause visions, it's often described as a heart-opening medicine, good for the relief of grief and other emotions. (Some describe it as more like MDMA than a classic psychedelic.) When done, it can give you the warm fuzzies and is activated by movement and bodywork. It also can focus the mind, increase physical stamina, and sharpen vision. For this reason, some people use it for creative pursuits, such as writing, composing music, and making art—or for taking long hikes. Unlike shrooms, LSD, and ayahuasca, which can take you completely under, San Pedro can offer a lucidity that some people describe as causing them to feel like a superhuman version of themselves.

San Pedro is also used an integration tool and for processing other kinds of psychedelic experiences. Some facilitators do retreats where ayahuasca or mushrooms are served in the evening and San Pedro is served the next day. Sounds intense, we know, but it can actually be quite a beautiful pairing that helps make the journey from the previous night come into more clarity.

San Pedro is legal in most countries, including the United States, as it is not scheduled. In fact, it grows native all over California and is even sold in gardening stores. However, extracting and using mescaline from San Pedro is illegal in many places—and mescaline is classified as a Schedule I controlled substance in the United States.

CHAPTER 12

MICRODOSING

In the last half decade, microdosing has been all the rage. From Silicon Valley to Wall Street, from middle-aged moms looking to dip their toes into the psychedelic waters to seasoned psychonauts who want to stay connected to their bigger journeys, people are reporting that this practice is transforming their lives for the better.

Microdosing is defined as the practice of consuming a small, subperceptual dose (a dose that does not induce significant alterations in perception) of a psychedelic substance, typically around one-tenth to one-twentieth of a standard recreational dose. The most common substances used in a microdosing regimen are LSD and psilocybin, although other psychedelics like mescaline, MDMA, or even cannabis may also be used.

In this chapter, we will delve into how you can decide between microdosing and macrodosing, the scientific perspectives behind both approaches, established protocols, dosing considerations, and tips for tracking your results effectively.

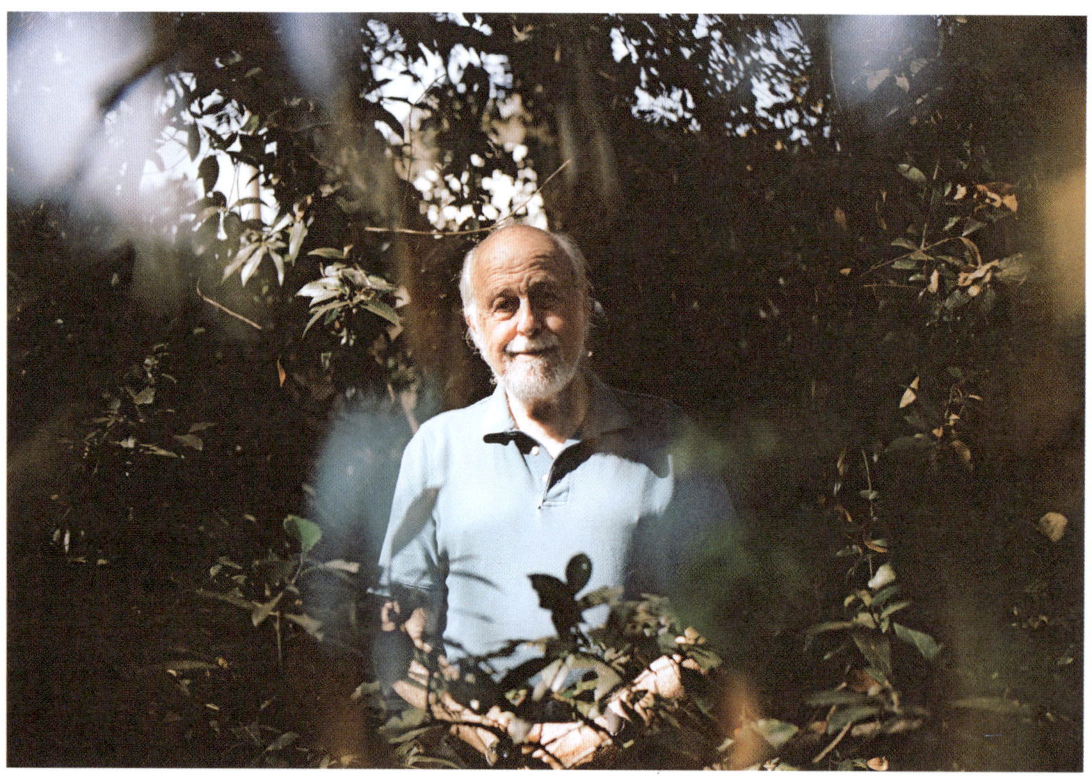

Microdosing vs. Macrodosing

The choice between microdosing and macrodosing (taking a full therapeutic dose of a psychedelic) depends on your intention, goals, and personal circumstances. Microdosing is often used to enhance creativity, improve mood, increase cognitive function, or alleviate anxiety and depression. It can be an appealing option for those seeking to integrate psychedelics into their daily routine without the possibility of an overwhelming experience. On the other hand, macrodosing induces profound shifts in consciousness, emotions, spirituality, somatic sensations, and introspection. This approach is better suited for those interested in exploring their psyche deeply, healing from trauma, or engaging in spiritual practices.

Lifestyle and scheduling considerations play a role, too. Microdosing typically doesn't disrupt daily activities, making it a practical choice for those juggling work, family, and other commitments. Macrodosing, however, requires more preparation and recovery time. Setting aside a day for the experience itself and ensuring that the days before and after allow for reflection and integration are crucial. While macrodosing can lead to transformative experiences, it may also bring unconscious material to the surface that needs to be processed. Ask yourself whether you have the time and space to handle this potential challenge.

---

hikrodosing
noun

hiking while microdosing

Your experience level is another factor to consider. Beginners may feel more comfortable starting with microdosing, which generally has subtle effects on mood and perception. This can help build confidence with psychedelics and ease any nervousness about trying larger doses in the future. However, some people advocate starting with a macrodose for a more significant shift. While microdosing might leave you questioning its effectiveness, a macrodose is more likely to bring about noticeable changes.

Last, personal health considerations are essential. Psychedelics can interact with mental and physical health conditions, so it's important to evaluate these factors before choosing any dose. Some individuals turn to microdosing as a way to transition off medications like SSRIs, but it's important to seek guidance from a professional when managing mental health challenges. While many doctors may be hesitant to discuss psychedelics, a qualified psychedelic integration therapist can offer valuable support and advice.

Jim Fadiman, a psychedelic researcher credited with popularizing microdosing, at his home in Menlo Park, California, in 2024

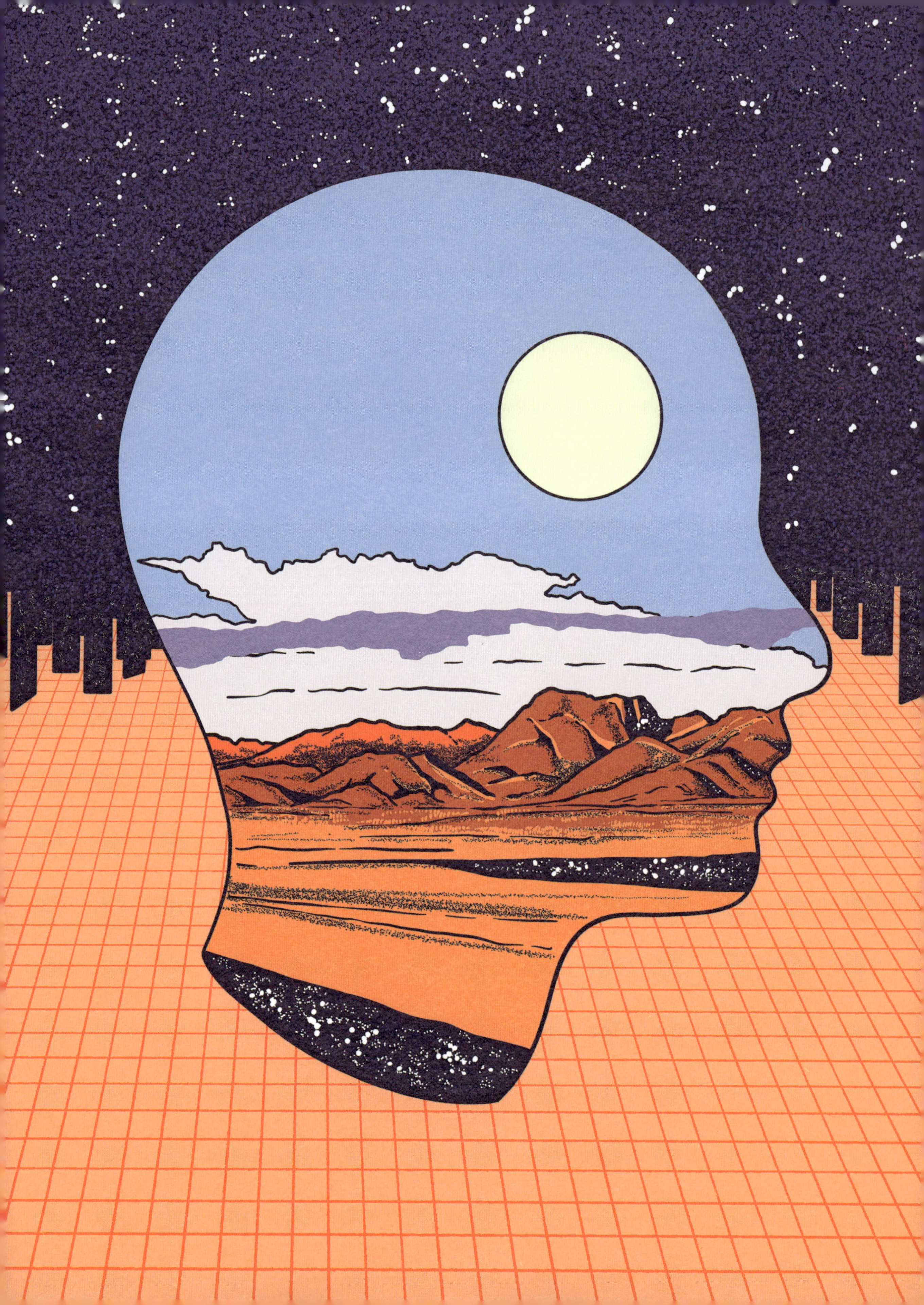

Dosage and Protocols

In general, a microdose of mushrooms ranges between 0.05 and 0.3 gram. Microdosers often take doses in the form of capsules of ground mushroom material, which may be mixed with other ingredients like certain herbs or functional mushrooms. In the case of LSD, a microdose is between 10 and 20 micrograms. This is equivalent to one-tenth to one-twentieth of a macrodose.

As is the case for all forms of psychedelics, it's important to be sure that whatever substance you're using is not adulterated or counterfeit. Use a drug testing kit (such as those from DanceSafe) to be sure that you're getting what you think you're getting.

Microdosing protocols can vary. One of the more common regimens is to take a microdose every two to three days over the course of several months, followed by a pause. Psychedelic researcher James Fadiman, cofounder of the Institute of Transpersonal Psychology, developed a methodology that calls for one day on, two days off, while the Microdosing Institute in the Netherlands calls for taking a dose every other day. The Stamets protocol, popularized by mycologist Paul Stamets, recommends a protocol of four days on and five days off, or five days on and four days off. (Some people with depression report that the Stamets protocol is most effective for them.) Other protocols for microdosing are more intuitive, based on when the user feels the "need" for the microdose. Some people microdose on a very occasional basis.

There isn't a definitive answer as to what protocol you should follow, what substance you should try, and what your dose should be. Generally, it's recommended that you figure out what works best for you via trial and error.

TRACK YOUR RESULTS

One of the keys to effective microdosing is maintaining a detailed record of your experiences. Tracking your results will help you understand how or if it's helping you. Consider the following techniques for tracking:

1. JOURNALING

Maintain a microdosing journal to document your dosages, feelings, emotional state, and any significant insights. Include notes about your daily life, interactions, and changes in productivity.

2. MOOD TRACKING APPS

Utilize smartphone applications designed for mood and mental health tracking that allow you to log your microdosing sessions alongside mood ratings and personal reflections.

3. SELF-REFLECTION

Take weekly stock of your experiences. Are you feeling more creative? Is your anxiety reduced? Reflecting critically will help you gauge the effectiveness and adapt your approach accordingly.

4. COMMUNITY CONNECTION

Engage with other people who follow microdosing practices to get tips and compare notes, which could help you gain further insights on your own journey.

Does Microdosing Actually Work?

While most evidence on the benefits of microdosing comes from anecdotal reports, research from institutions like Imperial College London suggests that the practice could enhance mood, creativity, mental clarity, emotional stability, and cognitive flexibility, over time. That is to say, taking one microdose won't necessarily do much, but having a practice of microdosing a few times a week could enable the substance to build up in your system and have a longer-term effect.

In addition to reports on microdosing's boost to creativity and mood, many athletes, from professional skiers to soccer players, have reported that small doses of psychedelics help with focus and stamina. Trust us, there's nothing quite like moving your body in nature with the glittery enhancement of a psychedelic. It's definitely a good baby step before full-on tripping in the woods.

It's worth noting, however, that alongside small yet promising studies on microdosing, the benefits could be attributable to the placebo effect. Some data, including a 2020 study published in the journal *eLife*, suggests that participants reported improvements in mood, creativity, and focus. However, these positive effects were also seen in placebo groups. Critics argue that many of the studies on microdosing are limited by small sample sizes and self-reported data, which can introduce bias. While anecdotal reports from users often highlight the benefits of microdosing, the scientific consensus remains inconclusive, calling for larger and more rigorously controlled trials. That said, there don't appear to be many risks to microdosing, especially in the short term, so if it's something you want to try, the barrier to entry is lower than it is with macrodosing, which may require support and therapy afterward.

---

stacking
noun

combining supplements or compounds

Stacking is a common practice with mushroom microdosing, for which psilocybin mushroom capsules are "stacked" with lion's mane, cacao, reishi, and B-complex vitamins, among other ingredients, to increase their efficacy. The Stamets stack, popularized by mycologist Paul Stamets, combines psilocybin mushrooms with niacin and lion's mane mushrooms. The goal of the Stamets stack is to encourage neurogenesis, improve brain health, and enhance cognitive function, although scientific evidence on it remains limited.

CHAPTER 13

TRIP SITTING

Once someone has had transformative experiences on psychedelics, often they begin to feel as though they want to help other people on their healing journeys, too. This can look like a call to support others while they are tripping, sometimes called "trip sitting" or "space holding." Holding space for another person who is journeying is a delicate dance of knowing when to step in and when to hold back, and of putting aside your own emotions, judgments, and personal needs for at least a few hours, if not all day long. It means being present with them, being a witness, and being able to help guide them, if necessary, without being heavy-handed or wielding too much influence. The idea is to allow and empower the person's own inner healer to take the lead. The role of the person holding the space is not to tell the psychonaut what to think or feel but rather to foster a safe, supportive environment for them to explore their own inner world. In this chapter, we'll cover the basics of how to do that.

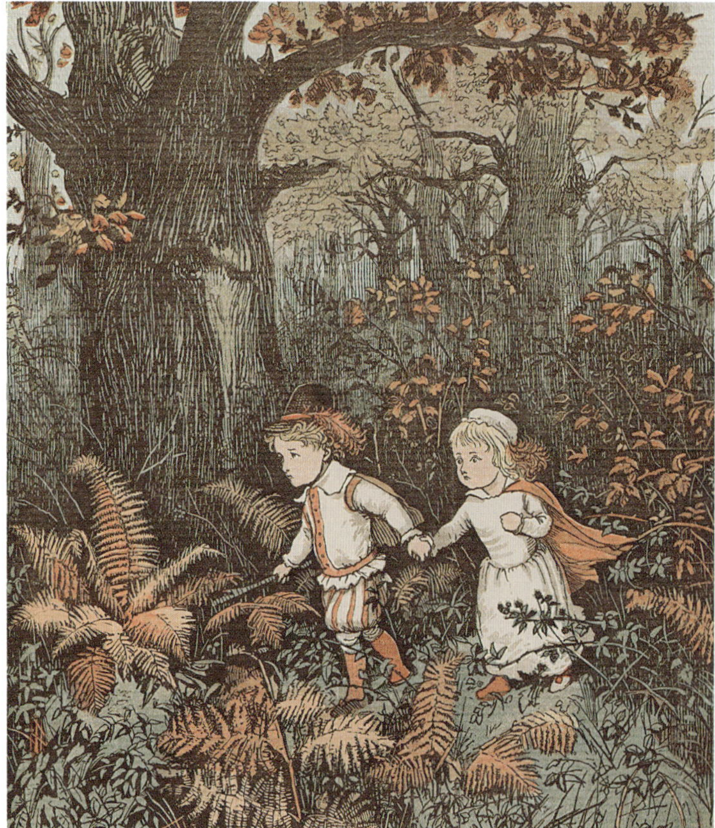

Do Your Own Work First

Facilitating someone else's psychedelic experience is like seeing them through the depths of the underworld and shepherding them back. To do so, you have to be able to hold yourself in such a way that you serve as a warm, grounded, compassionate, and, most of all, neutral presence in a situation that could be anywhere from fun to frightening, calm to chaotic, and anything in between.

That means you first need to be centered and comfortable with your own inner world, and have the ability to decenter yourself from the situation, in order to maintain emotional boundaries and give the journeyer enough space to heal and explore. How do you cultivate such a quality of presence? You might want to engage in practices like meditation, yoga, journaling, or breathwork, or reflect on your own personal relationship and past experiences with psychedelics, both positive and negative, easeful or challenging. Trip sitting is not about knowing everything or having the answers to someone's questions during their journey: It's about being a safe presence to help a person go deeper into their own process.

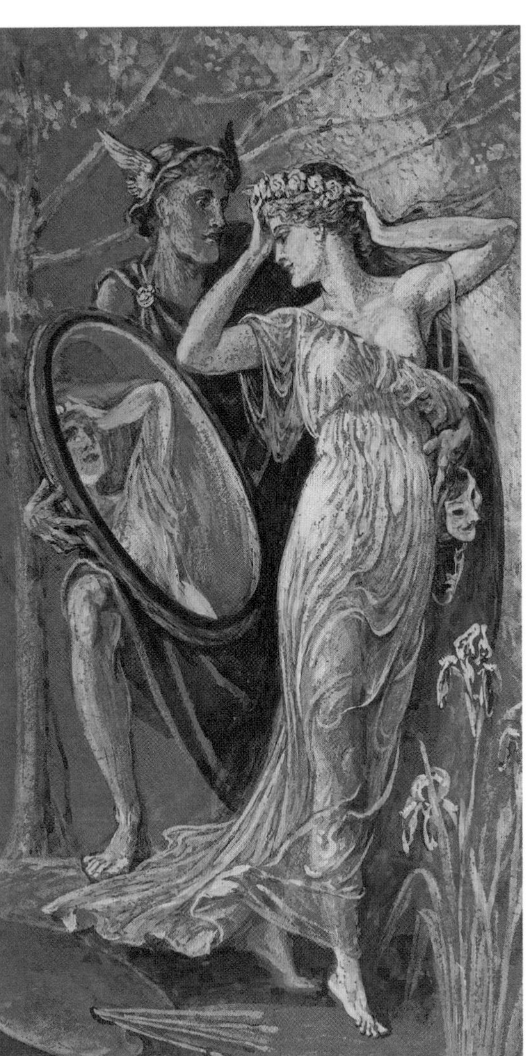

---

scope
noun

a person's capacity to hold space for a particular type of psychedelic experience

In the context of psychedelic sessions, scope is typically dependent on how many years of training a person has, what types of experiences they feel comfortable facilitating, and what types of psychedelics they know how to facilitate for. Someone who is trained to hold space for MDMA, for example, might tell a client that mushrooms are "beyond their scope." As a person new to trip sitting, it's important to be able to recognize what is beyond your scope so that the tripper has what they need to feel safe and supported.

Prepare for the Trip

Remember: The journey begins the moment someone decides they're doing it. The role of any space holder is to set the stage for a safe, successful experience, before, during, and after. There are a few different ways to approach trip sitting. Some people prefer to be actively involved, providing prompts, suggestions, and guidance throughout the experience. Others prefer to be more passive, providing a quiet and supportive presence and allowing the person on the journey to explore their own inner world without interference. Whichever approach you choose, here are some dos and don'ts.

PRIOR TO THE JOURNEY

Do:

- Discuss the person's intentions, goals, and expectations.
- Make sure they aren't on any contraindicated medications and that they don't have any underlying mental or physical health issues that may pose a risk. If there's any concern about the person's physical safety, they should consult with a professional who can review their medical history.
- Establish boundaries with regard to conversation topics and physical touch.
- Ask about their personal history and mental health background so you know what might come up for them.
- Help them curate a well-thought-out set and setting (more on this on page 42).
- Give them a vague idea of what the substance might feel like or bring up, but without setting firm expectations for how the experience will play out.

Do Not:

- Tell them exactly what the journey will be like.
- Guarantee them that they will heal.

DAY OF

Do:

- Limit unnecessary chatter.
- Be attentive to their needs (water, room temperature, blankets, scents, lighting, etc.).

Do Not:

- Try to guide the experience with a heavy hand.
- Push them to tell you what they are thinking or feeling.
- Bring up negative topics, news items, memories, or anything else that could be triggering or psychologically dangerous.
- Comment on how the substance appears to be affecting them.
- Dismiss anything they say.
- Make any sudden movements or sounds.

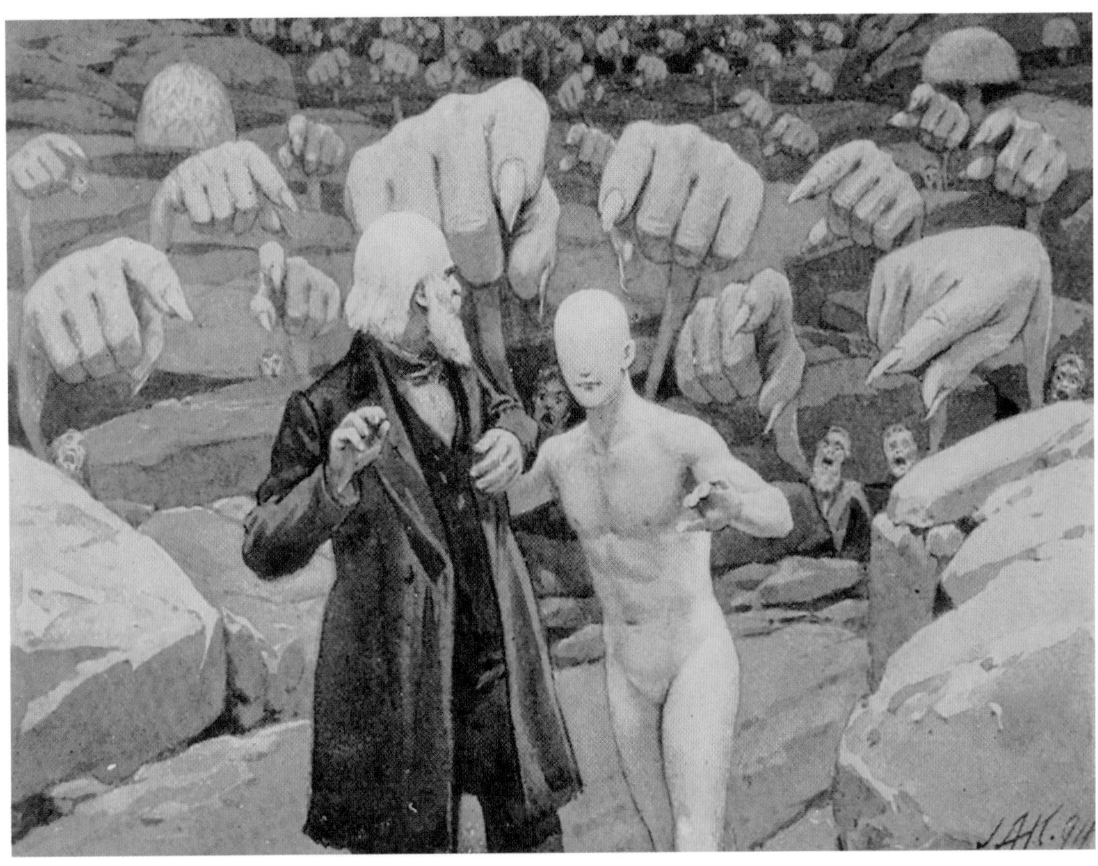

QUICK TIPS FOR TRIP SITTERS

- Make sure you're familiar with the risks of the psychedelic the person is choosing. If they have a personal or family history of bipolar disorder, schizophrenia, or any other serious mental health condition, it's best that they seek support from a trained guide. Amateur trip sitters are best for people who are experiencing only low-level distress or are interested in exploring their consciousness but otherwise are healthy.

- Be aware of your own triggers and boundaries. It's important to be mindful of your own emotional state and to set limits when necessary.

- Don't be afraid to ask for help. You don't have to do it alone. Join a peer support group, or let a friend know that you are holding space and ask them to be on call in case anything comes up during that time.

- Be patient and understanding. Challenging experiences may happen, and it's not necessarily your fault if the journeyer is struggling, but do engage techniques to help them feel better.

- Take care of yourself during the experience. It can be a long haul sitting with someone for five or more hours. Bring snacks, water, coffee, and whatever you may need to stay alert and on point for the journeyer.

What to Do If the Tripper Is Experiencing Something Uncomfortable

First things first: Don't call it a bad trip. Challenging experiences happen to the best of us, so make sure the journeyer knows that they are not alone.

In the event that the journeyer hits rocky waters, it's vital for the space holder to stay calm and grounded and to know what to say and do, and especially what not to. Try the following strategies.

- Validate their experience: Acknowledge their feelings and reassure them that whatever they are going through is okay.
- Employ grounding techniques: Guide them through grounding exercises, such as focusing on the breath (with the exhalation longer than the inhalation, which is a technique known to calm the nervous system), meditating, body scanning, conscious movement, or simply entering into the present moment.
- Prepare distractions ahead of time: Offer activities that can help take their mind off what's happening, such as switching the music; inviting them to dance, do yoga, or make art; or opening up a spiritual book such as *Be Here Now*.
- Change the environment: Bring them outside if you're inside, or vice versa. Perhaps go to another room or change the lighting.
- Offer something soothing: Try brewing them some chamomile tea, have them inhale the scent of lavender or another calming aroma, or offer them CBD or ghost pipe droplets, which have an anxiolytic effect.

Ultimately, the best approach to trip sitting is to be flexible, compassionate, and attentive to the needs of the journeyer. Listen to them, support them, and allow them to explore their own inner world without judgment. Remember: It is their trip, their own experience, and whatever they are going through is something that needs to come up. Your job is not to save them from their pain or discomfort, nor to control their journey, but simply to be a safe, grounding presence to support them through it.

It's important to note that trip sitting is not a substitute for professional medical care. If the tripper is experiencing a medical emergency, seek immediate medical attention.

Joining the Psychedelic Movement

It's not uncommon for people, whether they've journeyed once or many times, to start feeling like they want to devote a significant portion of their lives to psychedelics and helping others heal, too. If this is you, in addition to becoming a trip sitter, there are a number of ways to work in this burgeoning field. Many jobs that exist in other industries now also exist within the field of psychedelics. There's a psychedelic bar association for lawyers, psychedelic marketing agencies, trainings for doctors and therapists who want to pivot toward focusing on ketamine therapy, musicians who play during ceremony, and much more. The opportunities aren't yet vast because the market is still small, but they exist.

If you have another career but want to get involved in your community, you can volunteer to help raise awareness about and destigmatize psychedelics. If there's already a decriminalization measure underway in your city, you can join in the effort. If there's not, you can start one. At DoubleBlind, we often say that we're not trying to make psychedelics mainstream, but we're trying to make the mainstream more psychedelic. And that means, if you feel comfortable doing so, advocating for reform and opening up about your own transformative experiences. The simple act of sharing your story is one of the most powerful ways to support others in embarking on the psychedelic path. There are so many people who want to, but don't know where to begin. Beyond this, there's also the path of contributing to research and education, which are fundamental to changing minds and policy. Universities and independent labs are conducting clinical trials on psilocybin, MDMA, and other substances, and many of them welcome volunteers or research assistants—even those without formal science backgrounds. Writing, podcasting, and public speaking about psychedelics are other avenues that can ripple out to thousands of people, giving them context, resources, and hope.

Ultimately, the importance of creating and offering spaces for people to gather, connect, share, and learn cannot be overstated. Virtual spaces make people who live in remote areas and don't know others engaging with psychedelics feel less alone, while gathering in-person can be a beautiful opportunity for new initiatives and projects to take root. You might consider starting a community integration circle, organizing a book club around psychedelic literature, or hosting legal gatherings (such as cannabis ceremonies and breathwork) as a safe way to begin exploring altered states of consciousness. Whatever form it takes, this work is about using your gratitude for what this journey has offered you as fuel to support others and, hopefully, build a culture of care as psychedelics reenter the collective conversation.

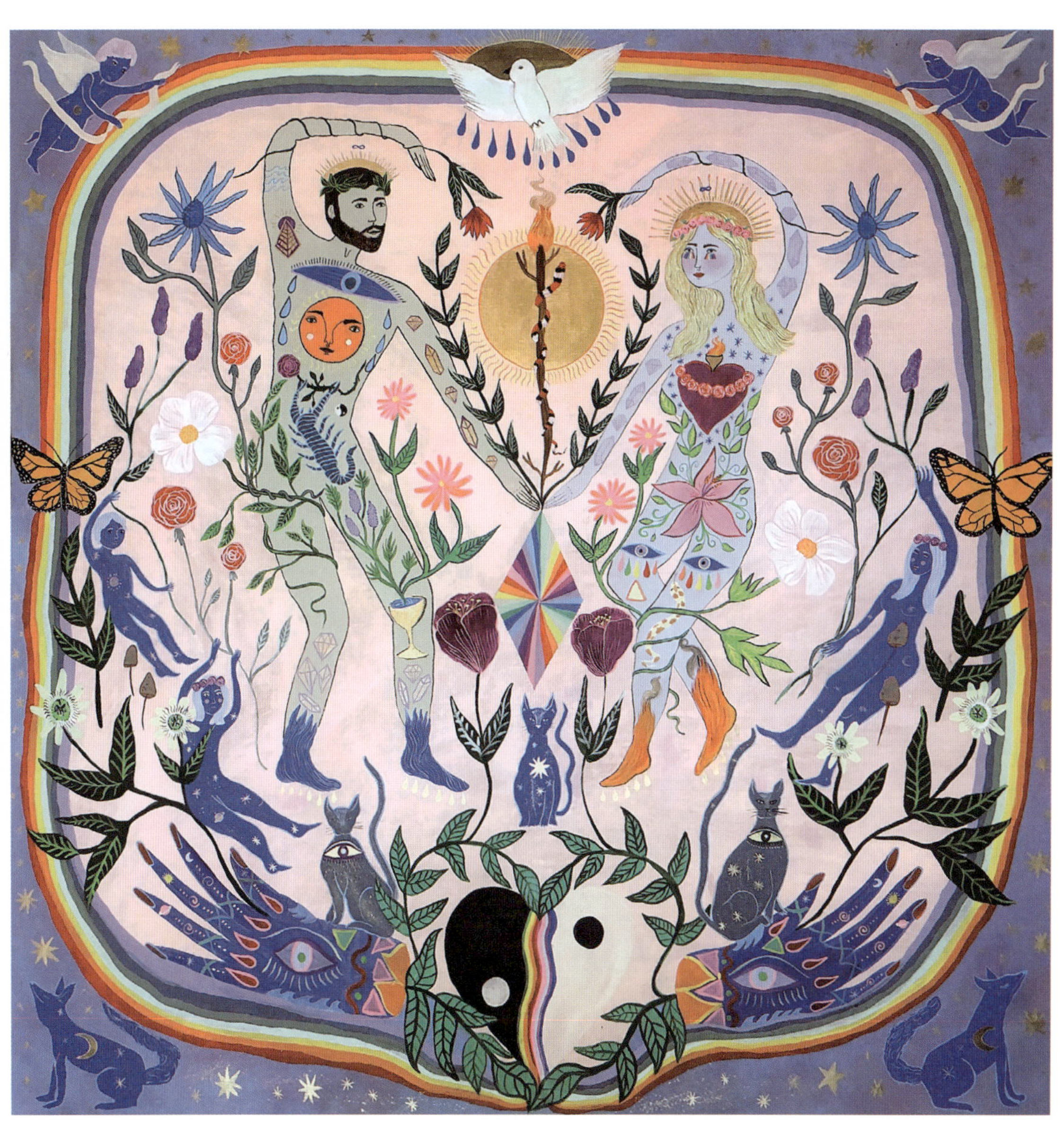

AFTERWORD

Many people have the expectation, based on documentaries and stories in the media, that they'll do a psychedelic once and then their life will transform. This does happen for some people. But for many others, their first experience with a psychedelic puts them on a lifelong path of journey work—journeying, integrating, journeying, and integrating again.

All of our problems, wounds, and traumas can't be healed overnight, with or without a psychedelic. But doing a psychedelic can catalyze a new understanding of our internal landscape—the depth of it and how we can navigate it.

Arguably one of the most beautiful consequences of doing a psychedelic—even for purely therapeutic reasons—is that the experience often connects people to a reality larger than themselves, something theologians sometimes call "unitive consciousness." From there, we find new questions, not just about our personal healing, but about profound existential issues and our place in it all. Can those questions prompt us to be more conscientious global citizens?

As a final nod to the traditional wisdom keepers of these plants and fungi, we will say that Indigenous cosmologies tend to see everything as connected, from the smallest organism to the colossal, invisible mycelial networks growing beneath our feet. Unlike in facilitated sessions run by Westerners, intentions for Indigenous ceremonies usually reflect this belief in interconnectivity. These ceremonies include everything from prayers for the land to visioning of political strategies for peace. As Miguel Evanjuanoy, an Inga from Colombia and member of UMIYAC, a collective preserving the traditional knowledge around yagé (a form of ayahuasca), told us, "Within . . . the cosmology of Indigenous communities of the Amazon rainforest, you do not separate the individual from the community, from the planet. That's fictitious. Individual health is collective health, [and] collective health includes the territory. We're talking about one ecosystem, which is inseparable, and it's very important to view it as one."

Might the experiences of unity that we have under psychedelics enable us not only to heal ourselves but to find a renewed commitment to collective well-being as well? We'll refrain from making any grandiose claims about the potential of the psychedelic movement at this complex moment in human history, but something worth considering after you've integrated the revelations about your own life is: Now what?

ADDITIONAL RESOURCES

At DoubleBlind, we often say we're standing on the shoulders of giants. By this, we mean that our work is made possible by every person who has preserved the knowledge around sacred plants and fungi for generations. We hope this book is just the beginning of your path—and if you'd like to go deeper, you'll check out some of the following resources.

We'd also like to note that this is not a definitive list, and that we offer hundreds of free articles and guides, as well as classes and workshops on microdosing, growing mushrooms, and beyond, at doubleblindmag.com.

ORGANIZATIONS SUPPORTING INDIGENOUS WISDOM AND RECIPROCITY

Many organizations are doing this good work. Here are just a few that DoubleBlind has supported throughout the years.

Amazon Sacred Headwaters Initiative
sacredheadwaters.org
This initiative focuses on protecting the Amazon Sacred Headwaters region in Ecuador and Peru. They work in partnership with Indigenous nations to safeguard biodiversity, promote sustainable development, and uphold cultural traditions.

ASCY (Associação Sociocultural Yawanawa)
@ascyawanawa
This organization represents Yawanawa councils and authorities in the Cauca region of Colombia. They work to preserve traditional culture, promote Indigenous rights, and protect sacred lands.

Ayahuasca Defense Fund
iceers.org/adf
This organization provides legal support and advocacy for individuals and groups involved in the responsible use of ayahuasca. They aim to protect Indigenous traditions while promoting safe and ethical practices.

Beneficial Plant Research Association
bpra.org
This association supports the study and conservation of plants with medicinal and nutritional properties. They focus on education, research, and promoting sustainable practices, with a particular focus on the coca plant.

Blessings of the Forest
blessingsoftheforest.org
BOTF works to protect the sacred iboga plant and support Indigenous communities in Gabon. They focus on sustainable harvesting, cultural preservation, and ensuring fair compensation for traditional healers.

Chacruna and the Indigenous Reciprocity Initiative
chacruna.net/indigenous-reciprocity-initiative
Chacruna is a nonprofit that has brought visibility to historically marginalized groups in psychedelics, including women, queer thought leaders, and Indigenous voices. Their Indigenous Reciprocity Initiative (IRI) is dedicated to supporting Indigenous peoples in the Americas by promoting equitable relationships and sustainable economic opportunities. The IRI helps fund grassroots projects that preserve traditional ecological knowledge and cultural practices.

Chaikuni Institute
chaikuni.org
The Chaikuni Institute is an organization based in Peru that supports regenerative development, conservation, and cultural preservation in the Amazon. They partner with local communities to foster sustainable practices.

Esperanza Mazateca
instagram.com/esperanza_mazateca20
This organization is dedicated to supporting the Mazatec people of Mexico in their efforts to

preserve their cultural heritage, including sacred mushroom ceremonies. They provide resources for community-led initiatives such as education and ecological conservation.

Fungi Foundation
ffungi.org
The Fungi Foundation is the first global organization dedicated to protecting fungi. They work on conservation, education, and research, ensuring that fungal biodiversity is preserved for future generations.

Global Psychedelic Society
globalpsychedelic.org
This global network connects psychedelic societies worldwide to promote education, harm reduction, and safe practices. They aim to create a supportive and inclusive community for those interested in psychedelics.

Grandmothers Wisdom Project
grandmotherswisdom.org
This initiative uplifts the voices of Indigenous grandmothers around the world, sharing their wisdom and cultural knowledge. They work to preserve oral traditions, promote intergenerational healing, and foster community connections.

Huachuma Collective
huachumacollective.org
The Huachuma Collective works to preserve and promote the traditional use of Huachuma (San Pedro cactus) by supporting Indigenous knowledge, sustainable cultivation, and public education about this sacred plant.

Indigenous Medicine Conservation Fund
imc.fund
This organization supports efforts to protect and sustain Indigenous medicine practices, including the conservation of sacred plants and the ecosystems where they grow. They work to ensure the continued cultural survival and self-determination of Indigenous communities.

Union of Indigenous Yagé Doctors of the Colombian Amazon
umiyac.org
This collective of Indigenous communities focuses on preserving and protecting the traditional use of yagé (ayahuasca) in the Colombian Amazon. They aim to safeguard ancestral practices and defend Indigenous land rights.

Urban Indigenous Collective
urbanindigenouscollective.org
Based in the United States, this collective addresses health inequities faced by urban Indigenous communities. They focus on mental health, community support, and advocating for policy changes to improve access to resources and health care.

PSYCHEDELIC BOOKS WE LOVE

Acid Dreams: The Complete Social History of LSD: The CIA, the Sixties, and Beyond **by Martin Lee and Bruce Shlain**
A thorough history of LSD, its cultural impact, and its role in politics and society

American Trip: Set, Setting, and the Psychedelic Experience in the Twentieth Century **by Ido Hartogsohn**
A historical analysis of the social, cultural, and psychological impact of psychedelics in the twentieth century

Be Here Now **by Ram Dass**
A spiritual classic blending psychedelic culture with Eastern philosophy, emphasizing mindfulness and presence

The Body Keeps the Score: Brain, Mind, and Body in the Healing of Trauma **by Bessel van der Kolk**
A seminal book explaining how trauma impacts the body and how to heal through various therapeutic approaches

***DMT and the Soul of Prophecy: A New Science of Spiritual Revelation in the Hebrew Bible* by Rick Strassman**
A study on the intersection of DMT experiences and ancient spiritual texts, offering insights into altered states

***The Doors of Perception* by Aldous Huxley**
A philosophical and poetic reflection on Huxley's experiences with mescaline, examining perception and reality

***Exile & Ecstasy: Growing Up with Ram Dass and Coming of Age in the Jewish Psychedelic Underground* by Madison Margolin**
A memoir exploring the intersection between Hasidic counterculture and the community surrounding Ram Dass, reconciling heritage with spiritual exploration and psychedelic escapades

***Food of the Gods: The Search for the Original Tree of Knowledge: A Radical History of Plants, Drugs, and Human Evolution* by Terence McKenna**
A bold exploration of humanity's relationship with psychoactive plants throughout history

***Good Chemistry: The Science of Connection from Soul to Psychedelics* by Julie Holland**
An exploration of how psychedelics and other practices foster connection, healing, and emotional balance

***The Harvard Psychedelic Club: How Timothy Leary, Ram Dass, Huston Smith, and Andrew Weil Killed the Fifties and Ushered in a New Age for America* by Don Lattin**
A lively account of four influential figures who shaped the psychedelic movement in the 1960s

***Heads: A Biography of Psychedelic America* by Jesse Jarnow**
A cultural history of the psychedelic movement in America, focusing on its music and counterculture roots

***Healing the Fragmented Selves of Trauma Survivors: Overcoming Internal Self-Alienation* by Janina Fisher**
A groundbreaking book offering insights into trauma recovery and integration using therapeutic techniques

***How to Change Your Mind: What the New Science of Psychedelics Teaches Us About Consciousness, Dying, Addiction, Depression, and Transcendence* by Michael Pollan**
A bestselling book examining the science and cultural impact of psychedelics in the modern world

***In the Realm of Hungry Ghosts: Close Encounters with Addiction* by Gabor Maté**
A compassionate exploration of addiction, its causes, and pathways to healing

***LSD: My Problem Child* by Albert Hofmann**
The autobiography of the chemist who discovered LSD, detailing its discovery, uses, and cultural implications

***Meditation: Waking Up to Life* by Americ Azevedo**
A guide to mindfulness and meditation as tools for presence and awareness in everyday life

***Microdosing for Health Healing and Enhanced Performance* by James Fadiman and Jordan Gruber**
An overview of the practice, benefits, and scientific basis of microdosing psychedelics for personal growth and mental health

***Mycelium Running: How Mushrooms Can Help Save the World* by Paul Stamets**
A practical guide on how fungi can revolutionize ecological restoration and human health

***The Natural Mind: A Revolutionary Approach to the Drug Problem* by Andrew Weil**
A visionary book challenging conventional views on drug use and advocating for natural states of consciousness

PiHKAL: A Chemical Love Story **by Alexander and Ann Shulgin**
Part memoir, part scientific catalog, exploring the creation and effects of psychedelic compounds

The Psychedelic Experience: A Manual Based on the Tibetan Book of the Dead **by Timothy Leary, Ralph Metzner, and Richard Alpert**
A classic manual for navigating the inner journey during a psychedelic experience, inspired by the Tibetan Book of the Dead

The Psychedelic Explorer's Guide: Safe, Therapeutic, and Sacred Journeys **by James Fadiman**
A comprehensive guide to safely and meaningfully engaging with psychedelics for personal growth

Psychedelic Medicine: The Healing Powers of LSD, MDMA, Psilocybin, and Ayahuasca **by Richard Louis Miller**
An overview of the therapeutic potential of various psychedelics in treating mental health issues and fostering personal transformation

Queering Psychedelics: From Oppression to Liberation in Psychedelic Medicine, edited **by Alex Belser, Clancy Cavnar, and Beatriz C. Labate**
A collection of essays exploring the intersection of queer identities and psychedelic medicine, addressing historical injustices and envisioning an inclusive future for psychedelic science and practice

A Really Good Day: How Microdosing Made a Mega Difference in My Mood, My Marriage, and My Life **by Ayelet Waldman**
A memoir recounting how microdosing helped the author improve her mental health and personal relationships

Sacred Knowledge: Psychedelics and Religious Experiences **by William A. Richards**
An exploration of the intersection of psychedelics and spirituality, drawing on decades of clinical research

Stealing Fire: How Silicon Valley, the Navy SEALs, and Maverick Scientists Are Revolutionizing the Way We Live and Work **by Steven Kotler and Jamie Wheal**
An investigation into how altered states of consciousness are unlocking human potential in unexpected ways

Tending Grief: Embodied Rituals for Holding Our Sorrow and Growing Cultures of Care in Community **by Camille Sapara Barton**
An embodied guide to being with grief individually and in community, with practical exercises, decolonized rituals, and Earth-based medicines for healing and processing loss

The Untethered Soul: The Journey Beyond Yourself **by Michael A. Singer**
A spiritual book exploring how to free oneself from mental barriers and achieve inner peace

The Way of the Psychonaut **by Stanislav Grof**
A deep dive into the potential of nonordinary states of consciousness for healing, creativity, and personal exploration

Your Psilocybin Mushroom Companion: An Informative, Easy-to-Use Guide to Understanding Magic Mushrooms **by Michelle Janikian**
A practical and friendly guide to safely using psilocybin mushrooms for therapeutic and personal purposes

ART CREDITS

Additional photo and art credits by page number:

Front and back cover, 2, 60, 216: Tyler Spangler; 18–19, 56, 57: Daniel Marin Medina; 20–21, 23: Roger Steffens; 24, 88, 89: Steve Koss; 25 (top), 135, 139 (top and bottom): Tony Hoare/Temple of the Way of Light; 25 (bottom), 187: Laurent Sazy; 26, 36, 62, 75, 204: Nick Potts; 32, 33: Aless MC; 42, 43, 44: Ieva Paliukaitytė; 52 (*Pride*), 53 (*Ashore*): Yue Li; 58, 59, 113: Kaya Blaze; 68–69 (*Net of Being*), 117 (*Albert Hofmann & the New Eleusis*), 127 (*Cosmic Christ*): Alex Grey; 70 (*El Encanto de las Piedras*, courtesy of Howard G. Charing & Peter Cloudsley, featured in *The Ayahuasca Visions of Pablo Amaringo*, published by Inner Traditions), 71 (*Huasi Yachana [Templo del Saber]*), 150–151 (*Amazonica Romantica*): Pablo Amaringo; 72 (*Moon Womb*), 73 (*Flowers of Fire–Kodkille Rayen*): Mariela de la Paz; 74: *Iman Al-Dabbagh;* 76, 100, 120, 130, 152, 164: Gina Kim; 79, 80–81 (courtesy of Tom Lane and the Tina & R. Gordon Wasson Ethnomycological Collection Archives at the Harvard University Herbaria): Alan B. Richardson; 90–91 (from *Brian Blomerth's Mycelium Wassonii*, published by Anthology Editions): Brian Blomerth; 93, 108, 109, 110–111, 157 (top and bottom): Jessica Chou; 94–95 (top), 95 (bottom), 96–97: Matt Reichel; 106–107: Alamy/Farmer Dodds; 112: NASA Ames Research Center; 114 (*Inwards*), 115 (*Good Vibrations*): Reza Hasni; 124: Requa Tolbert; 138: Matthew Watherson/Temple of the Way of Light; 140–141, 192: Paul Winner/Temple of the Way of Light; 142: Alienor de Sas/Temple of the Way of Light; 144 (top), 145: Christian Melchior/Living Gaia; 144 (bottom): Jakob Stolz/Living Gaia; 156: Jack Coddington; 159 (courtesy of Pure Ecstasy and M3 Films, LLC): Vernon Bryant; 163: Javier Palma; 167 (*Slices*): Jiayue Li; 170, 171: María Luque; 188, 189: Tui Anandi/Xapiri Ground; 196–197: Tracy L. Barnett/The Esperanza Project; 202: Matt Goff; 215: Meagan Boyd.

Bridgeman Images: Page 10: © Hazel Florez. All Rights Reserved 2025; Page 13: Godong; Page 129: © Carlo Alberto Giardina. All Rights Reserved 2025; Page 208: © Look and Learn.

Getty Images: 35: Bryan Bedder; 38–39, 40: Jan Sochor/LatinContent; 103: LMPC; 104–105: Ben Martin; 136–137: Ernesto Benavides; 148–149: Giulio Paletta/Education Images/Universal Images Group; 155: Rick Friedman/Corbis; 169: John Bryson; 195: Alan Hagman/*Los Angeles Times*.

Public Domain: 6, 49: Codex Magliabecchianus, via Wikimedia Commons; New York Public Library; 15, 47, 143: University of California Libraries; 29: Library of Congress; 51: Smithsonian Libraries; 48: John Tenniel, via Wikimedia Commons; 64–65, 179: University of Toronto; 67, 209: The Metropolitan Museum of Art; 78: Charles H. Peck, "Annual report of the state botanist," University of Albany, via Wikimedia Commons; 83: John Anster Fitzgerald, via Wikimedia Commons; 84–85 New York: Golden Press; 92: UMass Amherst Libraries; 118: Whitney Museum of American Art, Frances Mulhall Achilles Library; 128: Los Angeles County Museum of Art; 174: Wellesley College Library; 183: The Art Institute of Chicago, 1954.320; 185: Walther Otto Müller, Gera-Untermhaus, FE Köhlerp, via Wikimedia Commons; 190: Korthals: P. W., Public domain, via Wikimedia Commons; 199: Franz Eugen Köhler, Köhler's Medizinal-Pflanzen, via Wikimedia Commons; 210: Duke University Libraries.

Unsplash: 31, 119, 125, 127, 160, 175, 176, 198, 212.

ACKNOWLEDGMENTS

There are so many people who have helped us and DoubleBlind get to where we are, that it's impossible to list everyone here. This includes every writer, photographer, and artist who has contributed to the magazine; every advisor who has offered us their counsel; every psychedelic thought leader who has joined us for a webinar; and every community member who has lent us their spirit and desire to learn and grow together. Throughout it all, our community is what keeps us going.

At the top of our gratitude list is also the DoubleBlind team, past and present; they are the kindest and most talented humans we've ever met who helped us bring the magazine to life when we had nothing to give them but passion and vision. This includes: Sarah Schnur, Maxwell Josephson, Alex Field, David Good, Zoe Wilder, Mike Schurr, Ophelia Chong, David Carrico, Daníel Colón, Ba Minuzzi, Mary Carreon, Jenalle Dion, Michael Issac Stein, Georgia Love, Noelle Armstrong, Monica Cadena, Michael Wertheim, Jenay Rose, Daniel Klein, Jeremy Gardner, Emily and Yousef Al-Humaidhi, Ryan Frame, Zeeshan Hyder, Dr. K Mandrake, Virginia Haze, Caine Barlow, Anna Wilcox, Meghan Earl, Marissa Brinkman, Belle De Orta, and our family Elise and Carl Hartman, Ronald and Sylvia Hartman, and Bruce Margolin.

Thank you to the many experts who have helped make sure our reporting is accurate and credible in this book and the magazine, including: Zeus Tipado, Julie Holland, Rick Strassman, Aydin Mayers, Natalie Ginsberg, Rick Doblin, Matthew Stoltz, Charles Nichols, Jeffrey Becker, Michael Verbora, Shayla Love, Andy Letcher, Juliana Mulligan, Ivan Chocron, and Joel Brierre.

Thank you to our resident facilitators, who hold space for our community with such care: Skye Weaver, Ido Cohen, Deanna Rogers, and Ellen Wong.

Thank you to Bridget Monroe Itkin, Zach Greenwald, Lia Ronnen, Jack Dunnington, Suet Chong, Hillary Leary, Nancy Ringer, Julia Perry, Annie O'Donnell, Donna Brown, and the rest of the Artisan team for entrusting us to bring this into the world under your leadership, and to Charles Kim and Regina Brooks at Serendipity Literary Agency for supporting us throughout this process.

And lastly, to all the human and more-than-human life that has supported us on our own journeys such that we can seek to support others. The journey never ends, but we're grateful to have crossed paths with so many incredible beings along the way.

INDEX

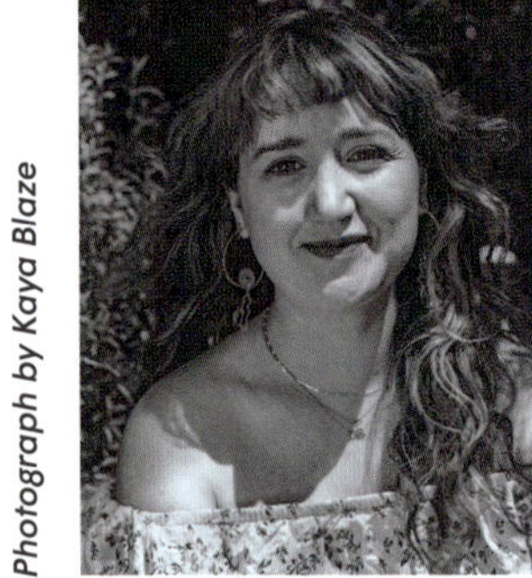

Photograph by Kaya Blaze

SHELBY HARTMAN is cofounder and publisher at DoubleBlind. Her work has been featured in *The New York Times*, *Business Insider*, and *Bustle*, among other media. She has reported for *Rolling Stone*, *VICE*, *Playboy*, and *Quartz*, and she has been invited to speak about psychedelics at SXSW, Horizons: Perspectives in Psychedelics, Harvard Law School, and more. In 2020, she was named by *Forbes* as a female leader in psychedelics and cannabis. Find all her work or get in touch at shelbyannehartman.com.

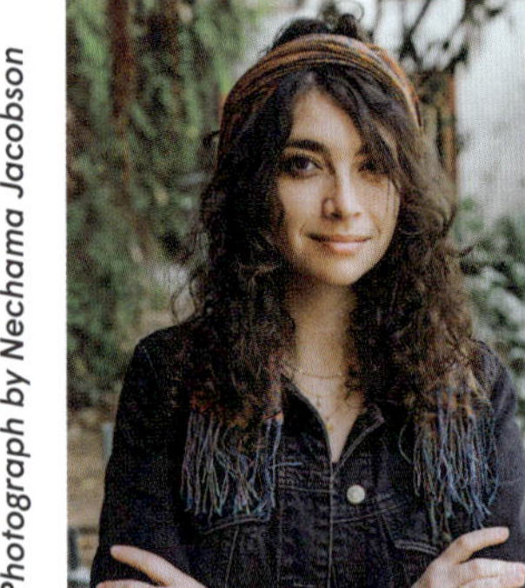

Photograph by Nechama Jacobson

MADISON MARGOLIN is cofounder of both DoubleBlind and the Jewish Psychedelic Summit and the author of *Exile & Ecstasy: Growing Up with Ram Dass & Coming of Age in the Jewish Psychedelic Underground*. Her work has been featured in *The New York Times*, *Forbes*, and *High Times*, among other outlets, and she has reported for *Playboy*, *Rolling Stone*, *VICE*, and more. Having presented on these topics at SXSW, Harvard Law School, MAPS Psychedelic Science, and other conferences, Madison now serves as an educator, writer, and guide to all things Jewish-psychedelic, blending Kabbalah, yoga, and other embodiment rituals with entheogenic practice. Find all her work at madisonmargolin.com.

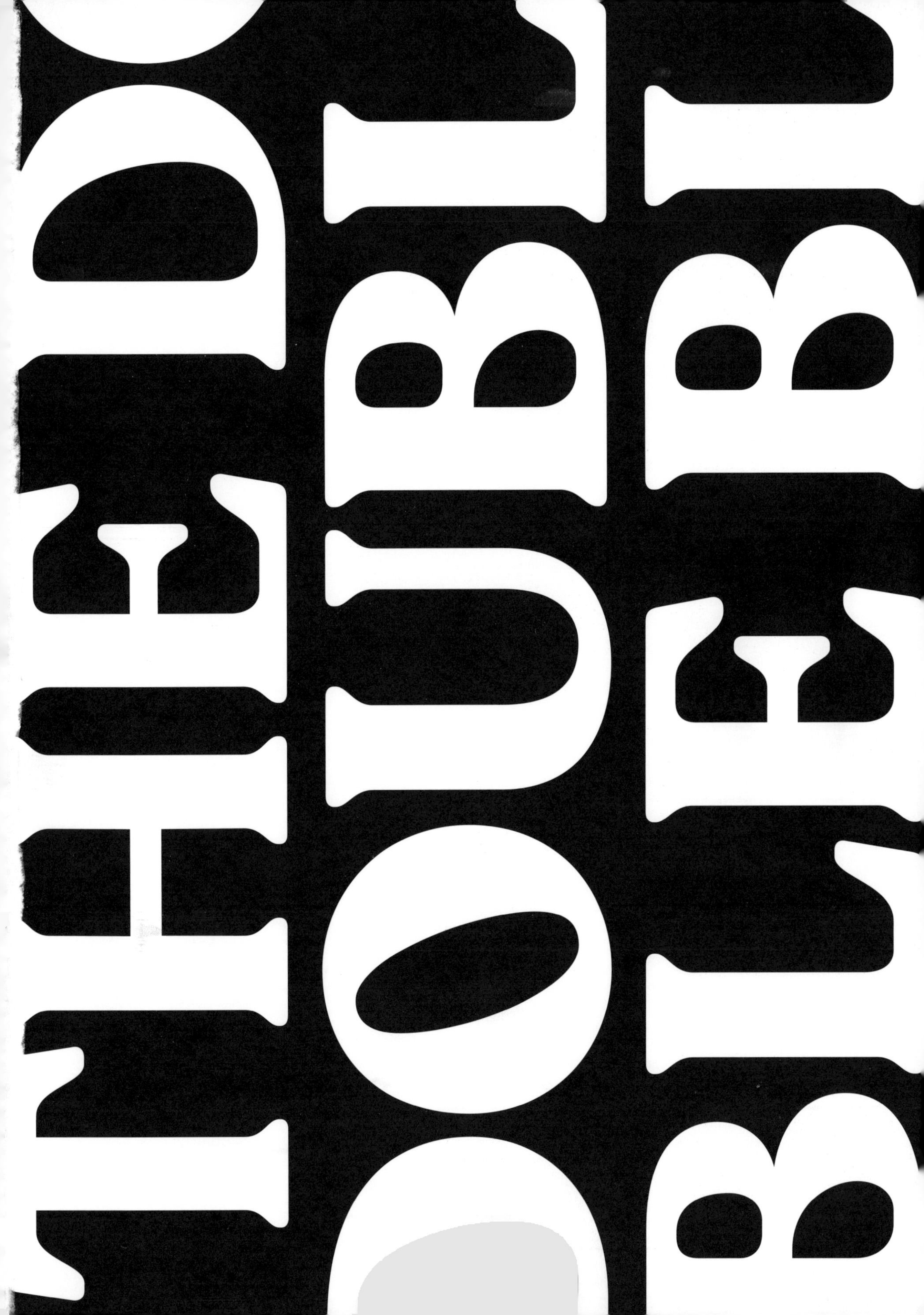

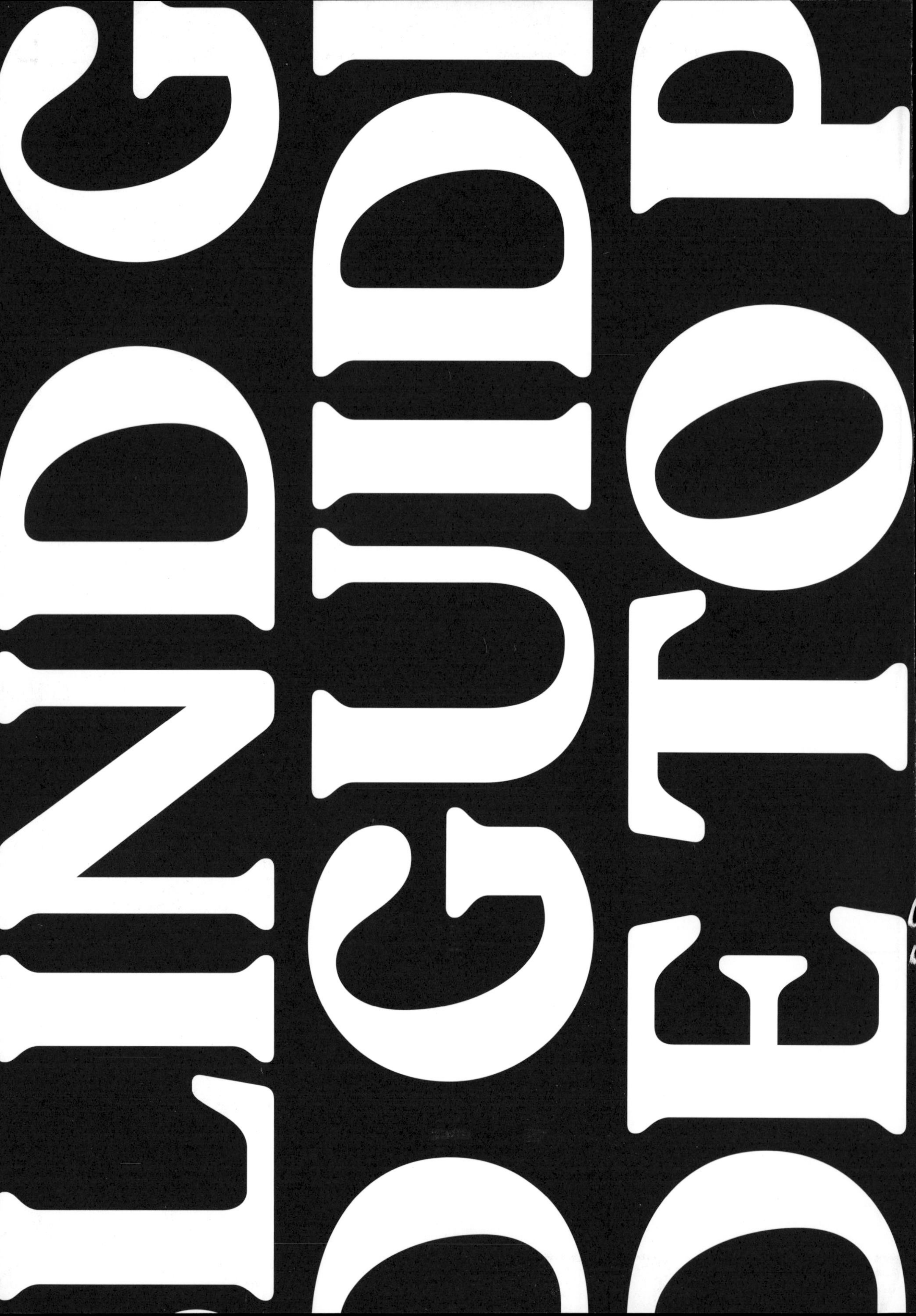